Surgical Treatment of Pancreatic Ductal Adenocarcinoma

Surgical Treatment of Pancreatic Ductal Adenocarcinoma

Editor

Sohei Satoi

MDPI • Basel • Beijing • Wuhan • Barcelona • Belgrade • Manchester • Tokyo • Cluj • Tianjin

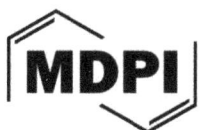

Editor
Sohei Satoi
Deparment of Surgery
Kansai Medical University
Hirakata
Japan, and
Division of Surgical Oncology
University of Colorado
Anschutz Medical Campus
Aurora
USA

Editorial Office
MDPI
St. Alban-Anlage 66
4052 Basel, Switzerland

This is a reprint of articles from the Special Issue published online in the open access journal *Cancers* (ISSN 2072-6694) (available at: www.mdpi.com/journal/cancers/special_issues/pancreatic_surgical).

For citation purposes, cite each article independently as indicated on the article page online and as indicated below:

LastName, A.A.; LastName, B.B.; LastName, C.C. Article Title. *Journal Name* **Year**, *Volume Number*, Page Range.

ISBN 978-3-0365-1866-4 (Hbk)
ISBN 978-3-0365-1865-7 (PDF)

© 2021 by the authors. Articles in this book are Open Access and distributed under the Creative Commons Attribution (CC BY) license, which allows users to download, copy and build upon published articles, as long as the author and publisher are properly credited, which ensures maximum dissemination and a wider impact of our publications.

The book as a whole is distributed by MDPI under the terms and conditions of the Creative Commons license CC BY-NC-ND.

Contents

About the Editor vii

Preface to "Surgical Treatment of Pancreatic Ductal Adenocarcinoma" ix

Sohei Satoi
Surgical Treatment of Pancreatic Ductal Adenocarcinoma
Reprinted from: *Cancers* **2021**, *13*, 4015, doi:10.3390/cancers13164015 1

Mirang Lee, Wooil Kwon, Hongbeom Kim, Yoonhyeong Byun, Youngmin Han, Jae Seung Kang, Yoo Jin Choi and Jin-Young Jang
The Role of Location of Tumor in the Prognosis of the Pancreatic Cancer
Reprinted from: *Cancers* **2020**, *12*, 2036, doi:10.3390/cancers12082036 5

Yuichi Nagakawa, Naoya Nakagawa, Chie Takishita, Ichiro Uyama, Shingo Kozono, Hiroaki Osakabe, Kenta Suzuki, Nobuhiko Nakagawa, Yuichi Hosokawa, Tomoki Shirota, Masayuki Honda, Tesshi Yamada, Kenji Katsumata and Akihiko Tsuchida
Reconsideration of the Appropriate Dissection Range Based on Japanese Anatomical Classification for Resectable Pancreatic Head Cancer in the Era of Multimodal Treatment
Reprinted from: *Cancers* **2021**, *13*, 3605, doi:10.3390/cancers13143605 19

Nana Kimura, Suguru Yamada, Hideki Takami, Kenta Murotani, Isaku Yoshioka, Kazuto Shibuya, Fuminori Sonohara, Yui Hoshino, Katsuhisa Hirano, Toru Watanabe, Hayato Baba, Kosuke Mori, Takeshi Miwa, Mitsuro Kanda, Masamichi Hayashi, Koshi Matsui, Tomoyuki Okumura, Yasuhiro Kodera and Tsutomu Fujii
Optimal Preoperative Multidisciplinary Treatment in Borderline Resectable Pancreatic Cancer
Reprinted from: *Cancers* **2020**, *13*, 36, doi:10.3390/cancers13010036 35

Kongyuan Wei and Thilo Hackert
Surgical Treatment of Pancreatic Ductal Adenocarcinoma
Reprinted from: *Cancers* **2021**, *13*, 1971, doi:10.3390/cancers13081971 51

Yosuke Inoue, Atushi Oba, Yoshihiro Ono, Takafumi Sato, Hiromichi Ito and Yu Takahashi
Radical Resection for Locally Advanced Pancreatic Cancers in the Era of New Neoadjuvant Therapy—Arterial Resection, Arterial Divestment and Total Pancreatectomy
Reprinted from: *Cancers* **2021**, *13*, 1818, doi:10.3390/cancers13081818 67

Yuko Mataki, Hiroshi Kurahara, Tetsuya Idichi, Kiyonori Tanoue, Yuto Hozaka, Yota Kawasaki, Satoshi Iino, Kosei Maemura, Hiroyuki Shinchi and Takao Ohtsuka
Clinical Benefits of Conversion Surgery for Unresectable Pancreatic Ductal Adenocarcinoma: A Single-Institution, Retrospective Analysis
Reprinted from: *Cancers* **2021**, *13*, 1057, doi:10.3390/cancers13051057 83

Hiroaki Yanagimoto, Sohei Satoi, Tomohisa Yamamoto, So Yamaki, Satoshi Hirooka, Masaya Kotsuka, Hironori Ryota, Mitsuaki Ishida, Yoichi Matsui and Mitsugu Sekimoto
Benefits of Conversion Surgery after Multimodal Treatment for Unresectable Pancreatic Ductal Adenocarcinoma
Reprinted from: *Cancers* **2020**, *12*, 1428, doi:10.3390/cancers12061428 99

Simone Serafini, Cosimo Sperti, Alberto Friziero, Alessandra Rosalba Brazzale, Alessia Buratin, Alberto Ponzoni and Lucia Moletta
Systematic Review and Meta-Analysis of Surgical Treatment for Isolated Local Recurrence of Pancreatic Cancer
Reprinted from: *Cancers* **2021**, *13*, 1277, doi:10.3390/cancers13061277 111

Jelena Milin-Lazovic, Petar Madzarevic, Nina Rajovic, Vladimir Djordjevic, Nikola Milic, Sonja Pavlovic, Nevena Veljkovic, Natasa M. Milic and Dejan Radenkovic
Meta-Analysis of Circulating Cell-Free DNA's Role in the Prognosis of Pancreatic Cancer
Reprinted from: *Cancers* **2021**, *13*, 3378, doi:10.3390/cancers13143378 121

Chang Moo Kang and Woo Jung Lee
Is Laparoscopic Pancreaticoduodenectomy Feasible for Pancreatic Ductal Adenocarcinoma?
Reprinted from: *Cancers* **2020**, *12*, 3430, doi:10.3390/cancers12113430 143

Sarah Powell-Brett, Rupaly Pande and Keith J. Roberts
Achieving 'Marginal Gains' to Optimise Outcomes in Resectable Pancreatic Cancer
Reprinted from: *Cancers* **2021**, *13*, 1669, doi:10.3390/cancers13071669 163

Wooil Kwon, Youngmin Han, Yoonhyeong Byun, Jae Seung Kang, Yoo Jin Choi, Hongbeom Kim and Jin-Young Jang
Predictive Features of Malignancy in Branch Duct Type Intraductal Papillary Mucinous Neoplasm of the Pancreas: A Meta-Analysis
Reprinted from: *Cancers* **2020**, *12*, 2618, doi:10.3390/cancers12092618 187

Y.H. Andrew Wu, Atsushi Oba, Laurel Beaty, Kathryn L. Colborn, Salvador Rodriguez Franco, Ben Harnke, Cheryl Meguid, Daniel Negrini, Roberto Valente, Steven Ahrendt, Richard D. Schulick and Marco Del Chiaro
Ductal Dilatation of 5 mm in Intraductal Papillary Mucinous Neoplasm Should Trigger the Consideration for Pancreatectomy: A Meta-Analysis and Systematic Review of Resected Cases
Reprinted from: *Cancers* **2021**, *13*, 2031, doi:10.3390/cancers13092031 205

About the Editor

Sohei Satoi

Dr. Sohei SATOI is a pancreatobiliary surgeon and surgical oncologist with more than 20 years of experience. He is internationally recognized as a leader in the surgical treatment of pancreatic ductal adenocarcinoma including unresectable disease as well as in multimodal treatment of peritoneal dissemination. Dr. Satoi is also keen on developing mitigation strategies for post-pancreatectomy complications. He is active in academic research, with more than 180 peer reviewed papers, and is a member of several scientific journal's editorial boards. His mission is to bring a "cure" to patients with pancreatic ductal adenocarcinoma and to have zero-mortality and less incidence of surgical complication after pancreatectomy.

Preface to "Surgical Treatment of Pancreatic Ductal Adenocarcinoma"

Dear Colleagues,

Surgical resection has been the only chance for a cure in patients with pancreatic ductal adenocarcinoma (PDAC) in recent decades, but the 5-year survival rate is still low (approximately 20%) in PDAC patients who have undergone margin-negative resection only.

A multimodal approach is widely accepted for treating PDAC in the modern era. The implementation of adjuvant chemotherapy or neo-adjuvant treatment has dramatically been enhanced to increase the long-term survival rate of patients with resectable, borderline resectable, and unresectable PDAC in the world. Margin-negative surgical resection still plays a pivotal role in multimodal treatment in patients with PDAC. Therefore, a growing amount of interest has focused on the optimization of the perioperative therapeutic strategy, including regimens of chemo(radio)therapy, the introduction of extended pancreatectomy, and advanced peri-operative management.

This Special Issue highlights the role of surgical resection during multimodal treatments in patients with PDAC from resectable to unresectable diseases to advance our understanding of the surgical treatment of PDAC.

Sohei Satoi
Editor

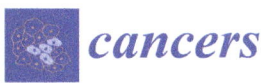

Editorial
Surgical Treatment of Pancreatic Ductal Adenocarcinoma

Sohei Satoi

Department of Surgery, Kansai Medical University, Hirakata 573-1010, Japan; satoi@hirakata.kmu.ac.jp

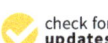

Citation: Satoi, S. Surgical Treatment of Pancreatic Ductal Adenocarcinoma. *Cancers* **2021**, *13*, 4015. https://doi.org/10.3390/cancers13164015

Received: 22 July 2021
Accepted: 6 August 2021
Published: 10 August 2021

Publisher's Note: MDPI stays neutral with regard to jurisdictional claims in published maps and institutional affiliations.

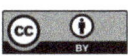

Copyright: © 2021 by the author. Licensee MDPI, Basel, Switzerland. This article is an open access article distributed under the terms and conditions of the Creative Commons Attribution (CC BY) license (https://creativecommons.org/licenses/by/4.0/).

This special issue, "Surgical Treatment of Pancreatic Ductal Adenocarcinoma" contains 13 articles (five original articles, five reviews, and three systematic reviews/meta-analyses) authored by international leaders and surgeons who treat patients with pancreatic ductal adenocarcinoma (PDAC).

Oncological pancreatic surgery requires a deep knowledge of multimodal treatment, accurate preoperative recognition of tumor extension—especially to adjacent major vessels—high-quality technical skills for margin-negative resection, and well-established perioperative management for the reduction of morbidity and mortality. In the modern era, it involves a two-sided advancement toward extended pancreatectomy, such as portal vein or major arterial resection for locally advanced PDAC, as well as minimally invasive surgery for resectable PDAC.

Surgical resection has provided the only chance for a cure in patients with PDAC, but the 5 year survival rate is still low (approximately 20%) in patients with margin-negative resection. The implementation of adjuvant chemotherapy or neoadjuvant therapy has dramatically increased the long term survival of patients with resectable, borderline resectable, and even unresectable PDAC. Margin-negative surgical resection still plays a pivotal role in multimodal treatment in patients with PDAC. Therefore, a growing amount of interest has focused on optimization of the perioperative therapeutic strategy, including multimodal treatment regimens, the introduction of extended pancreatectomy, and advanced perioperative management. Moreover, the introduction of minimally invasive surgery, such as laparoscopic and robotic pancreatic surgery, has been applied worldwide.

This special issue highlights the role of surgical resection in patients with PDAC to advance our understanding of the surgical treatment of PDAC.

With regard to the influence of tumor location on prognosis, among 2483 patients with all types of PDAC, long term survival was significantly better for patients with pancreatic head/uncinate PDAC than with body/tail PDAC, regardless of resectability [1]. Among patients who underwent curative resection, those with head/uncinate cancers had a higher number of T1/T2 tumors, but worse outcomes. Multivariate analysis identified tumor factors, preoperative CA 19-9 level, margin status, and adjuvant therapy, but not tumor location as independent prognostic factors. Margin-negative resection during multimodal treatment is mandatory for long term survival in patients with PDAC.

What can we do to optimize the rate of margin-negative resection? According to the "appropriate dissection range" identified with simulated use of high-quality computed tomography preoperatively, surgeons should carry out "dissection to achieve margin-negative resection", identifying anatomical structures, such as layers, arteries, and veins, as anatomical landmarks to determine the dissection region intraoperatively [2].

Neoadjuvant therapy has been implemented recently to achieve a high proportion of margin-negative resection and negative lymph node metastasis through anatomical and biological shrinkage of borderline resectable tumors. Neoadjuvant therapy followed by surgery, rather than upfront surgery, has been reported to offer clinical benefits to patients with borderline resectable PDAC [3]. Moreover, it is suggested that nutritional management during neoadjuvant therapy may lead to a better prognosis.

Given the multimodal approach with new chemotherapy regimens, such as fluorouracil plus leucovorin, irinotecan, oxaliplatin (FOLFIRINOX), or gemcitabine plus nab-paclitaxel, substantial progress has been made in surgical techniques to address advanced resections [4]. Margin-negative resection in patients with locally advanced PDAC usually requires portal vein or major arterial resection and reconstruction. These mainly vessel-oriented technical approaches of pancreatic head resection allow the removal of all putative tumor-infiltrated soft tissue with the utmost aim for an improved R0 resection rate [4].

Aggressive pancreatectomy, such as total pancreatectomy or combined arterial resection, for achieving margin-negative resection has become justified by the principle of total neoadjuvant therapy in recent decades [5]. Further technical standardization and an optimal neoadjuvant strategy are mandatory for the global adoption of aggressive pancreatectomy.

Recently, surgical resection in PDAC has been extended to patients with unresectable PDAC. Additional surgery during multimodal treatment is defined as "conversion surgery" in patients with unresectable PDAC (metastatic and locally advanced disease) which comprises 70–80% of the PDAC population. Although surgical resectability was less than 10% in 398 patients [6] and 469 patients [7] with unresectable PDAC, including metastatic disease, the median survival time after initial treatment was 37 months and 73.7 months in patients who underwent conversion surgery, respectively. The number of candidates for conversion surgery is now increasing with the introduction of modern chemotherapy regimens; however, the actual clinical benefits of resection have not yet been fully investigated. Prospective studies will be needed to explore the clinical benefit of conversion surgery.

A high rate of recurrence, even after margin-negative resection, has been reported in patients with PDAC. Recurrent PDAC, mainly containing liver or peritoneal metastasis, and local recurrence is commonly treated with systemic chemotherapy or best supportive care. The clinical role of surgical resection for patients with isolated local recurrent PDAC after initial pancreatectomy is still under investigation. Although there is a possibility of selection bias, meta-analysis revealed that surgical resection in selected patients with recurrent pancreatic cancer was safe and feasible and might offer a survival advantage [8]. This meta-analysis also suggested that surgery should be considered part of the multimodal management of relapsing pancreatic cancer, and a multidisciplinary approach is essential to choose the most appropriate treatment [8]. Thus, PDAC surgery in the modern era frequently requires extended pancreatectomy; therefore, appropriate patient selection is mandatory. The development of precise biological and anatomical assessments will be urgently needed.

Therefore, novel biomarkers predicting resectability, overall survival, and disease-free survival should be established promptly. Liquid biopsy involving cancer DNA and circulating tumor cells in the blood may be an additional tool for estimating disease course and outcome in patients with PDAC [9]. Clinical application of liquid biopsy may provide a cancer diagnosis at an earlier stage, enable optimal selection of treatment, and inform prediction of prognosis and recurrence.

While extended pancreatectomy has been developed safely and effectively in patients with locally advanced PDAC, minimally invasive pancreatic surgery has also evolved. Laparoscopic and robotic pancreatectomy are considered safe and feasible for experienced surgeons in well-selected patients with PDAC. With the advancement of minimally invasive techniques and experiences, laparoscopic distal pancreatectomy (LDP) and even laparoscopic pancreaticoduodenectomy (LPD) have been implemented successfully for treating PDAC [10]. However, due to a limited volume of evidence, without doubt, there is a strong need for more high-quality trials to confirm the potential advantages of minimally invasive pancreatic surgery [4].

Optimizing existing pathways for PDAC treatment so that patients realize the benefits of already proven treatments presents a clear opportunity to improve outcomes in the short term. The narrative review [11] focuses on treatments and interventions where there was a clear evidence base to improve outcomes in pancreatic cancer and where there was evidence of variation and undertreatment. The avoidance of preoperative biliary drainage, treatment of pancreatic exocrine insufficiency, prehabilitation and enhanced recovery after surgery, reduction of perioperative complications, optimization of opportunities for elderly patients to receive therapy, optimization of adjuvant chemotherapy, and regular surveillance after surgery are some of the strategies discussed. Each treatment or pathway change represents an opportunity for marginal gain, and the accumulation of marginal gains can result in a considerable benefit to patients. It is essential that surgeons understand that surgery is just one part of a complex pathway and that they are ideally placed to act as change agents to optimize broader pathway improvements.

Other concerns are risk factors for malignancy, defined as high-grade dysplasia and invasive carcinoma in patients with intraductal papillary mucinous neoplasm (IPMN). One meta-analysis revealed risk factors for malignancy as symptoms, size $\geq$ 3 cm, cystic wall thickening, mural nodule, main pancreatic duct dilatation, abrupt caliber change in the pancreatic duct, lymphadenopathy, elevated carbohydrate antigen 19-9 level, and elevated carcinoembryonic antigen level [12]. Among the above risk factors, the role of main pancreatic duct (MPD) dilatation is important for establishing a simple surgical indication. However, the degree of ductal dilatation that warrants pancreatectomy is still controversial across the existing guidelines. The other meta-analysis concluded that MPD dilatation was an important predictive factor of IPMN malignancy, and 5 mm was a highly sensitive cutoff for the detection of high-risk pre-cancerous or cancerous lesions in resected patients. The need for pancreatectomy should be thoroughly evaluated in patients with ductal dilatations of $\geq$5 mm for improving surgical patient selection and reducing overall IPMN malignancy mortality [13].

In conclusion, surgical treatment of PDAC has experienced a paradigm shift, from "the only way for cure" in the last century, to "the essential position during multimodal treatment" in the modern era. Pancreatic surgery for PDAC now has two-sided progress. Extended pancreatectomy with vessel resection and reconstruction has been performed safely and effectively in patients with locally advanced PDAC following multimodal treatment. In contrast, the implementation of minimally invasive surgery is also useful in selected patients with PDAC. The establishment of an appropriate surgical indication for predicting an acceptable prognosis is required in the era of multimodal treatment. Biomarkers that inform a surgical indication may be revealed by liquid biopsy in the near future. Sustainable efforts are warranted to establish a role for surgical treatment during multimodal treatment in patients with PDAC who still have high lethality.

Funding: This research received no external funding.

Conflicts of Interest: The author declares no conflict of interest.

References

1. Lee, M.; Kwon, W.; Kim, H.; Byun, Y.; Han, Y.; Kang, J.; Choi, Y.; Jang, J. The Role of Location of Tumor in the Prognosis of the Pancreatic Cancer. *Cancers* **2020**, *12*, 2036. [CrossRef] [PubMed]
2. Nagakawa, Y.; Nakagawa, N.; Takishita, C.; Uyama, I.; Kozono, S.; Osakabe, H.; Suzuki, K.; Nakagawa, N.; Hosokawa, Y.; Shirota, T.; et al. Reconsideration of the Appropriate Dissection Range Based on Japanese Anatomical Classification for Resectable Pancreatic Head Cancer in the Era of Multimodal Treatment. *Cancers* **2021**, *13*, 3605. [CrossRef] [PubMed]
3. Kimura, N.; Yamada, S.; Takami, H.; Murotani, K.; Yoshioka, I.; Shibuya, K.; Sonohara, F.; Hoshino, Y.; Hirano, K.; Watanabe, T.; et al. Optimal Preoperative Multidisciplinary Treatment in Borderline Resectable Pancreatic Cancer. *Cancers* **2021**, *13*, 36. [CrossRef] [PubMed]
4. Wei, K.; Hackert, T. Surgical Treatment of Pancreatic Ductal Adenocarcinoma. *Cancers* **2021**, *13*, 1971. [CrossRef] [PubMed]
5. Inoue, Y.; Oba, A.; Ono, Y.; Sato, T.; Ito, H.; Takahashi, Y. Radical Resection for Locally Advanced Pancreatic Cancers in the Era of New Neoadjuvant Therapy—Arterial Resection, Arterial Divestment and Total Pancreatectomy. *Cancers* **2021**, *13*, 1818. [CrossRef] [PubMed]
6. Mataki, Y.; Kurahara, H.; Idichi, T.; Tanoue, K.; Hozaka, Y.; Kawasaki, Y.; Iino, S.; Maemura, K.; Shinchi, H.; Ohtsuka, T. Clinical Benefits of Conversion Surgery for Unresectable Pancreatic Ductal Adenocarcinoma: A Single-Institution, Retrospective Analysis. *Cancers* **2021**, *13*, 1057. [CrossRef] [PubMed]
7. Yanagimoto, H.; Satoi, S.; Yamamoto, T.; Yamaki, S.; Hirooka, S.; Kotsuka, M.; Ryota, H.; Ishida, M.; Matsui, Y.; Sekimoto, M. Benefits of Conversion Surgery after Multimodal Treatment for Unresectable Pancreatic Ductal Adenocarcinoma. *Cancers* **2020**, *12*, 1428. [CrossRef] [PubMed]

8. Serafini, S.; Sperti, C.; Friziero, A.; Brazzale, A.; Buratin, A.; Ponzoni, A.; Moletta, L. Systematic Review and Meta-Analysis of Surgical Treatment for Isolated Local Recurrence of Pancreatic Cancer. *Cancers* **2021**, *13*, 1277. [CrossRef] [PubMed]
9. Milin-Lazovic, J.; Madzarevic, P.; Rajovic, N.; Djordjevic, V.; Milic, N.; Pavlovic, S.; Veljkovic, N.; Milic, N.M.; Radenkovic, D. Meta-Analysis of Circulating Cell-Free DNA's Role in the Prognosis of Pancreatic Cancer. *Cancers* **2021**, *13*, 3378. [CrossRef] [PubMed]
10. Kang, C.; Lee, W. Is Laparoscopic Pancreaticoduodenectomy Feasible for Pancreatic Ductal Adenocarcinoma? *Cancers* **2020**, *12*, 3430. [CrossRef] [PubMed]
11. Powell-Brett, S.; Pande, R.; Roberts, K. Achieving 'Marginal Gains' to Optimise Outcomes in Resectable Pancreatic Cancer. *Cancers* **2021**, *13*, 1669. [CrossRef] [PubMed]
12. Kwon, W.; Han, Y.; Byun, Y.; Kang, J.; Choi, Y.; Kim, H.; Jang, J. Predictive Features of Malignancy in Branch Duct Type Intraductal Papillary Mucinous Neoplasm of the Pancreas: A Meta-Analysis. *Cancers* **2020**, *12*, 2618. [CrossRef] [PubMed]
13. Wu, Y.; Oba, A.; Beaty, L.; Colborn, K.; Rodriguez Franco, S.; Harnke, B.; Meguid, C.; Negrini, D.; Valente, R.; Ahrendt, S.; et al. Ductal Dilatation of ≥ 5 mm in Intraductal Papillary Mucinous Neoplasm Should Trigger the Consideration for Pancreatectomy: A Meta-Analysis and Systematic Review of Resected Cases. *Cancers* **2021**, *13*, 2031. [CrossRef] [PubMed]

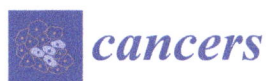

Article

The Role of Location of Tumor in the Prognosis of the Pancreatic Cancer

Mirang Lee †, Wooil Kwon †, Hongbeom Kim, Yoonhyeong Byun, Youngmin Han, Jae Seung Kang, Yoo Jin Choi and Jin-Young Jang *

Department of surgery, Seoul National University Hospital, Seoul 03080, Korea; rang5026@snu.ac.kr (M.L.); willdoc@snu.ac.kr (W.K.); surgeonkhb@snu.ac.kr (H.K.); yoonhyeong@snu.ac.kr (Y.B.); views@snu.ac.kr (Y.H.); 74398@snuh.org (J.S.K.); 74401@snuh.org (Y.J.C.)
* Correspondence: jangjy4@snu.ac.kr; Tel.: +822-2072-2194; Fax: +822-766-3975
† These authors contributed equally to this work as first authors.

Received: 9 June 2020; Accepted: 22 July 2020; Published: 24 July 2020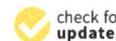

Abstract: Identification of prognostic factors is important to improve treatment outcomes in pancreatic cancer. This study aimed to investigate the effect of the location of pancreatic cancer on survival and to determine whether it was a significant prognostic factor. Altogether, 2483 patients diagnosed with pancreatic cancer were examined. Comparative analysis of clinicopathologic characteristics, survival analysis, and multivariate analysis were performed. Cancers of the pancreatic head or the uncinate process were present in 49.5% of patients. The head/uncinate cancers had more clinical T1/T2 tumors (59.4% vs. 35.5%, $p < 0.001$) and a significantly higher 5-year survival rate (8.9% vs. 7.3%, $p < 0.001$) than the body/tail cancers. The 5-year survival rate in patients with head/uncinate cancers was significantly lower in the resectable ($p = 0.014$) and the locally advanced groups ($p = 0.007$). In patients who underwent resection with curative intent, the 5-year survival rate was lower in the head/uncinate group ($p = 0.046$). The overall outcome of the head/uncinate cancers was better than the body/tail cancers, due to the high proportion of resectable cases. In patients who underwent curative resection, the head/uncinate cancers had a higher number of T1/T2 tumors, but worse outcomes. In the multivariate analysis, tumor location was not an independent prognostic factor for pancreatic cancer.

Keywords: pancreatic neoplasm/analysis; pancreatic neoplasm/surgery; tumor location; survival; clinical staging

1. Introduction

Pancreatic cancer is one of the leading causes of cancer-related mortality in developed countries and one of the most lethal malignant neoplasms worldwide [1]. Its prognosis might be poor, and accurate prediction of the prognosis is important for patients as well as clinicians in the management of pancreatic cancer.

Surgical approach to pancreatic cancer and its prognosis greatly differ according to the tumor location [2–4]. Some authors have argued that pancreatic body and tail cancers have a worse prognosis due to delayed diagnosis. Others have reported that according to the tumor stage at diagnosis, pancreatic body and tail cancers showed superior survival than pancreatic head cancers, in localized and resectable tumors. Despite these differences, tumor location was never taken into consideration in any edition of the American Joint Committee on Cancer (AJCC) staging system, since the first edition in 1978. Thus, the effect of location on pancreatic cancer needs to be highlighted.

Several issues related to tumor location need to be scrutinized in depth. One of them is to clarify whether tumor location affects the prognosis of pancreatic cancer and if it does, the manner in which it affects the prognosis. Furthermore, it should be examined whether tumor location affects the prognosis to such an extent that it should be reflected in the staging system of pancreatic cancer. With these questions in mind, the present study aimed to compare the survival outcomes and clinicopathological features of pancreatic cancer, according to its location.

2. Results

2.1. Patient Demographics and Survival Outcomes

Altogether, 2483 patients were identified. Among these, 1228 patients (49.5%) had tumors in the pancreatic head or the uncinate process (PHU group) and 1255 patients (50.5%) had tumors in the pancreatic body or the tail (PBT group). Demographics and clinicopathological features are summarized in Table 1. The mean age was comparable between the PHU and the PBT groups (64.3 years and 64.0 years, respectively $p = 0.468$). The sex ratio was also similar between the groups, showing male predominance (1:0.68 and 1:0.68, respectively; $p = 0.097$).

Table 1. Demographics and clinicopathological features of overall patients.

Variables	Total (N = 2483)	PHU (N = 1228)	PBT (N = 1255)	*p*-Value
Age (years)	64.1 (23–94)	64.3 (28–94)	64.0 (23–93)	0.468
Sex (Male:Female)	1:0.68	1:0.68	1:0.68	0.970
Tumor size (cm)	3.8 (0.1–15.5)	3.4 (0.1–8.5)	4.3 (0.1–15.5)	<0.001
Clinical T stage				
T1	192 (7.7%)	113 (9.2%)	79 (6.3%)	
T2	983 (39.6%)	616 (50.2%)	367 (29.2%)	<0.001
T3	495 (19.9%)	152 (12.4%)	343 (27.3%)	
T4	813 (32.7%)	347 (28.3%)	466 (37.1%)	
Resectability				
Resectable	677 (27.3%)	449 (36.6%)	228 (18.2%)	
Borderline	124 (5.0%)	85 (6.9%)	39 (3.1%)	<0.001
Locally advanced	615 (24.8%)	313 (25.5%)	302 (24.1%)	
Distant metastasis	1067 (43.0%)	381 (31.0%)	686 (54.7%)	
Operation				
Non-resectable	1778 (71.6%)	766 (62.4%)	1012 (80.6%)	<0.001
Preemptive-resectable	705 (28.4%)	462 (37.6%)	243 (19.4%)	

PHU—tumors in the pancreas head or uncinated process; PBT—tumors in the pancreas body and tail. Continuous variables were expressed as median (range). Statistical significance when *p* value < 0.05.

Mean tumor size was significantly different between the PHU group and the PBT group (3.4 cm and 4.3 cm, respectively; $p < 0.001$). The proportion of clinical T stages was significantly different ($p < 0.001$). The PHU group had a higher proportion of cT2 (50.2% in PHU vs. 29.2% in PBT) tumors. The PBT group had a higher proportion of cT3 and cT4 tumors than the PHU group (cT3: 27.3% vs. 12.4% and cT4: 37.1% vs. 28.3%, respectively).

The proportion of tumors was significantly different in terms of classification according to resectability between the PHU and the PBT groups ($p < 0.001$). The PHU group had a higher proportion of resectable and borderline resectable pancreatic cancers (resectable—36.6% vs. 18.2% and borderline resectable: 6.9% vs. 3.1%, respectively) and a lower proportion of metastatic pancreatic cancer (31.0% vs. 54.7%, respectively) than the PBT group. The proportion of locally advanced pancreatic cancers was similar between the groups (25.5% and 24.1% in the PHU and the PBT groups, respectively).

The median survival in all patients was 11 months and the 5-year survival rate was 8.1%. The PHU group demonstrated significantly better survival than the PBT group (median survival—12 vs. 10 months, and 5-year survival—8.9% vs. 7.3%, respectively; $p < 0.001$) (Figure 1).

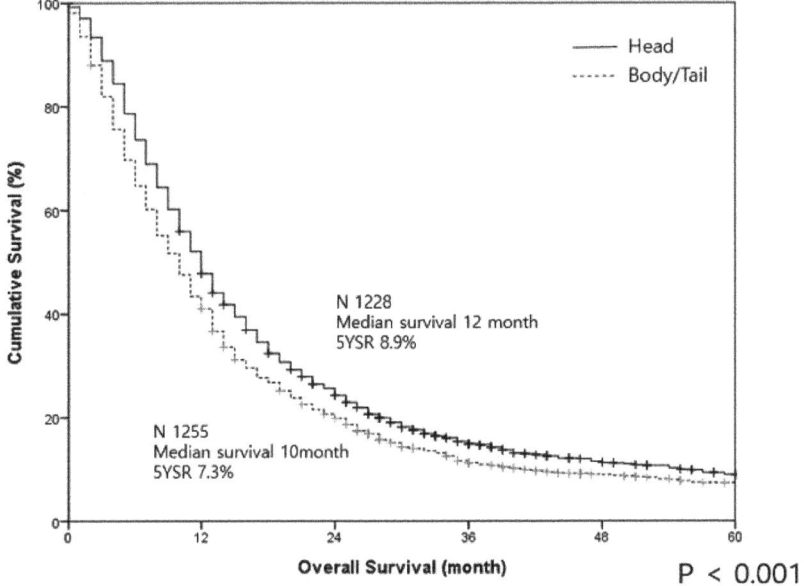

Figure 1. The survival curves of pancreatic cancer in the head/uncinate region and body/tail regions in all patients are illustrated.

2.2. Demographics of the Patients Who Underwent Resection

Among 705 patients who were advised to undergo curative resection, 28 patients who underwent neoadjuvant treatment and 31 patients who ended up having non-curative surgery were excluded. Thus, 646 patients underwent curative resection. Altogether, 432 (66.9%) patients in the PHU group and 214 (33.1%) patients in the PBT group underwent curative resection. The PHU group had a significantly smaller tumor size, more angiolymphatic invasion and perineural invasion, a lower proportion of T3 and T4 tumors, a higher proportion of N2 and a lower proportion of N0 tumors, greater recurrence, and lower incidence of systemic recurrence, when compared to the PBT group. There were no differences in carcinoembryonic antigen and carbohydrate antigen (CA) 19-9 levels, lymph node (LN) metastasis rate, and the proportion of patients who received adjuvant therapy. Demographics and clinicopathological features are summarized in Table 2.

Table 2. Demographics and clinicopathological features of resected patients.

Variables	Total (N = 646)	PHU (N = 432)	PBT (N = 214)	p-Value
Age (years)	64.6 (29–89)	63.7 (29–88)	66.4 (35–89)	0.001
Sex (Male:Female)	1:0.7	1:0.67	1:0.75	0.552
Preoperative CEA (ng/mL)	4.1 (0.5–179.1)	3.5 (0.5–63)	5.2 (0.5–179.1)	0.124
Preoperative CA19-9 (U/mL)	1040.7 (0.1–37800)	1109.2 (0.1–28700)	901.7 (1–37800)	0.421
Operation name				<0.001
PPPD	251 (38.9%)	251 (58.1%)	0	
Whipple's operation	163 (25.2%)	163 (37.7%)	0	
Distal pancreatectomy	190 (29.4%)	0	190 (88.8%)	
Subtotal pancreatectomy	17 (2.6%)	0	17 (7.9%)	
Total pancreatectomy	23 (3.6%)	17 (3.9%)	23 (3.6%)	
Central pancreatectomy	2 (0.3%)	1 (0.2%)	2 (0.3%)	

Table 2. Cont.

Variables	Total (N = 646)	PHU (N = 432)	PBT (N = 214)	p-Value
Complication	264 (40.9%)	199 (46.1%)	65 (30.4%)	<0.001
Adjuvant therapy				
Chemotherapy	516 (79.9%)	344 (79.6%)	172 (80.4%)	0.917
Radiotherapy	343 (53.1%)	231 (53.5%)	112 (52.3%)	0.802
Tumor size(cm)	3.3 (0.2–12.2)	3.1 (0.2–8.0)	3.5 (0.5–12.2)	0.008
Differentiation				
Well Differentiated	43 (7.1%)	23 (5.6%)	20 (10.2%)	0.053
Moderate Differentiated	488 (80.7%)	340 (83.1%)	148 (75.5%)	
Poorly Differentiated	74 (12.2%)	46 (11.2%)	28 (14.3%)	
Resection margin status				
Tumor free	549 (85.0%)	373 (86.3%)	176 (82.2%)	0.198
Presence of tumor	97 (15.0%)	59 (13.7%)	38 (17.8%)	
Angiolymphatic invasion				
Negative	354 (55.0%)	213 (49.4%)	141 (66.2%)	<0.001
Positive	290 (45.0%)	218 (50.6%)	72 (33.8%)	
Vascular invasion				
Negative	389 (60.3%)	252 (58.5%)	137 (64.0%)	0.200
Positive	256 (39.7%)	179 (41.5%)	77 (36.0%)	
Perineural invasion				
Negative	108 (16.7%)	61 (14.1%)	47 (22.0%)	0.014
Positive	538 (83.3%)	371 (85.9%)	167 (78.0%)	
T stage				
T1	96 (14.9%)	62 (14.4%)	34 (15.9%)	
T2	426 (65.9%)	299 (69.2%)	127 (59.3%)	0.041
T3	113 (17.5%)	66 (15.3%)	47 (22.0%)	
T4	11 (1.7%)	5 (1.2%)	6 (2.8%)	
N stage				
N0	252 (39.0%)	160 (37.0%)	92 (43.0%)	
N1	270 (41.8%)	177 (41.0%)	93 (43.5%)	0.033
N2	124 (19.2%)	95 (22.0%)	29 (13.6%)	
Stage				
Ia	65 (10.1%)	38 (8.8%)	27 (12.6%)	
Ib	150 (23.2%)	101 (23.4%)	49 (22.9%)	
IIa	34 (5.3%)	20 (4.6%)	14 (6.5%)	0.171
IIb	265 (41.0%)	175 (40.5%)	90 (42.1%)	
III	132 (20.4%)	98 (22.7%)	34 (15.9%)	
Recurrence				
No	211 (32.7%)	125 (29.0%)	86 (40.2%)	0.006
Yes	434 (67.3%)	306 (71.0%)	128 (59.8%)	
Recurrence type				
Local	66 (15.2%)	54 (17.7%)	12 (9.4%)	0.028
Systemic	367 (84.8%)	251 (82.3%)	116 (90.6%)	

PHU—tumors in the pancreas head or uncinated process; PBT—tumors in the pancreas body and tail; PPPD—pylorus-preserving pancreatoduodenectomy. Continuous variables were expressed as median (range). Statistically significant when p value < 0.05.

2.3. Survival Analysis of the Patients Who Underwent Resection

The median survival duration was 25 months and the 5-year survival was 23.6%. For the PHU group, the median survival duration was 23 months and the 5-year survival was 20.8%. For the PBT group, the median survival duration was 30 months and the 5-year survival was 29.7%. Thus, the survival outcome in the PBT group was significantly superior to that in the PHU group ($p = 0.046$) (Figure 2).

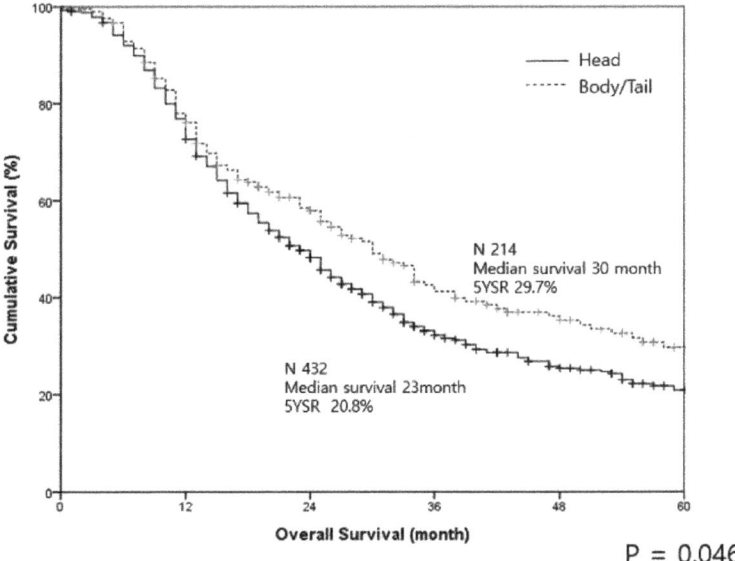

Figure 2. The survival curves of pancreatic cancer in the head/uncinate region and body/tail regions in resected patients are illustrated.

Survival outcomes were compared according to the T category. For T1, T2, and T4 tumors, the PHU group had worse outcomes compared to the PBT group. The difference was not significant for the T1 (median survival 34 vs. 41 months, respectively; $p = 0.288$) and T4 tumors (median survival 6 vs. 8 months, respectively; $p = 0.067$). A significant difference was found in T2 tumors with a median survival of 22 months for the PHU group (5-year survival 19.4%) and a median survival of 34 months for the PHU group (5-year survival 34.8%) ($p = 0.005$, Figure 3).

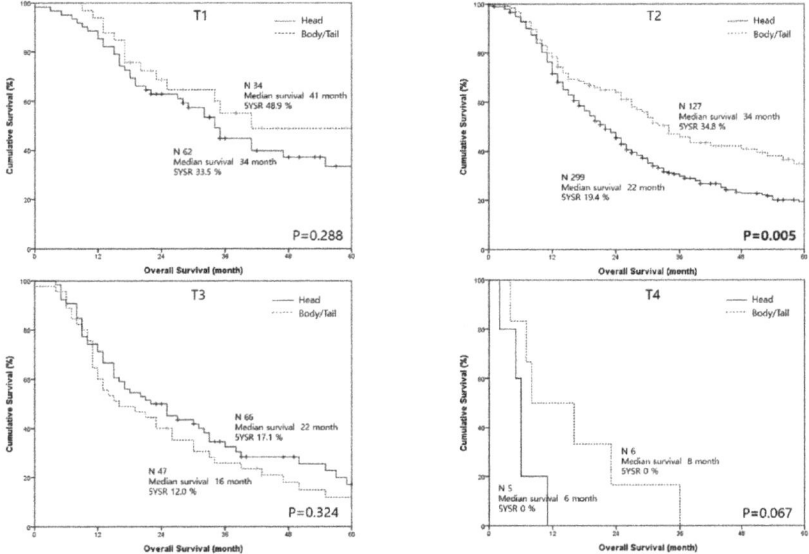

Figure 3. The survival curves of pancreas head/uncinate cancer and pancreas body cancer according to the T categories.

In node-negative disease, the PHU group had worse median survival than the PBT group, but the difference was not significant (33 vs. 39 months, respectively; $p = 0.454$). Similarly, in the node-positive disease, the PHU group had worse outcomes than the PBT group, but the difference lacked statistical significance (19 vs. 25 months, respectively; $p = 0.112$).

According to the prognostic groups of the AJCC cancer staging system (edition 8), there were no differences in survival outcomes between the PHU and the PBT groups, in all stages from stage Ia to stage III (Figure S1).

2.4. Prognostic Factors of Pancreatic Cancer

Tumor location, histological grade, margin status, angiolymphatic invasion, venous invasion, perineural invasion, T category, N category, adjuvant chemotherapy, adjuvant radiotherapy, and preoperative CA 19-9 were significantly associated with survival. In the multivariate analysis, tumor location did not reach statistical significance (vs. PBT: hazard ratio [HR] 1.174, confidence interval [CI] 0.932–1.478, $p = 0.173$). Histological grade, margin status, angiolymphatic invasion, venous invasion, T4 stage, lymph node metastasis, adjuvant chemotherapy, adjuvant radiotherapy, and preoperative CA 19-9 were independent prognostic factors (Table 3).

Table 3. Univariate and multivariate analysis comparing the 5-year survival rates in resected patients.

Variables	Univariate			Multivariate		
	n	5 YSR, %	p Value	HR	95%CI	p Value
Sex						
Male	380	21.2				
Female	266	27.3	0.269			
Age(years)						
<65	301	24.0				
≥65	345	23.6	0.070	1.095	0.881–1.362	0.414
Site of tumor						
Head	432	20.8				
Body, tail	214	29.7	0.046	1.174	0.932–1.478	0.173
Complication						
No	382	22.7				
Yes	264	24.9	0.986			
Histologic grade			<0.001			<0.001
Well differentiated	43	45.0				
Moderate differentiated	488	21.9	<0.001	2.092	1.306–3.351	0.002
Poorly differentiated	74	11.2	<0.001	3.133	1.834–5.354	<0.001
Margin						
Negative	549	26.5				
Positive	97	5.3	<0.001	1.471	1.126–1.923	0.005
Angiolymphatic invasion						
Negative	354	31.0				
Positive	290	13.7	<0.001	1.473	1.191-1.823	<0.001
Venous invasion						
Negative	389	30.1				
Positive	256	11.9	<0.001	1.309	1.059–1.618	0.013
Perineural invasion						
Negative	108	42.3				
Positive	538	19.7	<0.001	1.250	0.895–1.746	0.191

Table 3. Cont.

Variables	Univariate			Multivariate		
	n	5 YSR, %	p Value	HR	95%CI	p Value
T stage			<0.001			0.008
T1	96	37.9				
T2	426	23.7	0.001	1.143	0.814–1.604	0.440
T3	113	15.0	<0.001	1.278	0.858–1.902	0.227
T4	11	0.0	<0.001	4.874	2.228–10.664	<0.001
N stage			<0.001			0.005
N0	252	37.3				
N1	269	17.0	<0.001	1.271	1.002–1.613	0.048
N2	125	8.2	<0.001	1.611	1.207–2.150	0.001
Adjuvant Chemotherapy						
Yes	516	25.0				
No	130	18.4	<0.001	1.626	1.206–2.193	0.001
Adjuvant Radiotherapy						
Yes	343	27.3				
No	303	20.9	<0.001	1.417	1.103–1.821	0.006
Preoperative CEA						
<5.0 ng/mL	524	24.8				
≥5.0 ng/mL	94	21.9	0.061	1.168	0.884–1.544	0.274
Preoperative CA19-9						
<37.0 U/mL	187	38.9				
≥37.0 U/mL	446	18.1	<0.001	1.600	1.258–2.037	<0.001

YSR—year survival rate; HR—hazard ratio; CI—confidence interval. The variables with p-value less than 0.1 in univariate analysis were included in the multivariate analysis.

When analyzed separately for the PHU and the PBT groups, factors associated with survival in the univariate analysis were similar between the groups and similar to the factors associated with the overall patient population. For the PHU group, all associated categories were similar to those associated with the overall patient population. For the PBT group, T2 stage and preoperative CA 19-9 were not associated with survival, while age was associated with survival, when compared to the overall patient population.

Multivariate analysis showed that poorly differentiated histological grade, angiolymphatic invasion, perineural invasion, T4 stage, N2 stage, adjuvant chemotherapy, adjuvant radiotherapy, and preoperative CA 19-9 were significantly associated with survival in the PHU group. In the PBT group, histological grade, margin status, venous invasion, and adjuvant chemotherapy were significantly associated with survival (Table 4).

Table 4. Comparison of independent risk factors of pancreatic cancer in PHU and PBT.

Variables	PHU						PBT					
	Univariate			Multivariate			Univariate			Multivariate		
	n	5YSR, %	p Value	HR	95%CI	p Value	n	5YSR, %	p Value	HR	95%CI	p Value
Sex												
Male	258	16.6	0.254				122	31.2	0.968			
Female	174	26.9					92	27.0				
Age (years)												
<65	220	19.3	0.272				81	39.0	0.020	1.135	0.740–1.740	0.561
≥65	212	23.5					133	24.3				
Complication												
No	233	18.8	0.645				149	28.7	0.883			
Yes	199	22.8					65	33.1				
Histologic grade			<0.001			0.001			0.002			0.004
Well differentiated	23	27.7					20	69.1				
Moderate differentiated	340	19.7	0.035	1.368	0.781–2.396	0.273	148	27.5	0.003	3.632	1.503–8.777	0.004
Poorly differentiated	46	12.3	<0.001	2.692	1.419–5.108	0.002	28	9.0	<0.001	3.609	1.318–9.885	0.013
Margin												
Negative	373	22.5	0.006	1.165	0.823–1.649	0.388	176	35.8	<0.001	2.431	1.580–3.743	<0.001
Positive	59	5.8					38	4.4				
Angiolymphatic invasion												
Negative	213	29.0	<0.001	1.393	1.079–1.799	0.011	141	34.4	0.002	1.412	0.952–2.095	0.087
Positive	218	12.4					72	18.5				
Venous invasion												
Negative	252	26.5	<0.001	1.239	0.966–1.590	0.092	137	37.8	<0.001	1.523	1.014–2.288	0.042
Positive	179	11.1					77	14.3				
Perineural invasion												
Negative	61	40.7	<0.001	1.581	1.033–2.420	0.035	47	45.2	0.036	0.669	0.389–1.149	0.145
Positive	371	17.4					167	25.1				

Table 4. Cont.

Variables	PHU						PBT					
	Univariate			Multivariate			Univariate			Multivariate		
	n	5YSR, %	p Value	HR	95%CI	p Value	n	5YSR, %	p Value	HR	95%CI	p Value
T stage			<0.001			0.004			<0.001			0.034
T1	62	33.5					34	48.9				
T2	299	19.4	0.004	1.303	0.868–1.956	0.201	127	34.8	0.158	0.827	0.445–1.534	0.546
T3	66	17.1	0.034	1.215	0.734–2.012	0.448	47	12.0	0.001	1.433	0.749–2.742	0.278
T4	5	0.0	<0.001	13.539	4.519–40.565	<0.001	6	0.0	<0.001	2.336	0.769–7.096	0.134
N stage			<0.001			0.037			0.004			0.180
N0	160	33.2					92	45.3				
N1	177	16.4	<0.001	1.223	0.920–1.627	0.166	92	18.4	0.005	1.474	0.936–2.319	0.094
N2	95	7.3	<0.001	1.571	1.114–2.214	0.010	30	12.2	0.006	1.554	0.867–2.784	0.139
Adjuvant Chemotherapy												
Yes	344	22.5	<0.001	1.511	1.074–2.125	0.018	172	30.6	0.034	2.466	1.463–4.156	0.001
No	88	14.1					42	26.2				
Adjuvant Radiotherapy												
Yes	231	25.1	<0.001	1.482	1.108–1.983	0.008	112	32.1	0.080	1.279	0.793–2.064	0.313
No	201	17.0					102	29.2				
Preoperative CEA												
<5.0 ng/mL	354	22.1	0.053	1.277	0.917–1.778	0.148	170	30.9	0.459			
≥5.0 ng/mL	60	18.5					34	27.3				
Preoperative CA19-9												
<37.0 U/mL	177	39.9	<0.001	1.621	1.199–2.192	0.002	70	35.6	0.120			
≥37.0 U/mL	307	14.2					139	26.8				

PHU—tumors in the pancreas head or uncinated process; PBT—tumors in the pancreas body and tail; YSR—year survival rate; HR—hazard ratio; CI—confidence interval; The variables which p-value was less than 0.1 in univariate analysis were included in the multivariate analysis.

3. Discussion

The AJCC staging system was revised for the eighth time since its first edition in 2018. Its validity was demonstrated in several studies [5–7]. The AJCC staging system always considered pancreatic cancers in terms of the whole pancreas, without dividing the pancreas according to the location, since pancreatic cancers in the head/uncinate process and those in the body/tail share the same prognosis and have comparable tumor biology. However, pancreatic cancer is usually treated according to the location. Many studies investigated pancreatic cancers separately according to the location [2,4,8–12]. Furthermore, many studies investigated whether the subjects underwent distal pancreatectomy or pancreatoduodenectomy, which is a reflection of the location of the tumor [13–16]. Pancreatic cancer is often not looked at somewhat differently. In this light, it must be clarified whether pancreatic head cancers and pancreatic body or tail cancers have comparable outcomes and oncological behaviors.

Traditionally, pancreatic cancers in the body/tail are believed to have a worse prognosis compared to pancreatic head cancers. This finding was supported by several studies [2,8–10,17] and it was also reproduced in the present study. The 5-year survival percentages and the median survival durations were significantly better for the PHU group than for the PBT group, in all pancreatic cancers, regardless of their resectability. The poor outcome of pancreatic cancers in the body/tail is usually explained by their late detection.

While a pancreatic head cancer might cause obstructive jaundice as the tumor progresses, patients with pancreatic body/tail cancers do not show symptoms until the tumor size increases sufficiently to cause abdominal pain and colon obstruction. In the present cohort, the tumor size measured on the cross-sectional images was significantly greater in the PBT group. Larger tumors reduce the possibility of resectability, which is also reflected in the results of the present study. In the present study, 36.6% of the pancreatic head cancers were deemed resectable, while only 18.2% of the pancreatic body/tail cancers were deemed resectable.

Late detection of the pancreatic body and tail tumors allows them to grow, reducing their resectability. It also increases the possibility of systemic involvement. Other studies that investigated pancreatic cancers according to their locations showed that pancreatic body and tail cancers often present with distant metastases at the time of diagnosis [2,11]. The present study also confirmed a higher proportion of systemic spread at presentation (54.7% in the body/tail cancers and 31.0% in the head/uncinate region cancers).

A completely opposite set of findings was observed when only the resected cases were considered. In the resected cases, pancreatic cancers in the head/uncinate region demonstrated significantly worse survival than those in the body/tail region. Many studies found similar results in resectable pancreatic cancers in the head/uncinate regions [11,12,18], while some studies failed to show worse results for the head region when compared to the body/tail region [9,10,13–16,19]. However, none of these studies showed significantly worse outcomes in pancreatic body/tail cancers [12].

Studies that demonstrated comparable outcomes between resectable pancreatic cancers in the head and those in the body/tail should be noted for their study population. Studies conducted by Sohn et al. [13], Wade et al. [14], and Brennan et al. [19] published in 2000, 1995, and 1996, respectively, are considered the historic ones. Their study populations were collected from as early as 1984 and up to 1999. During this period, safety and oncological feasibility of pancreatic cancer surgery was more of an issue. Furthermore, adjuvant treatment, which is currently an important part of pancreatic cancer treatment, was not established. The studies from the late 2000s and the 2010s had similar problems regarding patient populations as those associated with the patient populations from the 1980s and the 1990s, even though they included more recent cohorts [9,15,16].

Only one study that included 351 patients showed superior outcomes in the resected pancreatic head cancers, when compared with the resected body/tail cancers [4]. The median survivals of patients with pancreatic head cancers and of those with pancreatic body/tail cancers were 16 and 11 months, respectively. This rather poor survival outcome in patients with resected tumors limited the value of this study. All the other studies reported comparable or superior outcomes in resected pancreatic body/tail cancers than in resected pancreatic head cancers. Therefore, based on the recent literature and the results of the present study, it could be safely concluded that resected pancreatic cancers in the body/tail region have better outcomes than those in the head region. As such is the case, resection of pancreatic body/tail cancers should not be discouraged because of the poor overall prognosis, but rather should be attempted, whenever deemed resectable.

When analyzed according to the T stages, significant difference was observed in survival between the groups for T2 tumors. The PHU group showed worse outcomes than the PBT group for T1 tumors, but the difference was not significant. This finding might perhaps be attributed to small-sized subgroups. Thus, earlier T categories (T1 and T2) demonstrated significantly worse median survival and 5-year survival (24 months and 21.8%) in the PHU group than in the PBT group (34 months and 37.2%) ($p = 0.003$). Meng et al. [12] also found that resected pancreatic head cancers had worse outcomes in the earlier T stages, but significant difference was observed only for the T1 stage.

When stratified according to the N stage and the prognostic groups, the survival rates were not significantly different. There was a tendency toward worse survival for pancreatic head/uncinate cancers in the N0 and LN metastasis groups. For the prognostic groups, pancreatic head/uncinate cancers in stages IB, IIB, and III tended to have worse survival. Re-evaluation using a larger cohort or meta-analysis might clarify the effect of cancer location in each stratified analysis.

There were varying results regarding whether the location of pancreatic cancer was an independent prognostic factor. The present study found that cancer location was not an independent risk factor (head vs. body/tail: HR 1.174, CI 0.932–1.478, $p = 0.173$). Similarly, Ruess et al. [16] and van Erning et al. [10] did not identify location as an independent risk factor. Several other studies suggested that location was a significant risk factor [2,4,9,11,12,18]. Therefore, the status of cancer location as an independent prognostic factor is still controversial and needs further high-level evidence.

The difference in survival outcomes between the locations might be due to plain anatomical differences causing symptoms at different time intervals. There might be additional differences in tumor biology and behavior. To investigate the differences in tumor biology and behavior, clinicopathological features of pancreatic cancers in the head/uncinate process and cancers in the body/tail region were analyzed and compared. Some differences were present, but common risk factors were also observed. Hence, the results are unclear and a definite conclusion cannot be obtained.

Additionally, differences on genetic and molecular levels should also be considered. The present study did not examine this aspect, but previous studies examined genetic profiles. Birnbaum et al. [20] found differences in 334-gene expression signature between tumors in the head and those in the body/tail. Dreyer et al. [8] reported that tumors might have different molecular pathology, according to their location and the body/tail tumors are enriched with gene programs involved in tumor invasion, epithelial-to-mesenchymal transition, and poor antitumor immune response. This is an important area of research, as the differences on genetic and molecular levels might open a new era of more tailored treatment approaches, according to the location.

The present study had some limitations. The study was retrospective in nature. In addition, the overall patient dataset was acquired through a clinical data warehouse. Hence, more specific variables could not be retrieved in detail. As the present study was performed at a tertiary hospital, many patients visited after being diagnosed at other primary or secondary hospitals, which might have resulted in bias regarding the date of diagnosis. The study population was insufficient for subgroup analyses after stratification.

4. Materials and Methods

4.1. Study Design

The study was approved by the ethical committee of the Institutional Review Board of Seoul National University Hospital (IRB No. H-1902-012-1006). Seoul National University Hospital's Clinical

Data Warehouse was searched for patients who were diagnosed with pancreatic ductal adenocarcinoma between 2005 and 2016. A retrospective cohort study was performed.

This research was supported by the Collaborative Genome Program for Fostering New Post-Genome Industry of the National Research Foundation funded by the Ministry of Science and ICT (NRF-2017M3C9A5031591), and by a grant from the Korean Health Technology R and D Project, Ministry of Health and Welfare, Republic of Korea (HI14C2640).

4.2. Patient Selection

After the identification of patients with pancreatic cancer from the database, those with multiple tumors in both the head and the body/tail were excluded. Patients who had tumors across the junction of the head and the body were also excluded, as grouping according to the location was ambiguous in these tumors. Data regarding age, sex, tumor location, tumor size on radiological images, clinical feature (T) classification, and classification based on resectability were collected.

Further subgroup analysis was performed for patients who underwent resection with curative intent. Among all patients, 646 patients who underwent resection of pancreatic cancer with curative intent were examined. Patients who underwent only palliative operation including bypass or open biopsy were excluded. Since neoadjuvant treatment can alter the final pathological staging, patients who received neoadjuvant therapy were also excluded. Detailed information about the demographic and clinicopathological factors of these patients was obtained through a thorough review of their electronic medical records.

4.3. Determination of Tumor Location and Clinical T Staging

Computed tomography (CT) or magnetic resonance imaging (MRI) records of all patients were reviewed. An imaginary tangential line over the left border of the superior mesenteric vein or the portal vein was drawn on the CT image. The head/uncinate pancreatic cancer group (PHU) was defined as patients with tumors on the right side of this line. The body/tail pancreatic cancer group (PBT) was defined as patients with tumors on the left side of this line.

Clinical T staging was performed according to the AJCC staging system (edition 8) for pancreatic cancer. Tumor size was measured using CT and MRI.

4.4. Definition of Survival and Data Collection

Overall survival was used for the analysis. It was defined as the interval between the date of diagnosis and the date of death or the last follow-up. Survival status was acquired from the Ministry of Interior and Safety of Korea. Patients who were alive on 20 February 2019 were censored.

4.5. Statistical Analysis

Fisher's exact test and chi-squared test were used to compare categorical variables and unpaired two-sided Student's t-test was used to compare continuous variables between patients with tumors located in the head/uncinate process and patients with tumors in the body/tail. The Kaplan-Meier method with log-rank test was used for survival analysis. Cox regression test was used for the univariate and the multivariate analyses. A p-value < 0.050 was considered to be statistically significant. IBM SPSS statistics for Windows version 24 (IBM Corp., Armonk, NY, USA) was used for statistical analyses.

5. Conclusions

The prognosis of pancreatic cancers differed according to the location of the tumors. Pancreatic head cancers showed a better overall prognosis than pancreatic body/tail cancers, which might be related to a higher proportion of systemic involvement in the latter. On the contrary, resected pancreatic head cancers showed a worse prognosis than resected pancreatic body/tail cancers, especially in the earlier T stages. Tumor location was not an independent risk factor for pancreatic cancer.

Supplementary Materials: The following are available online at http://www.mdpi.com/2072-6694/12/8/2036/s1. Figure S1: The survival curves of pancreas head/uncinate cancer and pancreas body cancer in terms of the prognostic group, according to the eighth edition of AJCC cancer staging system.

Author Contributions: Conceptualization, W.K. and J.-Y.J.; Data curation, M.L., W.K., H.K. and Y.H.; Formal analysis, M.L.; Funding acquisition, Y.H.; Investigation, M.L., J.S.K. and Y.J.C.; Methodology, Y.B.; Project administration, W.K., H.K. and J.-Y.J.; Resources, J.S.K. and Y.J.C.; Supervision, W.K.; Validation, W.K., H.K., Y.B., Y.H. and J.-Y.J.; Writing—original draft, M.L.; Writing—review & editing, M.L., W.K., Y.B. and J.-Y.J. All authors have read and agreed to the published version of the manuscript.

Funding: This study was supported by the Collaborative Genome Program for Fostering New Post-Genome Industry of the National Research Foundation, funded by the Ministry of Science and ICT (NRF-2017M3C9A5031591) and the Korean Health Technology R&D Project, Ministry of Health and Welfare (HI14C2640), Korea.

Conflicts of Interest: The authors declare no conflict of interest.

References

1. Ilic, M.; Ilic, I. Epidemiology of pancreatic cancer. *World J. Gastroenterol.* **2016**, *22*, 9694–9705. [CrossRef] [PubMed]
2. Lau, M.K.; Davila, J.A.; Shaib, Y.H. Incidence and survival of pancreatic head and body and tail cancers: A population-based study in the United States. *Pancreas* **2010**, *39*, 458–462. [CrossRef] [PubMed]
3. Sener, S.F.; Fremgen, A.; Menck, H.R.; Winchester, D.P. Pancreatic cancer: A report of treatment and survival trends for 100,313 patients diagnosed from 1985–1995, using the National Cancer Database. *J. Am. Coll. Surg.* **1999**, *189*, 1–7. [CrossRef]
4. Sheng, W.W.; Dong, M.; Wang, G.S.; Shi, X.Y.; Gao, W.; Wang, K.W.; Song, H.; Shi, G.; Tan, X.D. The diversity between curatively resected pancreatic head and body-tail cancers based on the 8th edition of AJCC staging system: A multicenter cohort study. *BMC Cancer* **2019**, *19*, 981. [CrossRef] [PubMed]
5. Van Roessel, S.; Kasumova, G.G.; Verheij, J.; Najarian, R.M.; Maggino, L.; de Pastena, M.; Malleo, G.; Marchegiani, G.; Salvia, R.; Ng, S.C.; et al. International Validation of the Eighth Edition of the American Joint Committee on Cancer (AJCC) TNM Staging System in Patients with Resected Pancreatic Cancer. *JAMA Surg.* **2018**, *153*, e183617. [CrossRef] [PubMed]
6. Allen, P.J.; Kuk, D.; Castillo, C.F.; Basturk, O.; Wolfgang, C.L.; Cameron, J.L.; Lillemoe, K.D.; Ferrone, C.R.; Morales-Oyarvide, V.; He, J.; et al. Multi-institutional Validation Study of the American Joint Commission on Cancer (8th Edition) Changes for T and N Staging in Patients with Pancreatic Adenocarcinoma. *Ann. Surg.* **2017**, *265*, 185–191. [CrossRef] [PubMed]
7. Kwon, W.; He, J.; Higuchi, R.; Son, D.; Lee, S.Y.; Kim, J.; Kim, H.; Kim, S.W.; Wolfgang, C.L.; Cameron, J.L.; et al. Multinational validation of the American Joint Committee on Cancer 8th edition pancreatic cancer staging system in a pancreas head cancer cohort. *J. Hepatobiliary Pancreat. Sci.* **2018**, *25*, 418–427. [CrossRef] [PubMed]
8. Dreyer, S.B.; Jamieson, N.B.; Upstill-Goddard, R.; Bailey, P.J.; McKay, C.J.; Australian Pancreatic Cancer Genome Initiative; Biankin, A.V.; Chang, D.K. Defining the molecular pathology of pancreatic body and tail adenocarcinoma. *Br. J. Surg.* **2018**, *105*, e183–e191. [CrossRef] [PubMed]
9. Artinyan, A.; Soriano, P.A.; Prendergast, C.; Low, T.; Ellenhorn, J.D.; Kim, J. The anatomic location of pancreatic cancer is a prognostic factor for survival. *HPB (Oxford)* **2008**, *10*, 371–376. [CrossRef] [PubMed]
10. van Erning, F.N.; Mackay, T.M.; van der Geest, L.G.M.; Groot Koerkamp, B.; van Laarhoven, H.W.M.; Bonsing, B.A.; Wilmink, J.W.; van Santvoort, H.C.; de Vos-Geelen, J.; van Eijck, C.H.; et al. Association of the location of pancreatic ductal adenocarcinoma (head, body, tail) with tumor stage, treatment, and survival: A population-based analysis. *Acta Oncol.* **2018**, *57*, 1655–1662. [CrossRef] [PubMed]
11. Winer, L.K.; Dhar, V.K.; Wima, K.; Morris, M.C.; Lee, T.C.; Shah, S.A.; Ahmad, S.A.; Patel, S.H. The Impact of Tumor Location on Resection and Survival for Pancreatic Ductal Adenocarcinoma. *J. Surg. Res.* **2019**, *239*, 60–66. [CrossRef]
12. Meng, Z.; Cao, M.; Zhang, Y.; Liu, Z.; Wu, S.; Wu, H. Tumor location as an indicator of survival in T1 resectable pancreatic ductal adenocarcinoma: A propensity score-matched analysis. *BMC Gastroenterol.* **2019**, *19*, 59. [CrossRef]

13. Sohn, T.A.; Yeo, C.J.; Cameron, J.L.; Koniaris, L.; Kaushal, S.; Abrams, R.A.; Sauter, P.K.; Coleman, J.; Hruban, R.H.; Lillemoe, K.D. Resected adenocarcinoma of the pancreas-616 patients: Results, outcomes, and prognostic indicators. *J. Gastrointest. Surg.* **2000**, *4*, 567–579. [CrossRef]
14. Wade, T.P.; Virgo, K.S.; Johnson, F.E. Distal pancreatectomy for cancer: Results in U.S. Department of Veterans Affairs hospitals, 1987–1991. *Pancreas* **1995**, *11*, 341–344. [CrossRef]
15. Toomey, P.; Hernandez, J.; Golkar, F.; Ross, S.; Luberice, K.; Rosemurgy, A. Pancreatic adenocarcinoma: Complete tumor extirpation improves survival benefit despite larger tumors for patients who undergo distal pancreatectomy and splenectomy. *J. Gastrointest. Surg.* **2012**, *16*, 376–381. [CrossRef] [PubMed]
16. Ruess, D.A.; Makowiec, F.; Chikhladze, S.; Sick, O.; Riediger, H.; Hopt, U.T.; Wittel, U.A. The prognostic influence of intrapancreatic tumor location on survival after resection of pancreatic ductal adenocarcinoma. *BMC Surg.* **2015**, *15*, 123. [CrossRef] [PubMed]
17. Watanabe, I.; Sasaki, S.; Konishi, M.; Nakagohri, T.; Inoue, K.; Oda, T.; Kinoshita, T. Onset symptoms and tumor locations as prognostic factors of pancreatic cancer. *Pancreas* **2004**, *28*, 160–165. [CrossRef] [PubMed]
18. Zheng, Z.; Wang, M.; Tan, C.; Chen, Y.; Ping, J.; Wang, R.; Liu, X. Disparities in survival by stage after surgery between pancreatic head and body/tail in patients with nonmetastatic pancreatic cancer. *PLoS ONE* **2019**, *14*, e0226726. [CrossRef] [PubMed]
19. Brennan, M.F.; Moccia, R.D.; Klimstra, D. Management of adenocarcinoma of the body and tail of the pancreas. *Ann. Surg.* **1996**, *223*, 506–511. [CrossRef] [PubMed]
20. Birnbaum, D.J.; Bertucci, F.; Finetti, P.; Birnbaum, D.; Mamessier, E. Head and Body/Tail Pancreatic Carcinomas Are Not the Same Tumors. *Cancers* **2019**, *11*, 497. [CrossRef] [PubMed]

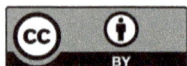

© 2020 by the authors. Licensee MDPI, Basel, Switzerland. This article is an open access article distributed under the terms and conditions of the Creative Commons Attribution (CC BY) license (http://creativecommons.org/licenses/by/4.0/).

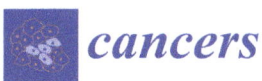

Review

Reconsideration of the Appropriate Dissection Range Based on Japanese Anatomical Classification for Resectable Pancreatic Head Cancer in the Era of Multimodal Treatment

Yuichi Nagakawa [1,*], Naoya Nakagawa [1], Chie Takishita [1], Ichiro Uyama [2], Shingo Kozono [1], Hiroaki Osakabe [1], Kenta Suzuki [1], Nobuhiko Nakagawa [1], Yuichi Hosokawa [1], Tomoki Shirota [1], Masayuki Honda [1], Tesshi Yamada [1,3], Kenji Katsumata [1] and Akihiko Tsuchida [1]

[1] Department of Gastrointestinal and Pediatric Surgery, Tokyo Medical University, Tokyo 160-8402, Japan; nao8nak@tokyo-med.ac.jp (N.N.); chie0428@tokyo-med.ac.jp (C.T.); s-kozono@tokyo-med.ac.jp (S.K.); osakabeh@tokyo-med.ac.jp (H.O.); ks_0828@tokyo-med.ac.jp (K.S.); nkgw_n1@tokyo-med.ac.jp (N.N.); yhosokaw@tokyo-med.ac.jp (Y.H.); but_ibshigin@tokyo-med.ac.jp (T.S.); masayuki@tokyo-med.ac.jp (M.H.); exk0009@tokyo-med.ac.jp (T.Y.); k-katsu@tokyo-med.ac.jp (K.K.); akihikot@tokyo-med.ac.jp (A.T.)

[2] Department of Advanced Robotic and Endoscopic Surgery, Fujita Health University, Toyoake 470-1192, Aichi, Japan; iuyama@fujita-hu.ac.jp

[3] Division of Chemotherapy and Clinical Research, National Cancer Center Research Institute, Tokyo 104-0045, Japan

* Correspondence: naga@tokyo-med.ac.jp; Tel.: +81-3-3342-6111

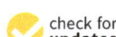

Simple Summary: Although the survival benefit of "regional lymph node dissection" for pancreatic head cancer remains unclear, the R0 resection rate is reportedly associated with prognosis. We reviewed the literature that could be helpful in determining the appropriate resection range. The recent development of high-quality computed tomography has made it possible to evaluate the extent of cancer infiltration. Even if the "dissection to achieve R0 resection" range is simulated based on the computed tomography evaluation, it is difficult to identify the range intraoperatively. It is necessary to be aware of the anatomical landmarks to determine the appropriate dissection range intraoperatively.

Abstract: Patients with resectable pancreatic cancer are considered to already have micro-distant metastasis, because most of the recurrence patterns postoperatively are distant metastases. Multi-modal treatment dramatically improves prognosis; thus, micro-distant metastasis is considered to be controlled by chemotherapy. The survival benefit of "regional lymph node dissection" for pancreatic head cancer remains unclear. We reviewed the literature that could be helpful in determining the appropriate resection range. Regional lymph nodes with no suspected metastases on preoperative imaging may become areas treated with preoperative and postoperative adjuvant chemotherapy. Many studies have reported that the R0 resection rate is associated with prognosis. Thus, "dissection to achieve R0 resection" is required. The recent development of high-quality computed tomography has made it possible to evaluate the extent of cancer infiltration. Therefore, it is possible to simulate the dissection range to achieve R0 resection preoperatively. However, it is often difficult to distinguish between areas of inflammatory changes and cancer infiltration during resection. Even if the "dissection to achieve R0 resection" range is simulated based on the computed tomography evaluation, it is difficult to identify the range intraoperatively. It is necessary to be aware of anatomical landmarks to determine the appropriate dissection range during surgery.

Keywords: pancreatic cancer; pancreaticoduodenectomy; mesopancreas; superior mesenteric artery; nerve and fibrous tissues; adjuvant chemotherapy; lymph node dissection; R0 resection

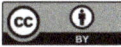

1. Introduction

Pancreatic ductal adenocarcinoma (PDAC) is recognized as having one of the poorest prognoses of all tumors. Resection is the only treatment that can result in long-term survival. Several randomized controlled trials have shown that extended lymph node dissection does not provide survival benefits in patients with pancreatic head cancer, despite a prolonged operative time and increased blood loss [1–5]. Regional lymph node dissection for pancreatic head cancer has been performed in many facilities, but its survival benefit remains unclear. On the other hand, pancreatic cancer treatment has dramatically changed recently owing to the development of effective chemotherapy. Adjuvant chemotherapy is essential for improving the prognosis of pancreatic cancer [6,7]. A randomized prospective study showed that the introduction of preoperative chemotherapy led to a prolonged prognosis in patients with pancreatic cancer [8]. Most of the recurrence patterns of resectable pancreatic cancer are distant metastases, and resectable pancreatic cancer is considered to be a systemic disease with micrometastasis. Thus, multimodal treatment is required to improve the prognosis of resectable pancreatic cancer, and pancreatic resection should be performed with consideration of preoperative and postoperative treatment.

However, many studies reported that the R0 resection rate is associated with prognosis. The recent development of high-quality high-resolution multi-detector computed tomography (MDCT) has made it possible to evaluate the extent of cancer progression, which makes it possible to simulate the appropriate dissection range to achieve R0 surgery before surgery. Even if the dissection range is simulated preoperatively, an accurate understanding of the anatomical structure is required to identify the dissection range during surgery. In the era of multidisciplinary treatment for resectable pancreatic cancer, we reviewed the literature that could be helpful in determining the appropriate resection range.

2. Is "Regional LYMPH Node Dissection" Required?

Patients with pancreatic cancer often have lymph node metastasis, and many studies have reported that lymph node metastasis is a prognostic factor [9–11]. Prior to the development of effective adjuvant chemotherapy, extended lymph node dissection, including para-aortic lymph nodes, was performed to prevent local recurrence [12,13]. However, several randomized controlled trials have shown that extended lymphadenectomy does not provide survival benefits in patients with pancreatic head cancer, despite a prolonged operative time and increased blood loss [1–5]. However, it has been reported that the number of retrieved lymph nodes is associated with R0 resection rates and survival [14].

The regional lymph nodes are numbered according to the Japanese Pancreatic Cancer classification [15]. Regional lymph nodes for pancreaticoduodenectomy are classified into Group 1 (8a, 8p, 13a, 13b, 17a and 17b) and Group 2 (5.6, 12a, 12b, 12p, 14p and 14d). The lymph node dissection in Group 1 is defined as D1 dissection, and the lymph node dissection of Group 1 and Group 2 is defined as D2 dissection (Figure 1A). However, it was reported that there was no significant difference in prognosis between D1 and D2 dissections in a randomized controlled trial [5] (Table 1), and it is still debated whether prophylactic dissection of regional lymph nodes improves prognosis [16]. Using surgical results of 495 patients with PDAC, Imamura et al. calculated the efficacy index for each lymph node station by multiplying the frequency of lymph node metastasis to the station and survival to clarify the optimal extent of lymph node dissection. Their results indicated that the efficacy of lymph node dissection differs between uncinate process cancer and pancreatic neck cancer, and the extent of dissection should be determined according to the location of the tumor. They also showed that the site of regional lymph node and lymph node recurrence pattern are different, indicating that it may be necessary to reconsider the need for regional lymph node dissection [15].

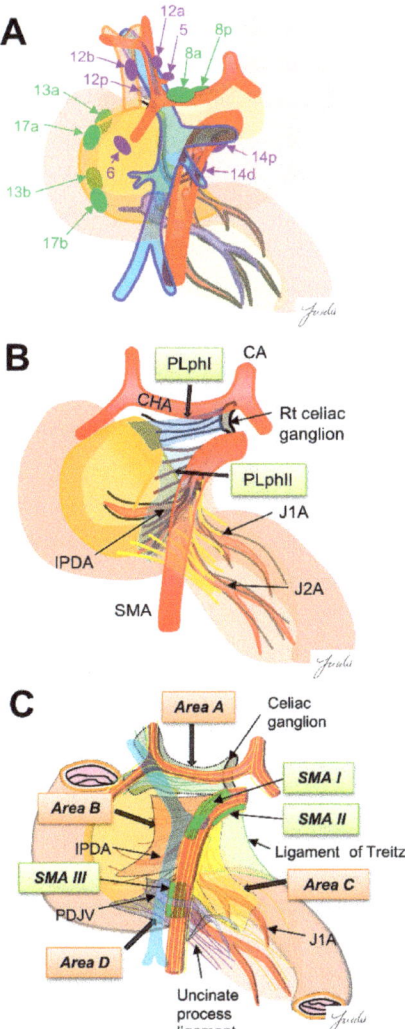

Figure 1. (**A**) The regional lymph nodes are numbered according to the Japanese Pancreatic Cancer classification. Green, D1 region, purple, D2 region. (**B**) Extra-pancreatic nerve plexus around the SMA nerve plexus in the Japanese pancreatic cancer classification. (**C**) Intensive NFTs spreading around the SMA are classified into four areas. Nagakawa et al. [16] classified "intensive NFTs" around the pancreatic head into areas A–D. They also found the three SMA regions (SMAI-III) that can be easily exposed. These regions become anatomical landmarks as "dissection-guiding points" to uniformly dissect each area A–D. PLphI, pancreatic head nerve plexus I; PLphII, pancreatic head nerve plexus II; CA, celiac artery; CHA, common hepatic artery; SMA, superior mesenteric artery; IPDA, inferior pancreaticoduodenal artery; J1A, first jejunal artery; J2A, second jejunal artery; PDJV, proximal dorsal jejunal vein.

Table 1. Dissection area in randomized controlled trials of extended lymph node dissection and standard dissection for pancreatic head cancer.

Author	Year	Country	Number of Cases	Standard Dissection	Extended Dissection	Standard Dissection	Extended Dissection	Prognosis	
				Lymph Node Dissection *		SMA Nerve Plexus Dissection			
Pedrazzoli S et al. [1]	1998	Italy	81	5, 6, 12b, 13, 17	5, 6, 9, 12b, 13, 14, 17, 16a2, 16b1	Not described		MST	
								Standard: 335 days	
								Extended: 500 days	
Yeo C et al. [2]	2002	United States	299	12b2, 12c, 13, 14b, 14v, 17	3, 4, 5, 6, 9, 12b2, 12c, 13, 14b, 14v, 16a2, 16b1, 17	Not described		5-year survival rate	
								Standard: 23%	
								Extended: 29%	
Farnell M et al. [3]	2005	United States	132	3, 4, 6, 8a, 12b1, 12b2, 12c, 13a, 13b, 14a, 14b, 17a, 17b	3, 4, 6, 8a, 8p, 9, 12a1, 12a2, 12b1, 12b2, 12p1, 12p2, 12c, 13a, 13b, 14a, 14b, 14c, 14d, 14v, 16a2, 16b, 17a, 17b	Not described		5-year survival rate	
								Standard: 17%	
								Extended: 16%	
Nimura Y et al. [4]	2012	Japan	112	13a, 13b, 17a, 17b	8a, 8p, 9, 14p, 1416a2, 16b112a, 12b, 12p	None	full circumference dissection	5-year survival rate	
								Standard: 15.7%	
								Extended: 6.0%	
Jang JY et al. [5]	2014	Korea	244	12c, 13, 17	9, 12, 13, 14, 16, 17	None	right half-circumferential dissection	5-year survival rate	
								Standard: 44.5%	
								Extended: 35.7%	

*: Lymph node numbers are listed according to the Japanese Pancreatic Cancer classification. MST: median survival time.

In the area around the superior mesenteric artery (SMA), "regional lymph node dissection" also dissects the adipose and connective tissues around the regional lymph nodes, which is almost the same dissection range as "dissection to achieve R0 resection." On the other hand, the 14p, 14d, and 8p lymph nodes, which are located around the CHA and the SMA, cannot be identified during resection because the lymph nodes are covered with many nerves and fibers. These regional lymph nodes may be confused with other numbers of lymph nodes. Thus, it is difficult to identify the precise location of each regional lymph node during surgery. Novel criteria may be needed to determine the appropriate lymph node dissection area [17].

Here, it should be noted that "regional lymph node dissection" and "dissection to achieve R0 resection" have different purposes. "Dissection to achieve R0 resection" is performed to avoid residual cancer infiltration, whereas "regional lymph node dissection" is performed to prevent recurrence of the lymph nodes. Thus, "regional lymph node dissection" and "dissection to achieve R0 resection" should be separately when considering the appropriate dissection range for resectable PDAC. Multimodal treatment, including neoadjuvant therapy and postoperative adjuvant chemotherapy, dramatically improve prognosis. Regional lymph nodes with no suspected metastases on preoperative imaging may become areas treated with preoperative and postoperative adjuvant chemotherapy. Further discussion is needed to clarify the necessity of "regional lymph node dissection."

3. Is "Dissection to Achieve R0 RESECTION" Required?

Many studies have described the need for R0 resection to achieve long-term survival, and the results of most studies have shown that R0 resection improves the survival rate of patients with resectable PDAC who have undergone pancreaticoduodenectomy (PD) [18,19]. Ghaneh et al. [20] analyzed data from the European Study Group for Pancreatic Cancer-3 randomized controlled trial and found that R1 (direct) resections were associated with significantly reduced overall and recurrence-free survival following pancreatic cancer resection. Resection margin involvement was also associated with an increased risk of local recurrence. Based on these results, the National Comprehensive Cancer Network (NCCN) guidelines have described that the goals of surgical extirpation of pancreatic carcinoma focus on the achievement of an R0 resection, as a margin-positive specimen is associated with poor long-term survival. In contrast, Schmocke et al. [21] retrospectively examined 468 patients with resectable pancreatic cancer or borderline resectable pancreatic cancer who received preoperative treatment. They reported that margin status was not a significant predictor of overall survival or relapse-free survival in multivariate analysis, but the clinical stage, duration of N-acetyl cysteine treatment, nodal status, histopathologic treatment response score, and receipt of adjuvant chemotherapy were factors associated with overall survival. In contrast, in pancreaticoduodenectomy with a complicated cutting surface, the R0 resection rate may differ depending on the evaluation and slicing methods [18]. Additionally, the inking of the cut surface according to a defined color code leads to an accurate R0/R1 evaluation [22]. Two definitions have been reported in assessing R1 [23]. American and Japanese classifications define R1 as direct microscopic involvement at the resection margin (0 mm rule) [15,24], and the Royal University of Pathologists classification defines R1 as the presence of cancer cells within 1 mm of the resection margin (1 mm rule) [25]. It is still unclear which classification reflects the prognosis [26]. To clarify the need to achieve R0 resection to prolong the prognosis in the era of multimodal treatments, the pathological evaluation should be standardized. Currently, there is little evidence that "R0 resection is not needed" to improve prognosis. Therefore, even in the era of multimodal treatment, resectable pancreatic cancer may require surgery to achieve R0 resection.

4. The Issue Regarding Tumor Infiltration of Nerve and Fibrous Tissues

Dense connective tissues exist around the pancreatic head, which is composed of intensive nerve and fibrous tissues (NFTs). It has been reported that dissection of the NFTs around the pancreatic head is important for achieving R0 resection because PDAC often infiltrate these NFTs [27,28]. However, the appropriate dissection range of NFTs has not been fully discussed, and a common classification showing the anatomical structure of NFTs around the pancreatic head is needed to determine the dissection range. Several classifications have been shown for the anatomy of NFTs. The Japanese classification for pancreatic cancer shows the anatomy of NFTs around the pancreatic head. In this classification, the major NFTs connecting to the pancreatic head are classified into two pathways. One is the pathway from the right celiac ganglion to the posterior side of the pancreas head (pancreatic head plexus I; PLph I), and the other is the pathway from the SMA nerve plexus to the left side of the uncinate process (pancreatic head nerve plexus II; PLph II) [15]. Nagakawa et al. [29] classified the intensive NTFs spreading around the SMA into four areas based on the autopsy findings. Area A: NFTs spreading from the right celiac ganglion and the superior side of the pancreatic head and the posterior side of the hepatoduodenal ligament. Area B: NFTs spreading from the SMA nerve plexus and the uncinate process. Area C: NFTs spreading from the SMA nerve plexus to the anterior side of the jejunal mesentery. Area D: NFTs spreading from the inferior side of the uncinate process to the posterior side of the jejunal mesentery. They also found three SMA nerve plexus regions without branching nerves (SMA I-III) and described that these regions become good anatomical landmarks to identify the SMA nerve plexus before stating these NFTs areas. These anatomical classifications may become good criteria for determining the appropriate dissection range of NFTs.

5. Determination of the Appropriate Dissection Range

Intraoperative pathological diagnosis using frozen section is generally performed to determine the pancreatic cutting line to avoid positive pancreatic neck margins. Additionally, resectability status is also evaluated using frozen sections of the SMA margin in some facilities. Nirsgke et al. reported that long-term survival was improved by re-resecting the positive surgical margin found using frozen section to achieve R0 resection [30]. However, many studies reported that intraoperative frozen section-based re-resection of R1 margins does not improve overall survival for patients with PDAC [31–33].

In patients with pancreatic head cancer, the extent of cancer infiltration varies depending on the tumor position (e.g., the difference between the pancreatic head and uncinate process) [34–37]. The development of MDCT has made it possible to confirm the accurate infiltration range of pancreatic head cancer, which can simulate the dissection range preoperatively to achieve R0 resection [38–41]. However, the extent of tumor infiltration cannot be accurately confirmed during surgery. It is often difficult to distinguish between areas of inflammatory changes and cancer infiltration during resection. Even if the "dissection to achieve R0 resection" range is simulated based on the MDCT evaluation, it is difficult to identify the range intraoperatively. Therefore, anatomical structures, such as layers, arteries, and veins, are commonly identified during surgery as anatomical landmarks to determine the dissection region [29,42].

6. Anatomical Landmarks Used to Determine the Appropriate Dissection Range at Each Surgical Site

We summarize below the anatomical structures that can be used as landmarks at each surgical site for achieving R0 resection based on preoperative diagnostic imaging.

6.1. Dissection around the Hepatoduodenal Ligament and Common Hepatic Artery

The dissection range around the hepatoduodenal mesentery and common hepatic artery (CHA) may need to be altered according to the tumor location. Uncinate process cancer invades the SMA mainly through the second part of the PLph II (equivalent to Area B) [29,34,36,43] (Figure 1B). However, in pancreatic head cancer, infiltration and lymph node metastasis around the CHA and hepatoduodenal ligament are observed [17,36]. There are 8a lymph nodes on the anterior side of the CHA, which must be removed to expose the CHA, proper hepatic artery (PHA), gastroduodenal artery (GDA), and portal vein (PV) at the superior border of the pancreas.

There is a left celiac ganglion on the right side of the root of the CHA and SMA, and nerve and fibrous tissues (NFTs) spread from the left celiac ganglion to the head of the pancreas and hepatoduodenal ligament (Area A, Figure 1C). These NFTs are divided into NFTs (PLph I) that pass through the dorsal side of the GDA (Figure 1B) and toward the upper edge of the head of the pancreas, and NFTs that pass through the dorsal side of the PHA and extend to the hepatoduodenal ligament [44] (Figure 1C). NFTs spreading to the hepatoduodenal ligament include 8p, 12p, and lymph nodes wrapped in adipose tissue [44]. These NFT regions need to be dissected when attempting complete skeletonization of the PV around the hepatic arteries around the hepatoduodenal ligament. If uncinate process cancer infiltrates around the SMA root and exposure of the CHA root is attempted, these NFT regions also need to be dissected. On the other hand, if no tumor extension is observed around the hepatoduodenal ligament and/or SMA root and CHA root, it is anatomically possible to preserve these NTF regions (Figure 2A–E).

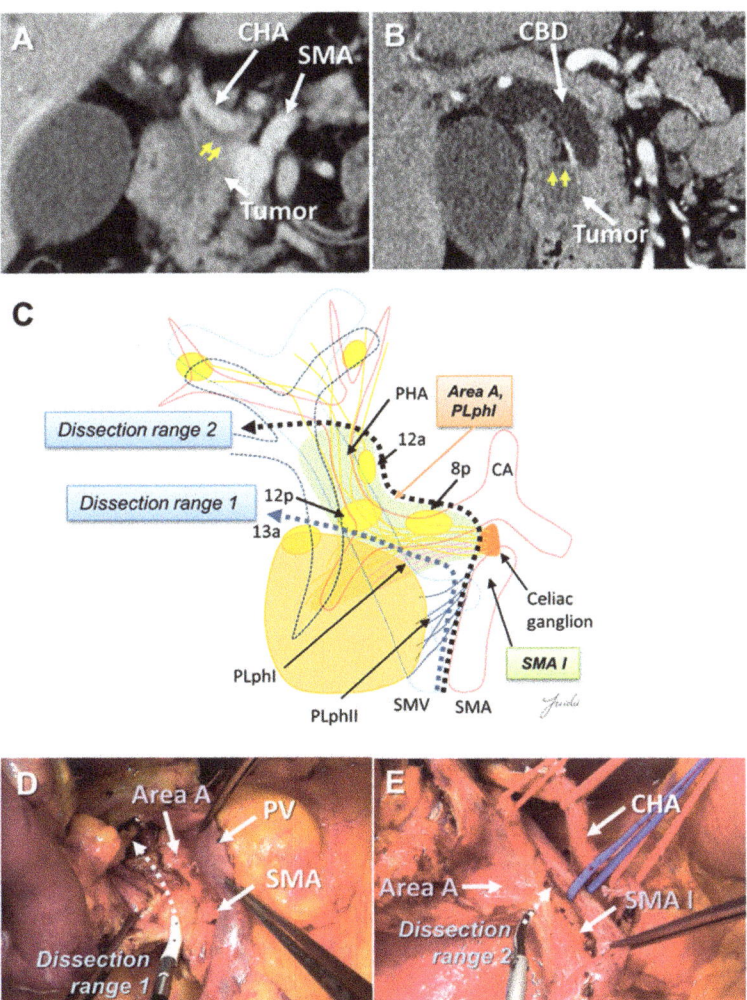

Figure 2. (**A**) Tumor extension is observed near the CHA root and SMA root on the preoperative MDCT findings. (**B**) Tumor extension is observed near the hepatoduodenal ligament. (**C**) Determination of the dissection range based on the MDCT findings. Dissection ranges 1 and 2 can be selected based on the anatomical structure, depending on tumor extension toward to the hepatoduodenal ligament, CHA root, and SMA root. (**D**) Cutting line for dissection range 1. (**E**) Cutting line for dissection range 2. MDCT: multi-detector computed tomography; CBD: common bile duct; CA: celiac artery; CHA: common hepatic artery; SMA: superior mesenteric artery; SMV: superior mesenteric vein.

6.2. Posterior Dissection

Few studies have described the appropriate range of posterior dissection for pancreatic head cancer. In extended lymph node dissection, including the para-aortic lymph nodes, the inferior vena cava, left renal vein, and anterior surface of the aorta are exposed. However, periaortic lymph node metastasis is now categorized as distant metastasis [15]. Prophylactic periaortic lymph node dissection is not generally performed for resectable PDAC. Delpero et al. investigated the association between each margin status and prognosis in a multicenter prospective study of 150 patients who underwent macroscopic margin-free PD. They showed that the R1 rate was 23%, while only 7% had R1 at the posterior margin; in addition, they reported that posterior R1 was not a prognostic factor [45]. Therefore, "dissection to achieve R0 resection" may not be necessary.

There is a fusion fascia between the posterior side of the pancreatic head and the anterior side of the vena cava and the aorta, which is called the fusion fascia of Treitz [46]. There is loose connective tissue at the anterior surface of this fusion fascia, which can be easily peeled off. If posterior infiltration is not found on the preoperative computed tomography image, this fusion fascia becomes a good anatomical landmark for indicating the range of posterior dissection. If posterior infiltration is suspected before resection and dissection with a surgical margin is needed, the anterior surface of the vena cava, renal vein, and aorta become anatomical landmarks (Figure 3A–E).

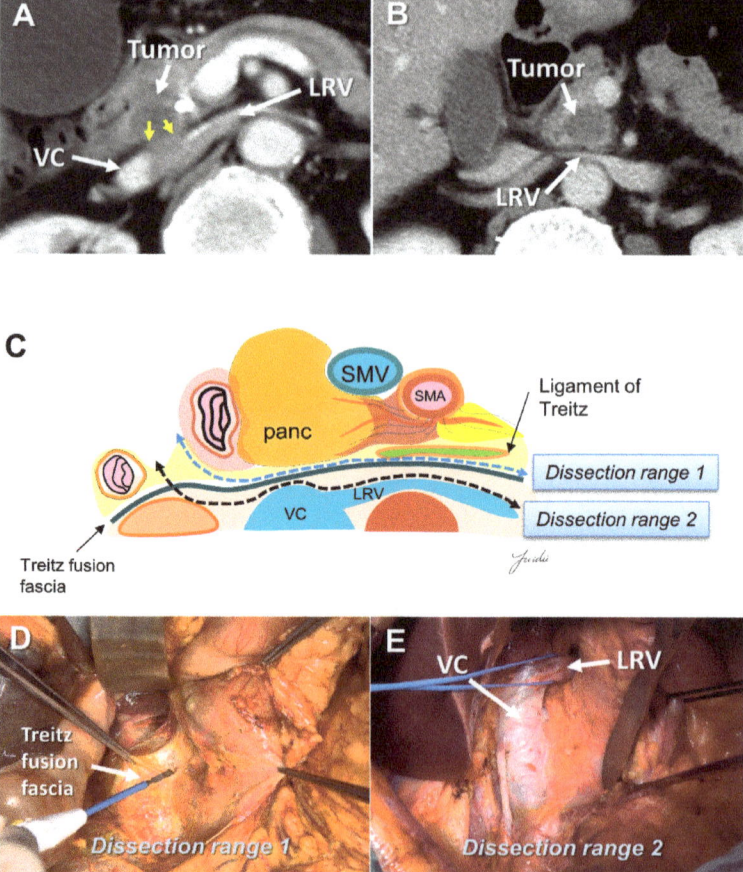

Figure 3. (**A**) Tumor extension to the posterior side of the pancreatic head is observed on the preoperative MDCT findings. (**B**) Tumor extension to the posterior side of the pancreatic head is not observed. (**C**) Determination of the dissection range based on the MDCT findings. Dissection ranges 1 and 2 can be selected based on the anatomical structure, depending on the range of posterior infiltration. (**D**) Surgical findings at dissection range 1. (**E**) Surgical findings at dissection range 2. MDCT: multi-detector computed tomography; VC: vena cava; LRV: left renal vein; SMA: superior mesenteric artery; SMV: superior mesenteric vein.

6.3. Dissection around the Superior Mesenteric Artery

The SMA margin is the most important factor for achieving R0 resection, especially in uncinate process cancer, because the tumor mainly spreads behind the SMA [42,47,48]. It is difficult to understand the anatomy around the SMA during surgery because it is very complex. Recently, region between the SMA and the uncinate process has been called the "mesopancreas" [49–51]. Many surgical procedures for complete dissection of the mesopancreas have been reported [41,52–57]. However, the range of dissection varies, and the standard dissection range remains unclear. Dense connective tissues exist around the pancreatic head, which is composed of intensive nerve and fibrous tissues (NFTs). It is generally considered that cancer spreads in these areas.

The SMA is covered with NFTs called the SMA nerve plexus. The hard NFTs spread to the uncinate process from the SMA nerve plexus, which is termed as the "pancreatic head plexus II" in the Japanese Classification of Pancreatic Carcinoma [15,43]. Previously, right half-circumferential dissection of the SMA nerve plexus was performed at many facilities [54]. However, extensive dissection of the nerve plexus around the SMA often causes severe diarrhea, which may lead to delays in the induction of adjuvant chemotherapy. Jang et al. conducted a randomized clinical trial comparing extended surgery with right half-circumferential dissection of the SMA nerve plexus and standard surgery without dissection, and revealed that there was no difference in prognosis between the two groups [5]. In their study, the number 14 lymph node was not dissected in the standard group, and the dissection range around the SMA was not clearly described [58,59].

Recently, PD with complete preservation of the SMA nerve plexus has been commonly performed to avoid severe postoperative diarrhea. However, no criteria have been established to indicate an appropriate dissection range for achieving R0 resection in PD with preservation of the SMA nerve plexus. The inferior pancreaticoduodenal artery (IPDA) becomes a good anatomical landmark during the dissection around the SMA [60–63]. The IPDA forms a common trunk with the first jejunal artery in most cases (J1A) [61,64]. The dissection range can be determined during surgery based on the path of this artery. Various approaches using the IPDA, J1A, and their common arteries as landmarks have been reported for dissection around the SMA [42,56,65,66]. Inoue et al. [42] standardized the anatomical range at levels I–III, depending on the type of tumor, based on the position of the IPDA as an anatomical landmark. They reported that standardizing the dissection range reduced the operative time and blood loss in a study of 162 patients who underwent PD. Of note, the IPDA is covered with intensive NFTs and cannot be identified before initiating the SMA dissection [29,43,49]. In contrast, uncinate process cancer spreads in these intensive NFTs [17,29]. Therefore, alternative anatomical landmarks are needed for the complete dissection of these intensive NFTs in PD with preserving the SMA nerve plexus. Nagakawa et al. [29] evaluated the cancer extension of these areas using pathological specimens from 78 patients who underwent PD for resectable PDAC. According to their results, cancer invasion and/or lymph node metastasis was observed in 14.1% of NFTs (Area C) spreading to the left side of the IPDA root and in 44.9% of NFTs (Area D) spreading between the inferior side of the uncinate process and the posterior side of the jejunal mesentery (Figures 4A–E and 5A–E).

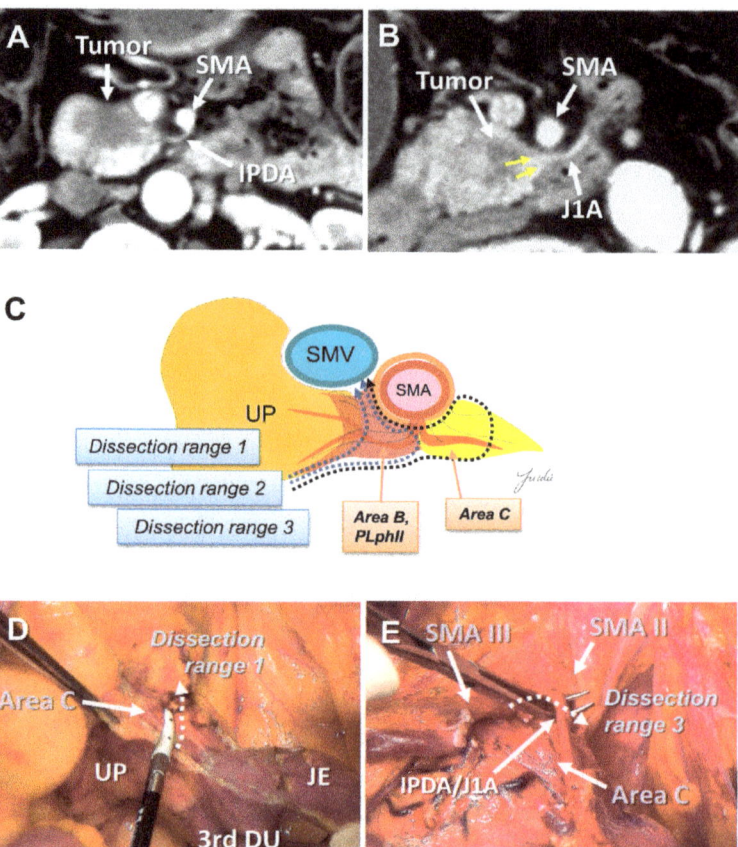

Figure 4. (**A**) Tumor extension to the SMA is not observed on the preoperative MDCT findings. (**B**) Tumor extension to the posterior side of the SMA is observed. (**C**) Determination of the dissection range based on the MDCT findings. Dissection ranges 1, 2, and 3 can be selected based on the anatomical structure, depending on the range of posterior infiltration. (**D**) Cutting line for dissection range 1. (**E**) Cutting line for dissection range 3. MDCT: multi-detector computed tomography; SMA: superior mesenteric artery; IPDA: inferior pancreaticoduodenal artery; J1A: first jejunal artery; UP: uncinate process; 3rd DU: third portion of duodenum; JE: jejunum.

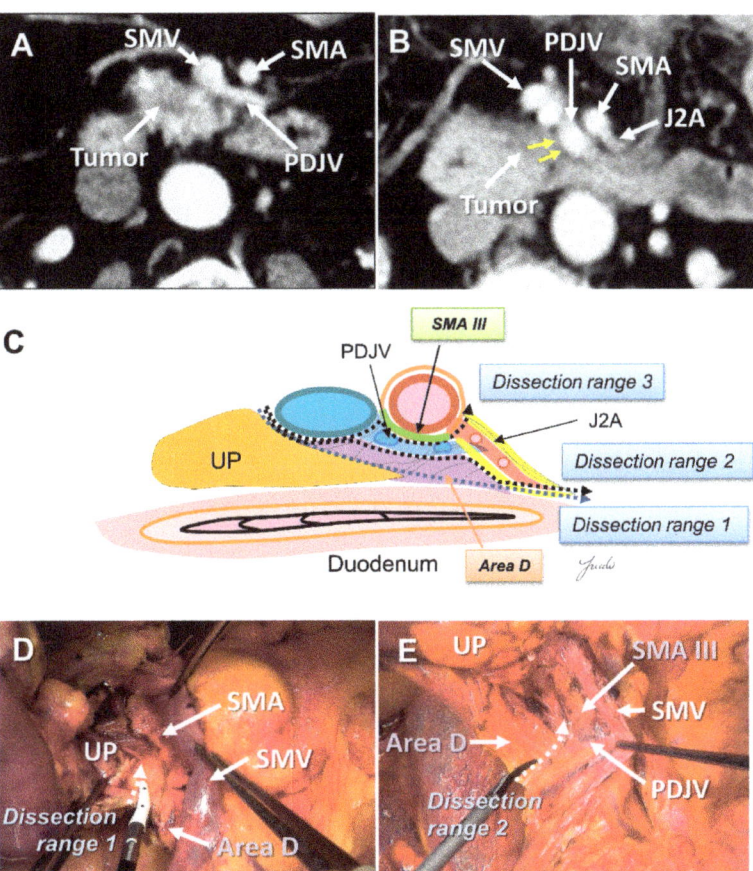

Figure 5. (**A**) Tumor extension on the dorsal side of the jejunal mesentery is not observed on the preoperative MDCT findings. (**B**) Tumor extension on the dorsal side of the jejunal mesentery is observed. (**C**) Determination of the dissection range based on the MDCT findings. Dissection ranges 1, 2, and 3 can be selected based on the anatomical structure, depending on the range of posterior infiltration. (**D**) Cutting line for dissection range 1. (**E**) Cutting line for dissection range 2. MDCT: multi-detector computed tomography; UP: uncinate process; SMA: superior mesenteric artery; SMV: superior mesenteric vein; PDJV: proximal dorsal jejunal vein; J2A: second jejunal artery.

6.4. Portal Vein and/or Superior Mesenteric Vein Resection

PV and/or superior mesenteric vein (SMV) resection for patients with PV involvement has been generally accepted with survival benefit of pancreatic cancer [41,67–73]. The extent of PV infiltration can be diagnosed by preoperative MDCT, and the need for preoperative resection of the PV can be predicted in advance. However, there are cases in which portal vein infiltration is suspected during surgery, even if MDCT does not show tumor infiltration. In addition, it is difficult to distinguish between tumor-related fibrosis and tumor infiltration in the venous wall, and the NCCN guidelines recommend performing PV resections if tumor infiltration is suspected [74].

PDAC often extends to the periphery of the SMV trunk, and the first jejunal vein (J1V) and second jejunal vein (JV) or later branches (J2, 3V) are involved with the tumor. Nevertheless, the resectability of PDAC with JV involvement remains unclear. The NCCN guidelines indicated that "unreconstructible PV/SMV due to tumor involvement or occlusion" is classified as unresectable pancreatic cancer [74]. Some surgeons choose to perform aggressive treatment such as PV/SMV resection with J1V and J2, 3V resection in patients with PDAC [75,76]. However, since the JV is thin, there is concern about the risk of complications, such as portal vein stenosis after portal vein reconstruction [77,78]. Additionally, the survival benefit of PV/SMV resection with JV resection remains unclear. Therefore, it is necessary to clarify the surgical safety and survival benefits of PV/SMV resection with JV resection (Figure 6).

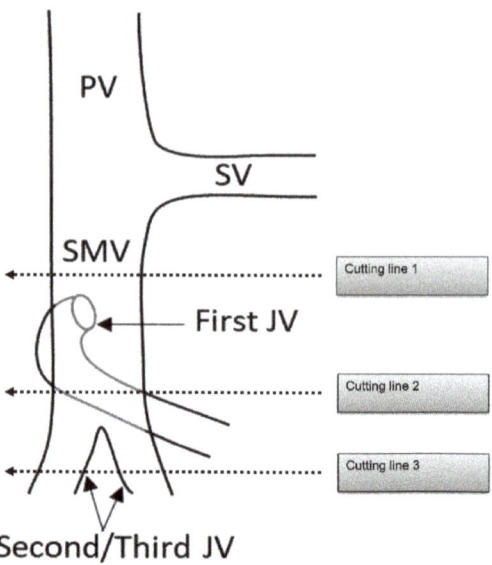

Figure 6. Cutting line for portal vein, superior mesenteric vein, and jejunal vein resection. PV: portal vein; SV: splenic vein; SMV: superior mesenteric vein; JV: jejunal vein.

Several running patterns of the J1V have been reported. In 74–99% of J1Vs, the JV flows out from the dorsal side of the SMV, branches off several IPDVs along the uncinate process, passes through the dorsal side of the superior mesenteric artery, and extends to the jejunal mesentery [56,75,79,80]. It is also termed the proximal dorsal JV (PDJV) [56,75]. As the PDJV is in contact with the uncinate process, some surgeons routinely resect the PDJV without reconstruction to ensure a surgical margin, even if combined PV/SMV resection is not required [75,76] (Figure 5).

7. Conclusions

The role of surgery has changed dramatically in the current treatment, where multi-modal treatment has become important to improve the prognosis of resectable PDAC. Now that effective preoperative and postoperative chemotherapy has been established, it may be necessary to reconsider the areas treated with chemotherapy and the areas treated with surgery. On the other hand, many studies have described that R0 resection is needed even in patients receiving adjuvant therapy. The appropriate dissection range for R0 resection can be simulated preoperatively with MDCT imaging. Therefore, surgeons need to perform a more accurate dissection, balancing both R0 resection and the introduction of adjuvant therapy, based on the precise anatomy.

Author Contributions: Details on the design of this review were discussed with Y.N.; N.N. (Naoya Nakagawa); C.T.; S.K.; H.O.; K.S.; N.N. (Nobuhiko Nakagawa); Y.H.; T.S. and M.H. The literature was searched and reviewed by Y.N.; N.N. (Naoya Nakagawa), and C.T. The draft of the manuscript was critiqued by Y.N.; I.U. and T.Y. This review was validated by K.K. and A.T. All authors have read and agreed to the published version of the manuscript.

Funding: This research received no external funding.

Conflicts of Interest: The authors declare no conflict of interest.

References

1. Pedrazzoli, S.; DiCarlo, V.; Dionigi, R.; Mosca, F.; Pederzoli, P.; Pasquali, C.; Klöppel, G.; Dhaene, K.; Michelassi, F. Standard Versus Extended Lymphadenectomy Associated with Pancreatoduodenectomy in the Surgical Treatment of Adenocarcinoma of the Head of the Pancreas: A Multicenter, Prospective, Randomized Study. Lymphadenectomy Study Group. *Ann. Surg.* **1998**, *228*, 508–517. [CrossRef]
2. Yeo, C.J.; Cameron, J.L.; Lillemoe, K.D.; Sohn, T.A.; Campbell, K.A.; Sauter, P.K.; Coleman, J.; Abrams, R.A.; Hruban, R.H. Pancreaticoduodenectomy with or without Distal Gastrectomy and Extended Retroperitoneal Lymphadenectomy for Periampullary Adenocarcinoma, Part 2: Randomized Controlled Trial Evaluating Survival, Morbidity, and Mortality. *Ann. Surg.* **2002**, *236*, 355–366. [CrossRef]
3. Farnell, M.B.; Pearson, R.K.; Sarr, M.G.; DiMagno, E.P.; Burgart, L.J.; Dahl, T.R.; Foster, N.; Sargent, D.J.; Pancreas Cancer Working Group. A Prospective Randomized Trial Comparing Standard Pancreatoduodenectomy with Pancreatoduodenectomy with Extended Lymphadenectomy in Resectable Pancreatic Head Adenocarcinoma. *Surgery* **2005**, *138*, 618–628. [CrossRef]
4. Nimura, Y.; Nagino, M.; Takao, S.; Takada, T.; Miyazaki, K.; Kawarada, Y.; Miyagawa, S.; Yamaguchi, A.; Ishiyama, S.; Takeda, Y.; et al. Standard Versus Extended Lymphadenectomy in Radical Pancreatoduodenectomy for Ductal Adenocarcinoma of the Head of the Pancreas: Long-Term Results of a Japanese Multicenter Randomized Controlled Trial. *J. Hepato-Bil. Pancreat. Sci.* **2012**, *19*, 230–241. [CrossRef]
5. Jang, J.Y.; Kang, M.J.; Heo, J.S.; Choi, S.H.; Choi, D.W.; Park, S.J.; Han, S.S.; Yoon, D.S.; Yu, H.C.; Kang, K.J.; et al. A Prospective Randomized Controlled Study Comparing Outcomes of Standard Resection and Extended Resection, Including Dissection of the Nerve Plexus and Various Lymph Nodes, in Patients with Pancreatic Head Cancer. *Ann. Surg.* **2014**, *259*, 656–664. [CrossRef]
6. Oettle, H.; Neuhaus, P.; Hochhaus, A.; Hartmann, J.T.; Gellert, K.; Ridwelski, K.; Niedergethmann, M.; Zülke, C.; Fahlke, J.; Arning, M.B.; et al. Adjuvant Chemotherapy with Gemcitabine and Long-Term Outcomes Among Patients with Resected Pancreatic Cancer: The CONKO-001 Randomized Trial. *JAMA* **2013**, *310*, 1473–1481. [CrossRef] [PubMed]
7. Ueno, H.; Ioka, T.; Ikeda, M.; Ohkawa, S.; Yanagimoto, H.; Boku, N.; Fukutomi, A.; Sugimori, K.; Baba, H.; Yamao, K.; et al. Randomized phase III Study of Gemcitabine plus S-1, S-1 Alone, or Gemcitabine Alone in Patients with Locally Advanced and Metastatic Pancreatic Cancer in Japan and Taiwan: GEST Study. *J. Clin. Oncol.* **2013**, *31*, 1640–1648. [CrossRef] [PubMed]
8. Motoi, F.; Kosuge, T.; Ueno, H.; Yamaue, H.; Satoi, S.; Sho, M.; Honda, G.; Matsumoto, I.; Wada, K.; Furuse, J.; et al. Randomized phase II/III Trial of Neoadjuvant Chemotherapy with Gemcitabine and S-1 Versus Upfront Surgery for Resectable Pancreatic Cancer (Prep-02/JSAP05). *Jpn. J. Clin. Oncol.* **2019**, *49*, 190–194. [CrossRef]
9. Lim, J.E.; Chien, M.W.; Earle, C.C. Prognostic Factors Following Curative Resection for Pancreatic Adenocarcinoma: A Population-Based, Linked Database Analysis of 396 Patients. *Ann. Surg.* **2003**, *237*, 74–85. [CrossRef] [PubMed]
10. Tarantino, I.; Warschkow, R.; Hackert, T.; Schmied, B.M.; Büchler, M.W.; Strobel, O.; Ulrich, A. Staging of Pancreatic Cancer Based on the Number of Positive Lymph Nodes. *Br. J. Surg.* **2017**, *104*, 608–618. [CrossRef] [PubMed]
11. Lowder, C.Y.; Metkus, J.; Epstein, J.; Kozak, G.M.; Lavu, H.; Yeo, C.J.; Winter, J.M. Clinical Implications of Extensive Lymph Node Metastases for Resected Pancreatic Cancer. *Ann. Surg. Oncol.* **2018**, *25*, 4004–4011. [CrossRef] [PubMed]
12. Fortner, J.G. Regional Pancreatectomy for Cancer of the Pancreas, Ampulla, and Other Related Sites. Tumor Staging and Results. *Ann. Surg.* **1984**, *199*, 418–425. [CrossRef] [PubMed]
13. Nagakawa, T.; Nagamori, M.; Futakami, F.; Tsukioka, Y.; Kayahara, M.; Ohta, T.; Ueno, K.; Miyazaki, I. Results of Extensive Surgery for Pancreatic Carcinoma. *Cancer* **1996**, *77*, 640–645. [CrossRef]
14. Contreras, C.M.; Lin, C.P.; Oster, R.A.; Reddy, S.; Wang, T.; Vickers, S.; Heslin, M. Increased Pancreatic Cancer Survival with Greater Lymph Node Retrieval in the National Cancer Data Base. *Am. J. Surg.* **2017**, *214*, 442–449. [CrossRef]
15. Japan Pancreas Society. *Classification of Pancreatic Carcinoma*, 4th ed.; Kanehara Press: Tokyo, Japan, 2017. Available online: http://www.suizou.org/pdf/Classification_of_Pancreatic_Carcinoma_4th_Engl_ed.pdf (accessed on 17 June 2021).
16. Tol, J.A.; Gouma, D.J.; Bassi, C.; Dervenis, C.; Montorsi, M.; Adham, M.; Andrén-Sandberg, A.; Asbun, H.J.; Bockhorn, M.; Büchler, M.W.; et al. Definition of a Standard Lymphadenectomy in Surgery for Pancreatic Ductal Adenocarcinoma: A Consensus Statement by the International Study Group on Pancreatic Surgery (ISGPS). *Surgery* **2014**, *156*, 591–600. [CrossRef]
17. Imamura, T.; Yamamoto, Y.; Sugiura, T.; Okamura, Y.; Ito, T.; Ashida, R.; Ohgi, K.; Uesaka, K. Reconsidering the Optimal Regional Lymph Node Staion According to Tumor Location for Pancreatic Cancer. *Ann. Surg. Oncol.* **2021**, *28*, 1602–1611. [CrossRef] [PubMed]
18. Bilimoria, K.Y.; Talamonti, M.S.; Sener, S.F.; Bilimoria, M.M.; Stewart, A.K.; Winchester, D.P.; Ko, C.Y.; Bentrem, D.J. Effect of Hospital Volume on Margin Status After Pancreaticoduodenectomy for Cancer. *J. Am. Coll. Surg.* **2008**, *207*, 510–519. [CrossRef] [PubMed]
19. Winter, J.M.; Cameron, J.L.; Campbell, K.A.; Arnold, M.A.; Chang, D.C.; Coleman, J.; Hodgin, M.B.; Sauter, P.K.; Hruban, R.H.; Riall, T.S.; et al. 1423 Pancreaticoduodenectomies for Pancreatic Cancer: A Single-Institution Experience. *J. Gastrointest. Surg.* **2006**, *10*, 1199–1210. [CrossRef]

20. Ghaneh, P.; Kleeff, J.; Halloran, C.M.; Raraty, M.; Jackson, R.; Melling, J.; Jones, O.; Palmer, D.H.; Cox, T.F.; Smith, C.J.; et al. The Impact of Positive Resection Margins on Survival and Recurrence Following Resection and Adjuvant Chemotherapy for Pancreatic Ductal Adenocarcinoma. *Ann. Surg.* **2019**, *269*, 520–529. [CrossRef]
21. Schmocker, R.K.; Delitto, D.; Wright, M.J.; Ding, D.; Cameron, J.L.; Lafaro, K.J.; Burns, W.R.; Wolfgang, C.L.; Burkhart, R.A.; He, J. Impact of Margin Status on Survival in Patients with Pancreatic Ductal Adenocarcinoma Receiving Neoadjuvant Chemotherapy. *J. Am. Coll. Surg.* **2021**, *232*, 405–413. [CrossRef]
22. Verbeke, C.S. Resection Margins and R1 Rates in Pancreatic Cancer—Are We There Yet? *Histopathology* **2008**, *52*, 787–796. [CrossRef] [PubMed]
23. Strobel, O.; Hank, T.; Hinz, U.; Bergmann, F.; Schneider, L.; Springfeld, C.; Jäger, D.; Schirmacher, P.; Hackert, T.; Büchler, M.W. Pancreatic Cancer Surgery: The New R-status Counts. *Ann. Surg.* **2017**, *265*, 565–573. [CrossRef] [PubMed]
24. Hruban, R.H.; Pitman, M.B.; Klimstra, D. Tumors of the pancreas. In *Fascicle 6, Atlas of Tumor Pathology*, 4th ed.; American Registry of Pathology, Armed Forces Institutes of Pathology: Washington, DC, USA, 2007.
25. The Royal College of Pathologists. Standards and Datasets for Reporting Cancers. In *Dataset for the Histopathological Reporting of Carcinomas of the Pancreas, Ampulla of Vater and Common Bile Duct*, 2nd ed.; The Royal College of Pathologists: London, UK, 2019.
26. Markov, P.; Satoi, S.; Kon, M. Redefining the R1 resection in patients with pancreatic ductal adenocarcinoma. *J. Hepatobiliary Pancreat. Sci.* **2016**, *23*, 523–532. [CrossRef] [PubMed]
27. Takahashi, H.; Ohigashi, H.; Ishikawa, O.; Gotoh, K.; Yamada, T.; Nagata, S.; Tomita, Y.; Eguchi, H.; Doki, Y.; Yano, M. Perineural invasion and lymph node involvement as indicators of surgical outcome and pattern of recurrence in the setting of preoperative gemcitabine-based chemoradiation therapy for resectable pancreatic cancer. *Ann. Surg.* **2012**, *255*, 95–102. [CrossRef] [PubMed]
28. Chen, J.W.; Bhandari, M.; Astill, D.S.; Wilson, T.G.; Kow, L.; Brooke-Smith, M.; Toouli, J.; Padbury, R.T. Predicting patient survival after pancreatoduodenectomy for malignancy: Histopathological criteria based on perineural infiltration and lymphovascular invasion. *HPB (Oxford)* **2010**, *12*, 101–108. [CrossRef] [PubMed]
29. Nagakawa, Y.; Yi, S.Q.; Takishita, C.; Sahara, Y.; Osakabe, H.; Kiya, Y.; Yamaguchi, H.; Miwa, Y.; Sato, I.; Tsuchida, A. Precise Anatomical Resection Based on Structures of Nerve and Fibrous Tissue Around the Superior Mesenteric Artery for Mesopancreas Dissection in Pancreaticoduodenectomy for Pancreatic Cancer. *J. Hepato-Bil. Pancreat. Sci.* **2020**, *27*, 342–351. [CrossRef] [PubMed]
30. Nitschke, P.; Volk, A.; Welsch, T.; Hackl, J.; Reissfelder, C.; Rahbari, M.; Distler, M.; Saeger, H.D.; Weitz, J.; Rahbari, N.N. Impact of Intraoperative Re-resection to Achieve R0 Status on Survival in Patients with Pancreatic Cancer: A Single-center Experience with 483 Patients. *Ann. Surg.* **2017**, *265*, 1219–1225. [CrossRef]
31. Yin, Z.; Zhou, Y.; Hou, B.; Ma, T.; Yu, M.; Zhang, C.; Lu, X.; Jian, Z. Revision of Surgical Margin under Frozen Section to Achieve R0 Status on Survival in Patients with Pancreatic Cancer. *J. Gastrointest. Surg.* **2018**, *22*, 1565–1575. [CrossRef]
32. Hernandez, J.; Mullinax, J.; Clark, W.; Toomey, P.; Villadolid, D.; Morton, C.; Ross, S.; Rosemurgy, A. Survival after Pancreaticoduodenectomy is not Improved by Extending Resections to Achieve Negative Margins. *Ann. Surg.* **2009**, *250*, 76–80. [CrossRef]
33. Barreto, S.G.; Pandanaboyana, S.; Ironside, N.; Windsor, J.A. Does Revision of Resection Margins Based on Frozen Section Improve Overall Survival Following Pancreatoduodenectomy for Pancreatic Ductal Adenocarcinoma? A Meta-analysis. *HPB (Oxford)* **2017**, *19*, 573–579. [CrossRef]
34. Kang, M.J.; Jang, J.Y.; Lee, S.E.; Lim, C.S.; Lee, K.U.; Kim, S.W. Comparison of the Long-Term Outcomes of Uncinate Process Cancer and non-Uncinate Process Pancreas Head Cancer: Poor Prognosis Accompanied by Early Locoregional Recurrence. *Langenbecks Arch. Surg.* **2010**, *395*, 697–706. [CrossRef]
35. El Nakeeb, A.; Roshdy, S.; Ask, W.; Sonbl, A.; Ali, M.; Abdelwahab, K.; Shams, N.; Abdelwahab, M. Comparative Study Between Uncinate Process Carcinoma and Pancreatic Head Carcinoma After Pancreaticodudenectomy (Clincopathological Features and Surgical Outcomes). *Hepato-Gastroenterology* **2014**, *61*, 1748–1755.
36. Padilla-Thornton, A.E.; Willmann, J.K.; Jeffrey, R.B. Adenocarcinoma of the Uncinate Process of the Pancreas: MDCT Patterns of Local Invasion and Clinical Features at Presentation. *Eur. Rad.* **2012**, *22*, 1067–1074. [CrossRef] [PubMed]
37. Liu, C.; Tian, X.; Xie, X.; Gao, H.; Zhuang, Y.; Yang, Y. Comparison of Uncinate Process Cancer and Non-Uncinate Process Pancreatic Head Cancer. *J. Cancer* **2016**, *7*, 1242–1249. [CrossRef] [PubMed]
38. Tian, H.; Mori, H.; Matsumoto, S.; Yamada, Y.; Kiyosue, H.; Ohta, M.; Kitano, S. Extrapancreatic Neural Plexus Invasion by Carcinomas of the Pancreatic Head Region: Evaluation Using Thin-Section Helical CT. *Radiat. Med.* **2007**, *25*, 141–147. [CrossRef]
39. Mochizuki, K.; Gabata, T.; Kozaka, K.; Hattori, Y.; Zen, Y.; Kitagawa, H.; Kayahara, M.; Ohta, T.; Matsui, O. MDCT Findings of Extrapancreatic Nerve Plexus Invasion by Pancreas Head Carcinoma: Correlation with en Bloc Pathological Specimens and Diagnostic Accuracy. *Eur. Rad.* **2010**, *20*, 1757–1767. [CrossRef]
40. Bae, J.S.; Kim, J.H.; Joo, I.; Chang, W.; Han, J.K. MDCT Findings Predicting Post-Operative Residual Tumor and Survival in Patients with Pancreatic Cancer. *Eur. Rad.* **2019**, *29*, 3714–3724. [CrossRef]
41. Hirono, S.; Kawai, M.; Tani, M.; Okada, K.; Miyazawa, M.; Shimizu, A.; Kitahata, Y.; Yamaue, H. Indication for the Use of an Interposed Graft During Portal Vein and/or Superior Mesenteric Vein Reconstruction in Pancreatic Resection Based on Perioperative Outcomes. *Langenbecks Arch. Surg.* **2014**, *399*, 461–471. [CrossRef]
42. Inoue, Y.; Saiura, A.; Yoshioka, R.; Ono, Y.; Takahashi, M.; Arita, J.; Takahashi, Y.; Koga, R. Pancreatoduodenectomy with Systematic Mesopancreas Dissection Using a Supracolic Anterior Artery-First Approach. *Ann. Surg.* **2015**, *262*, 1092–1101. [CrossRef]

43. Sharma, D.; Isaji, S. Mesopancreas Is a Misnomer: Time to Correct the Nomenclature. *J. Hepato-Bil. Pancreat. Sci.* **2016**, *23*, 745–749. [CrossRef] [PubMed]
44. Nagakawa, Y.; Yi, S.Q.; Sahara, Y.; Hosokawa, Y.; Takishita, C.; Shirota, T.; Hijikata, Y.; Osakabe, H.; Nishino, H.; Akashi, M.; et al. *Anatomical Structures of Nerve and Fibrous Tissues Around the Pancreatic Head -Pancreaticoduodenectomy Based on These Running Patterns for Pancreatic Cancer-, Overcoming Pancreatic Cancer -Focusing on Retro-Pancreatic Invasion-*; Tanaka & Shobundo Graphic, Art. Co., Ltd: Kanazawa, Japan, 2019.
45. Delpero, J.R.; Jeune, F.; Bachellier, P.; Regenet, N.; Le Treut, Y.P.; Paye, F.; Carrere, N.; Sauvanet, A.; Adham, M.; Autret, A.; et al. Prognostic Value of Resection Margin Involvement After Pancreaticoduodenectomy for Ductal Adenocarcinoma: Updates from a French Prospective Multicenter Study. *Ann. Surg.* **2017**, *266*, 787–796. [CrossRef]
46. Kimura, W. Surgical Anatomy of the Pancreas for Limited Resection. *J. Hepato-Bil. Pancreat. Surg.* **2000**, *7*, 473–479. [CrossRef] [PubMed]
47. Nagakawa, Y.; Hosokawa, Y.; Osakabe, H.; Sahara, Y.; Takishita, C.; Nakajima, T.; Hijikata, Y.; Kasahara, K.; Kazuhiko, K.; Saito, K.; et al. Pancreaticoduodenectomy with Right-Oblique Posterior Dissection of Superior Mesenteric Nerve Plexus Is Logical Procedure for Pancreatic Cancer with Extrapancreatic Nerve Plexus Invasion. *Hepato-Gastroenterology* **2014**, *61*, 2371–2376. [PubMed]
48. Patel, B.N.; Giacomini, C.; Jeffrey, R.B.; Willmann, J.K.; Olcott, E. Three-Dimensional Volume-Rendered Multidetector CT Imaging of the Posterior Inferior Pancreaticoduodenal Artery: Its Anatomy and Role in Diagnosing Extrapancreatic Perineural Invasion. *Cancer Imaging* **2013**, *13*, 580–590. [CrossRef] [PubMed]
49. Gockel, I.; Domeyer, M.; Wolloscheck, T.; Konerding, M.A.; Junginger, T. Resection of the Mesopancreas (RMP): A New Surgical Classification of a Known Anatomical Space. *World J. Surg. Oncol.* **2007**, *5*, 44. [CrossRef] [PubMed]
50. Gaedcke, J.; Gunawan, B.; Grade, M.; Szöke, R.; Liersch, T.; Becker, H.; Ghadimi, B.M. The Mesopancreas Is the Primary Site for R1 Resection in Pancreatic Head Cancer: Relevance for Clinical Trials. *Langenbecks Arch. Surg.* **2010**, *395*, 451–458. [CrossRef] [PubMed]
51. Peparini, N.; Chirletti, P. Mesopancreas: A Boundless Structure, Namely R1 Risk in Pancreaticoduodenectomy for Pancreatic Head Carcinoma. *Eur. J. Surg. Oncol.* **2013**, *39*, 1303–1308. [CrossRef] [PubMed]
52. Adham, M.; Singhirunnusorn, J. Surgical Technique and Results of Total Mesopancreas Excision (TMpE) in Pancreatic Tumors. *Eur. J. Surg. Oncol.* **2012**, *38*, 340–345. [CrossRef]
53. Welsch, T.; Bork, U.; Distler, M.; Weitz, J. Top-Down Approach to the Superior Mesenteric Artery and the Mesopancreas During Pancreatoduodenectomy for Pancreatic Cancer. *J. Surg. Oncol.* **2016**, *113*, 668–671. [CrossRef]
54. Kimura, W. Strategies for the Treatment of Invasive Ductal Carcinoma of the Pancreas and How to Achieve Zero Mortality for Pancreaticoduodenectomy. *J. Hepato-Bil. Pancreat. Surg.* **2008**, *15*, 270–277. [CrossRef]
55. Sugiyama, M.; Suzuki, Y.; Nakazato, T.; Yokoyama, M.; Kogure, M.; Matsuki, R.; Abe, N. Vascular Anatomy of Mesopancreas in Pancreatoduodenectomy Using an Intestinal Derotation Procedure. *World J. Surg.* **2020**, *44*, 3441–3448. [CrossRef] [PubMed]
56. Nagakawa, Y.; Hosokawa, Y.; Sahara, Y.; Takishita, C.; Hijikata, Y.; Osakabe, H.; Nakajima, T.; Shirota, T.; Katsumata, K.; Nakamura, M.; et al. Approaching the Superior Mesenteric Artery from the Right Side Using the Proximal-Dorsal Jejunal Vein Preisolation Method During Laparoscopic Pancreaticoduodenectomy. *Surg. Endosc.* **2018**, *32*, 4044–4051. [CrossRef] [PubMed]
57. Nagakawa, Y.; Watanabe, Y.; Kozono, S.; Boggi, U.; Palanivelu, C.; Liu, R.; Wang, S.E.; He, J.; Nishino, H.; Ohtsuka, T.; et al. Surgical Approaches to the Superior Mesenteric Artery During Minimally Invasive Pancreaticoduodenectomy: A Systematic Review. *J. Hepato-Bil. Pancreat. Sci.* **2021**. [CrossRef] [PubMed]
58. Paiella, S.; Butturini, G.; Bassi, C. Different Ideas of Nodal Grouping in Standard and Extended Lymphadenectomy During Pancreaticoduodenectomy for Pancreatic Head Cancer. *Ann. Surg.* **2017**, *265*, E73–E74. [CrossRef] [PubMed]
59. Jang, J.Y.; Kang, M.J.; Kim, S.W. Reply to "Different Ideas of Nodal Grouping in Standard and Extended Lymphadenectomy During Pancreaticoduodenectomy for Pancreatic Head Cancer". *Ann. Surg.* **2017**, *265*, E74–E75. [CrossRef] [PubMed]
60. Horiguchi, A.; Ishihara, S.; Ito, M.; Nagata, H.; Shimizu, T.; Furusawa, K.; Kato, R.; Katada, K.; Miyakawa, S. Pancreatoduodenectomy in Which Dissection of the Efferent Arteries of the Head of the Pancreas Is Performed First. *J. Hepato-Bil. Pancreat. Surg.* **2007**, *14*, 575–578. [CrossRef]
61. Horiguchi, A.; Ishihara, S.; Ito, M.; Asano, Y.; Yamamoto, T.; Miyakawa, S. Three-Dimensional Models of Arteries Constructed Using Multidetector-Row CT Images to Perform Pancreatoduodenectomy Safely Following Dissection of the Inferior Pancreaticoduodenal Artery. *J. Hepato-Bil. Pancreat. Sci.* **2010**, *17*, 523–526. [CrossRef] [PubMed]
62. Negoi, I.; Beuran, M.; Hostiuc, S.; Negoi, R.I.; Inoue, Y. Surgical Anatomy of the Superior Mesenteric Vessels Related to Pancreaticoduodenectomy: A Systematic Review and Meta-Analysis. *J. Gastrointest. Surg.* **2018**, *22*, 802–817. [CrossRef]
63. Onda, S.; Okamoto, T.; Kanehira, M.; Suzuki, F.; Ito, R.; Fujioka, S.; Suzuki, N.; Hattori, A.; Yanaga, K. Identification of Inferior Pancreaticoduodenal Artery During Pancreaticoduodenectomy Using Augmented Reality-Based Navigation System. *J. Hepato-Bil. Pancreat. Sci.* **2014**, *21*, 281–287. [CrossRef]
64. Tomimaru, Y.; Tanaka, K.; Noguchi, K.; Morita, S.; Imamura, H.; Dono, K. The Branching Pattern of the Inferior Pancreaticoduodenal Artery in Patients with a Replaced Right Hepatic Artery. *Am. Surg.* **2018**, *84*, 796–800. [CrossRef]
65. Nagakawa, Y.; Hosokawa, Y.; Sahara, Y.; Takishita, C.; Nakajima, T.; Hijikata, Y.; Tago, T.; Kasuya, K.; Tsuchida, A. A Novel "Artery First" Approach Allowing Safe Resection in Laparoscopic Pancreaticoduodenectomy: The Uncinate Process First Approach. *Hepato-Gastroenterology* **2015**, *62*, 1037–1040.

66. Sanjay, P.; Takaori, K.; Govil, S.; Shrikhande, S.V.; Windsor, J.A. 'Artery-first' Approaches to Pancreatoduodenectomy. *Br. J. Surg.* **2012**, *99*, 1027–1035. [CrossRef]
67. Nakao, A.; Harada, A.; Nonami, T.; Kaneko, T.; Inoue, S.; Takagi, H. Clinical Significance of Portal Invasion by Pancreatic Head Carcinoma. *Surgery* **1995**, *117*, 50–55. [CrossRef]
68. Chua, T.C.; Saxena, A. Extended Pancreaticoduodenectomy with Vascular Resection for Pancreatic Cancer: A Systematic Review. *J. Gastrointest. Surg.* **2010**, *14*, 1442–1452. [CrossRef]
69. Ravikumar, R.; Sabin, C.; Abu Hilal, M.; Bramhall, S.; White, S.; Wigmore, S.; Imber, C.J.; Fusai, G.; UK Vascular Resection in Pancreatic Cancer Study Group. Portal Vein Resection in Borderline Resectable Pancreatic Cancer: A United Kingdom Multicenter Study. *J. Am. Coll. Surg.* **2014**, *218*, 401–411. [CrossRef] [PubMed]
70. Kulemann, B.; Hoeppner, J.; Wittel, U.; Glatz, T.; Keck, T.; Wellner, U.F.; Bronsert, P.; Sick, O.; Hopt, U.T.; Makowiec, F.; et al. Perioperative and Long-Term Outcome After Standard Pancreaticoduodenectomy, Additional Portal Vein and Multivisceral Resection for Pancreatic Head Cancer. *J. Gastrointest. Surg.* **2015**, *19*, 438–444. [CrossRef] [PubMed]
71. Murakami, Y.; Satoi, S.; Motoi, F.; Sho, M.; Kawai, M.; Matsumoto, I.; Honda, G.; Multicentre Study Group of Pancreatobiliary Surgery (MSG-PBS). Portal or Superior Mesenteric Vein Resection in Pancreatoduodenectomy for Pancreatic Head Carcinoma. *Br. J. Surg.* **2015**, *102*, 837–846. [CrossRef] [PubMed]
72. Delpero, J.R.; Boher, J.M.; Sauvanet, A.; Le Treut, Y.P.; Sa-Cunha, A.; Mabrut, J.Y.; Chiche, L.; Turrini, O.; Bachellier, P.; Paye, F. Pancreatic Adenocarcinoma with Venous Involvement: Is Up-Front Synchronous Portal-Superior Mesenteric Vein Resection Still Justified? A Survey of the Association Française de Chirurgie. *Ann. Surg. Oncol.* **2015**, *22*, 1874–1883. [CrossRef]
73. Giovinazzo, F.; Turri, G.; Katz, M.H.; Heaton, N.; Ahmed, I. Meta-Analysis of Benefits of Portal-Superior Mesenteric Vein Resection in Pancreatic Resection for Ductal Adenocarcinoma. *Br. J. Surg.* **2016**, *103*, 179–191. [CrossRef] [PubMed]
74. National Comprehensive Cancer Network. Practice Guidelines for Pancreatic Cancer. Available online: https://www.nccn.org/professionals/physician_gls/pdf/pancreatic.pdf (accessed on 17 June 2021).
75. Hosokawa, Y.; Nagakawa, Y.; Sahara, Y.; Takishita, C.; Nakajima, T.; Hijikata, Y.; Osakabe, H.; Shirota, T.; Saito, K.; Yamaguchi, H.; et al. Surgical Outcomes of Pancreaticoduodenectomy for Pancreatic Cancer with Proximal Dorsal Jejunal Vein Involvement. *J. Gastrointest. Surg.* **2018**, *22*, 1179–1185. [CrossRef]
76. Honda, M.; Nagakawa, Y.; Akashi, M.; Hosokawa, Y.; Osakabe, H.; Takishita, C.; Nishino, H.; Tsuchida, A. Clinical Impact of Pancreaticoduodenectomy for Pancreatic Cancer with Resection of the Secondary or Later Branches of the Superior Mesenteric Vein. *J. Hepato-Bil. Pancreat. Sci.* **2020**, *27*, 731–738. [CrossRef] [PubMed]
77. Kang, M.J.; Jang, J.Y.; Chang, Y.R.; Jung, W.; Kim, S.W. Portal Vein Patency after Pancreatoduodenectomy for Periampullary Cancer. *Br. J. Surg.* **2015**, *102*, 77–84. [CrossRef] [PubMed]
78. Ohgi, K.; Sugiura, T.; Yamamoto, Y.; Okamura, Y.; Ito, T.; Ashida, R.; Aramaki, T.; Uesaka, K. Benign Portal Vein Stenosis After Pancreaticoduodenectomy. *World J. Surg.* **2019**, *43*, 2623–2630. [CrossRef]
79. Ishikawa, Y.; Ban, D.; Matsumura, S.; Mitsunori, Y.; Ochiai, T.; Kudo, A.; Tanaka, S.; Tanabe, M. Surgical Pitfalls of Jejunal Vein Anatomy in Pancreaticoduodenectomy. *J. Hepato-Bil. Pancreat. Sci.* **2017**, *24*, 394–400. [CrossRef]
80. Nakamura, M.; Nakashima, H.; Tsutsumi, K.; Matsumoto, H.; Muta, Y.; Ueno, D.; Yoshida, K.; Hino, K.; Urakami, A.; Tanaka, M. First Jejunal Vein Oriented Mesenteric Excision for Pancreatoduodenectomy. *J. Gastroenterol.* **2013**, *48*, 989–995. [CrossRef] [PubMed]

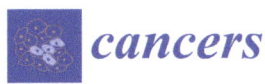

Article

Optimal Preoperative Multidisciplinary Treatment in Borderline Resectable Pancreatic Cancer

Nana Kimura [1,†], Suguru Yamada [2,†], Hideki Takami [2], Kenta Murotani [3], Isaku Yoshioka [1], Kazuto Shibuya [1], Fuminori Sonohara [2], Yui Hoshino [1], Katsuhisa Hirano [1], Toru Watanabe [1], Hayato Baba [1], Kosuke Mori [1], Takeshi Miwa [1], Mitsuro Kanda [2], Masamichi Hayashi [2], Koshi Matsui [1], Tomoyuki Okumura [1], Yasuhiro Kodera [2] and Tsutomu Fujii [1,*]

1. Department of Surgery and Science, Faculty of Medicine, Academic Assembly, University of Toyama, Toyama 9300194, Japan; nana@med.u-toyama.ac.jp (N.K.); isaku@med.u-toyama.ac.jp (I.Y.); chopper@med.u-toyama.ac.jp (K.S.); yui@hoshi-co.jp (Y.H.); hrnkths21@yahoo.co.jp (K.H.); toruwatanabetoru@yahoo.co.jp (T.W.); h881088@med.u-toyama.ac.jp (H.B.); mori0824@med.u-toyama.ac.jp (K.M.); tmiwa@med.u-toyama.ac.jp (T.M.); kmatsui@med.u-toyama.ac.jp (K.M.); okumura@med.u-toyama.ac.jp (T.O.)
2. Department of Gastroenterological Surgery (Surgery II), Nagoya University Graduate School of Medicine, Nagoya 4668550, Aichi, Japan; suguru@med.nagoya-u.ac.jp (S.Y.); takamihideki@med.nagoya-u.ac.jp (H.T.); fsonohara@med.nagoya-u.ac.jp (F.S.); m-kanda@med.nagoya-u.ac.jp (M.K.); m-hayashi@med.nagoya-u.ac.jp (M.H.); ykodera@med.nagoya-u.ac.jp (Y.K.)
3. Biostatistics Center, Graduate School of Medicine, Kurume University, Kurume, Fukuoka 8300011, Japan; kmurotani@med.kurume-u.ac.jp
* Correspondence: fjt@med.u-toyama.ac.jp; Tel.: +81-76-434-7331
† These authors contributed equally to this paper.

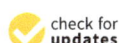

Citation: Kimura, N.; Yamada, S.; Takami, H.; Murotani, K.; Yoshioka, I.; Shibuya, K.; Sonohara, F.; Hoshino, Y.; Hirano, K.; Watanabe, T.; Baba, H.; et al. Optimal Preoperative Multidisciplinary Treatment in Borderline Resectable Pancreatic Cancer. Cancers 2021, 13, 36. https://dx.doi.org/10.3390/cancers 13010036

Received: 14 December 2020
Accepted: 21 December 2020
Published: 24 December 2020

Publisher's Note: MDPI stays neutral with regard to jurisdictional claims in published maps and institutional affiliations.

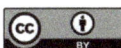

Copyright: © 2020 by the authors. Licensee MDPI, Basel, Switzerland. This article is an open access article distributed under the terms and conditions of the Creative Commons Attribution (CC BY) license (https://creativecommons.org/licenses/by/4.0/).

Simple Summary: For borderline pancreatic cancer, upfront surgery was standard in the past, and the usefulness of neoadjuvant treatment has been reported in recent years. However, few studies have been conducted to date on whether there is a difference in optimal treatment between borderline resectable pancreatic cancer invading the portal vein (BR-PV) or abutting major arteries (BR-A). The objective of this study was to investigate the optimal neoadjuvant therapy for BR-PV or BR-A. We retrospectively analyzed 88 patients with BR-PV and 111 patients with BR-A. In this study, we found that neoadjuvant treatment using new chemotherapy (FOLFIRINOX or gemcitabine along with nab-paclitaxel) is essential for improving the prognosis of BR pancreatic cancer. These findings suggest that prognosis may be prolonged by maintaining good nutritional status during preoperative treatment.

Abstract: *Background:* The objective of this study was to investigate the optimal neoadjuvant therapy (NAT) for borderline resectable pancreatic cancer invading the portal vein (BR-PV) or abutting major arteries (BR-A). *Methods:* We retrospectively analyzed 88 patients with BR-PV and 111 patients with BR-A. *Results:* In BR-PV patients who underwent upfront surgery ($n = 46$)/NAT ($n = 42$), survival was significantly better in the NAT group (3-year overall survival (OS): 5.8%/35.5%, $p = 0.004$). In BR-A patients who underwent upfront surgery ($n = 48$)/NAT ($n = 63$), survival was also significantly better in the NAT group (3-year OS:15.5%/41.7%, $p < 0.001$). The prognosis tended to be better in patients who received newer chemotherapeutic regimens, such as FOLFIRINOX and gemcitabine with nab-paclitaxel. In 36 BR-PV patients who underwent surgery after NAT, univariate analysis revealed that normalization of tumor marker (TM) levels ($p = 0.028$) and preoperative high prognostic nutritional index (PNI) ($p = 0.022$) were significantly associated with a favorable prognosis. In 39 BR-A patients who underwent surgery after NAT, multivariate analysis revealed that preoperative PNI > 42.5 was an independent prognostic factor (HR: 0.15, $p = 0.014$). *Conclusions:* NAT using newer chemotherapy is essential for improving the prognosis of BR pancreatic cancer. These findings suggest that prognosis may be prolonged by maintaining good nutritional status during preoperative treatment.

Keywords: pancreatic cancer; borderline resectable; neoadjuvant treatment; chemoradiotherapy; prognostic nutritional index

1. Introduction

Despite considerable improvements in diagnostic and therapeutic options, pancreatic ductal adenocarcinoma (PDAC) mostly remains a fatal disease worldwide [1]. Radical resection without residual tumor remains the only established curative treatment for PDAC. However, much more intervention is required beyond resection alone. A simple explanation for the poor consequences after resection is that almost every patient has microscopic disease remaining [2]. When a patient is diagnosed with PDAC and the optimal treatment strategy is considered, it is common to make a decision based on the resectable classification rather than the stage classification. The National Comprehensive Cancer Network (NCCN), an alliance of 25 cancer centers in the United States, have proposed a resectable classification for pancreatic cancer [3]. However, the NCCN guidelines are revised and updated annually and are considered to be very complex; thus, utilizing the NCCN classification system for resectability in clinical practice is difficult. Therefore, the Japan Pancreas Society (JPS) proposed novel and simplified resectability criteria in 2016 [4] based on the most recent NCCN guidelines [3].

The JPS published the 7th edition of the Classification of Pancreatic Carcinoma, and a unique resectable classification for borderline resectable (BR) was proposed (BR-A: BR-PDAC due to the infiltration of celiac and/or superior mesentery arteries, BR-PV: due only to the infiltration of the portal system). BR pancreatic cancer is a distinct subset of locally advanced pancreatic cancer first identified by Varadhachary et al. in 2006 [5]. It was hoped that the BR group would represent a subset of pancreatic cancer whose outcomes might be intermediate between the outcomes of patients with radiologically and technically resectable (R) and unresectable (UR) disease. With currently available operative techniques, patients with BR cancer are at high risk for margin-positive resection [6]. Therefore, the criteria for resectability are clinically important for determining the need for preoperative (neoadjuvant) systemic therapy and/or local-regional chemoradiation to maximize the potential for R0 resection and to avoid R2 resection [7]. For BR pancreatic cancer, upfront surgery was standard in the past, and the usefulness of neoadjuvant treatment (NAT) has been reported in recent years [8–10]. However, few studies have been conducted to date on whether there is a difference in optimal treatment between BR-PV and BR-A.

The objective of this study was to investigate the optimal preoperative multidisciplinary treatment for BR pancreatic cancer. Patients who had received treatment for BR-PDAC at two regional high-volume centers were reviewed retrospectively, and we analyzed survival differences among subgroups defined based on this novel classification system of resectability.

2. Results

2.1. Cohort Outline

We identified 199 patients who were diagnosed with BR-PDAC (Figure 1). Among them, 88 patients were diagnosed with BR-PV PDAC, and 111 patients were diagnosed with BR-A PDAC.

Of 88 BR-PV patients, 46 patients underwent upfront surgery, and 36 patients underwent resection after NAT. The other 6 patients did not undergo surgery because of chemotherapeutic failure or best supportive care. Of 111 BR-A patients, 48 patients underwent upfront surgery, and 39 patients underwent resection after NAT. The other 24 patients did not undergo surgery because of chemotherapeutic failure or best supportive care.

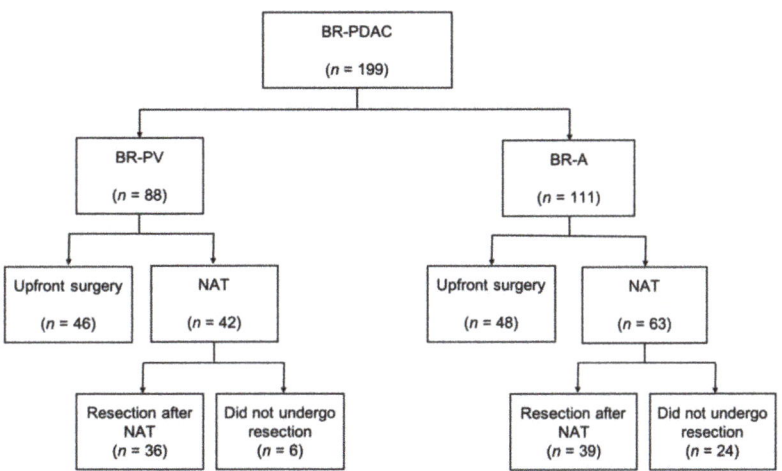

Figure 1. Study profiles and clinical courses of the enrolled patients. BR, borderline resectable; PDAC, pancreatic ductal adenocarcinoma; NAT, neoadjuvant treatment.

2.2. The Clinical Characteristics of BR-PDAC Patients

For patients who were enrolled in this study, detailed cohort demographics are summarized in Table 1. The median age was 66 years in BR-PV patients and 67 years in BR-A patients. Preoperative image examination revealed that the location of the tumor was dominant (BR-PV: 95%, BR-A: 75%) on the head side in both BR-PV and BR-A; thus, pancreatic head resection tended to be more frequent (BR-PV: 84%, BR-A: 60%).

In the BR-PV patients, 26 (30%) patients were treated with newer chemotherapeutic regimens such as FOLFIRINOX (FFX) and gemcitabine along with nab-paclitaxel (GnP). The median length of therapy was 2.1 months. In the BR-A patients, 36 (32%) patients were treated with newer chemotherapeutic regimens with a median length of 2.7 months.

The median baseline CA19-9 level at diagnosis was higher than the median at surgery. Additionally, both the BR-PV and BR-A groups had lower median CA19-9 levels at operation in patients who underwent surgery after NAT than in those who underwent upfront surgery. In both BR-PV and BR-A patients, approximately 20% of patients had a $\geq$90% decrease in CA19-9 levels compared to that before NAT. This suggests that preoperative NAT may be expected to significantly reduce tumor markers (TMs), as in previous reports [11].

The median baseline nutritional parameters at operation were as follows (in BR-PV/BR-A): controlling nutritional status (CONUT): 2/2, Glasgow prognostic score (GPS): 0/0, modified GPS (mGPS): 0/0, neutrophil/lymphocyte ratio (NLR): 2.4/2.5, platelet/lymphocyte ratio (PLR): 129.2/83.0, prognostic nutritional index (PNI): 46.0/44.5, lymphocyte/monocyte ratio (LMR): 3.6/3.8, systemic immune inflammation index (SII): 380.1/482.8, and C-reactive protein (CRP)/albumin ratio: 0.07/0.03.

For patients with BR-PDAC who were underwent surgery, detailed cohort demographics are summarized in Table 2. The median age was 65 years in BR-PV patients and 67 years in BR-A patients. In operation, venous resection was performed in 72 (88%) patients with BR-PV and 62 (71%) patients with BR-A. Moreover, arterial resection was performed in 5 (6%) patients with BR-PV and 12 (14%) patients with BR-A.

In addition, we compared the backgrounds of patients who underwent upfront surgery and those who underwent NAT. Details are shown in Table 3. For both BR-A and BR-PV, the CA19-9 level at operation was lower in the NAT group. There was no significant difference in preoperative nutritional status.

Table 1. Baseline characteristics of patients with BR-PV and BR-A.

Variable	BR-PV (n = 88)	BR-A (n = 111)	Variable	BR-PV (n = 88)	BR-A (n = 111)
Sex (male/female)	51/37	55/56	Surgical procedures		
Age, years *	66 (39–83)	67 (42–83)	Pancreatoduodenectomy	74 (84%)	67 (60%)
Body mass index *	21.1 (15.4–43.6)	21.2 (11.6–30.7)	Distal pancreatectomy	1 (1%)	13 (12%)
Tumor location			Total pancreatectomy	7 (8%)	6 (5%)
Head/Uncinate	84 (95%)	83 (75%)	Operative time, min *	508 (308–960)	501 (193–808)
Body/Tail	4 (5%)	28 (25%)	Blood loss volume, mL *	1075 (258–6000)	1090 (80–9845)
CA19-9 at diagnosis, U/mL *	179 (1–2900)	150 (1–6340)	Operative PRBC transfusion	34 (41%)	30 (34%)
Chemotherapy			Vascular resection		
no	46 (52%)	48 (43%)	Any venous resection	72 (82%)	62 (56%)
FFX/GnP	26 (30%)	36 (32%)	Any arterial resection	5 (6%)	12 (14%)
GS	2 (2%)	27 (24%)	Celiac axis	0	5
GS + Radiation	14 (16%)	14 (13%)	Hepatic artery	4	8
Length of therapy, mo *	2.1 (1.1–6.6)	2.7 (0.2–12.9)	Splenic artery	1	0
Tumor size at operation, mm *	30 (9–100)	30 (10–100)	Both venous and arterial	5 (6%)	8 (9%)
CA19-9 at operation, U/mL *	93 (1–9869)	102 (1–7316)	Positive lymph nodes	54 (66%)	58 (67%)
in upfront surgery group	196 (1–9869)	321.5 (1–7316)	R0 margin status	59 (72%)	49 (56%)
in resection after NAT group	41 (1–1500)	34 (1–2690)	90-day operative mortality	1 (1%)	1 (1%)
CA19-9 normalized	17 (47%)	17 (27%)	Adjuvant chemotherapy	56 (68%)	75 (86%)
CA19-9 decrease rate ≥90%	7 (19%)	9 (19%)	Recurrent disease	42 (51%)	58 (67%)
Nutrition at operation			Vital status at last follow-up		
CONUT *	2 (0–11)	2 (0–11)	Alive, no evidence of recurrence	32 (36%)	34 (31%)
GPS *	0 (0–2)	0 (0–2)	Alive, with recurrence	7 (8%)	19 (17%)
mGPS *	0 (0–2)	0 (0–2)	Not alive	49 (56%)	58 (52%)
NLR *	2.4 (0.8–20.4)	2.5 (0.7–15)			
PLR *	129.2 (0.1–416.5)	83.0 (0.05–522.5)			
PNI *	46.0 (28.5–56.2)	44.5 (26.3–55.5)			
LMR *	3.6 (1.0–40.4)	3.8 (1.0–10.9)			
SII *	380.1 (0.2–2180.5)	482.8 (0.1–3669.2)			
CRP/Alb *	0.07 (0–2.0)	0.03 (0.002–2.2)			

* values are median (range). CA19-9, carbohydrate antigen 19-9; FFX, FOLFIRINOX; GnP, gemcitabine along with nab-paclitaxel; GS, gemcitabine along with S-1; CONUT, controlling nutritional status; GPS, Glasgow prognostic score; mGPS, modified Glasgow prognostic score; NLR, neutrophil/lymphocyte ratio; PLR, platelet/lymphocyte ratio; PNI, prognostic nutritional index; LMR, lymphocyte/monocyte ratio; SII, systemic immune inflammation index; CRP, C-reactive protein; Alb, albumin; PRBC, packed red blood cells.

Table 2. Baseline characteristics of patients with BR-PDAC who underwent resection.

Variable	BR-PV (n = 82)	BR-A (n = 87)
Sex (male/female)	47/35	44/43
Age, years *	65 (39–83)	67 (42–83)
Chemotherapy		
no	46 (56%)	48 (55%)
FFX/GnP	26 (32%)	36 (30%)
GS	2 (2%)	27 (31%)
GS + Radiation	14 (17%)	14 (16%)
Tumor size at operation, mm *	30 (9–100)	30 (10–100)
CA19-9 at operation, U/mL *	93 (1–9869)	102 (1–7316)
in upfront surgery group	196 (1–9869)	321.5 (1–7316)
in resection after NAT group	41 (1–1500)	34 (1–2690)

Table 2. Cont.

Variable	BR-PV (n = 82)	BR-A (n = 87)
CA19-9 normalized	17 (21%)	17 (20%)
Surgical procedures		
Pancreatoduodenectomy	74 (90%)	67 (77%)
Distal pancreatectomy	1 (1%)	13 (15%)
Total pancreatectomy	7 (10%)	6 (7%)
Operative time, min *	508 (308–960)	501 (193–808)
Blood loss volume, mL *	1075 (258–6000)	1090 (80–9845)
Operative PRBC transfusion	34 (41%)	30 (34%)
Vascular resection		
Any venous resection	72 (88%)	62 (71%)
Any arterial resection	5 (6%)	12 (14%)
Celiac axis	0	5
Hepatic artery	4	8
Splenic artery	1	0
Both venous and arterial	5 (6%)	8 (9%)
Positive lymph nodes	54 (66%)	58 (67%)
R0 margin status	59 (72%)	49 (56%)
90-day operative mortality	1 (1%)	1 (1%)
Adjuvant chemotherapy	56 (68%)	75 (86%)

* values are median (range). CA19-9, carbohydrate antigen 19-9; FFX, FOLFIRINOX; GnP, gemcitabine along with nab-paclitaxel; GS, gemcitabine along with S-1; PRBC, packed red blood cells.

Table 3. Baseline characteristics of patients with BR-PDAC who underwent upfront surgery or NAT.

Variable	BR-PV (n = 88)		BR-A (n = 111)	
	UFS (n = 46)	NAT (n = 42)	UFS (n = 48)	NAT (n = 63)
Sex (male/female)	27/19	24/18	27/22	28/35
Age, years *	64 (39–83)	66 (40–81)	66 (42–83)	68 (45–82)
Body mass index *	20.1 (15.5–32.1)	21.4 (15.4–43.6)	20.9 (17.1–27.5)	21.4 (11.6–30.7)
Tumor location				
Head/Uncinate	44 (96%)	40 (95%)	38 (79%)	45 (71%)
Body/Tail	2 (4%)	2 (5%)	10 (21%)	18 (29%)
CA19-9 at diagnosis, U/mL *	N/A	178.5 (1–2900)	N/A	150 (1–6340)
CA19-9 at operation, U/mL *	196 (1–9869)	41 (1–5661)	321 (1–7316)	65 (1–5870)
Comorbidity (yes/no)				
Diabetes	20/26	11/26	23/25	13/34
History of other cancers	6/40	1/36	5/43	8/40
Pancreatitis	5/41	0/37	11/37	1/47
Hepatitis	2/44	1/36	4/44	3/45
Hypertension	11/35	12/25	13/35	19/29
Renal dysfunction	1/45	0/37	0/48	0/48
Nutrition at operation				
CONUT *	1.5 (0–10)	3 (0–11)	2 (0–11)	2 (0–10)
GPS *	0 (0–2)	0 (0–1)	0 (0–2)	0 (0–1)
mGPS *	0 (0–2)	0 (0–2)	0 (0–2)	0 (0–2)
NLR *	2.2 (1.1–20.4)	2.9 (0.8–8.6)	2.6 (1.0–9.7)	2.5 (0.7–15)
PLR *	97.7 (0.1–325.5)	166 (67.4–416.5)	104.2 (0.05–290)	184.9 (57.9–522.5)
PNI *	46.3 (29.5–56.2)	44.8 (28.5–52.5)	44.5 (26.3–55.5)	43 (32–51.5)
LMR *	4.1 (2.2–6.5)	3.1 (1.0–40.4)	5.4 (1.4–10.9)	3.5 (1–6.1)
SII *	300 (0.2–2180.5)	600 (168.4–1786.9)	376.9 (0.1–1944.4)	530.8 (95.1–3669.2)
CRP/Alb *	0.07 (0–2.0)	0.07 (0–3.3)	0.02 (0.002–1.0)	0.03 (0.002–2.2)

* Values are median (range). CA19-9, carbohydrate antigen 19-9; CONUT, controlling nutritional status; N/A, not available; GPS, Glasgow prognostic score; mGPS, modified Glasgow prognostic score; NLR, neutrophil/lymphocyte ratio; PLR, platelet/lymphocyte ratio; PNI, prognostic nutritional index; LMR, lymphocyte/monocyte ratio; SII, systemic immune inflammation index; CRP, C-reactive protein; Alb, albumin.

2.3. Comparison of Prognosis of Upfront Surgery vs. Neoadjuvant Treatment by Intention to Treat Analysis

In BR-PV patients who underwent upfront surgery ($n = 46$)/NAT ($n = 42$), survival was significantly better in the NAT group ($p = 0.004$) (Figure 2). In BR-A patients who underwent upfront surgery ($n = 48$)/NAT ($n = 63$), survival was significantly better in the NAT group ($p < 0.001$). This analysis was performed by intention-to-treat analysis.

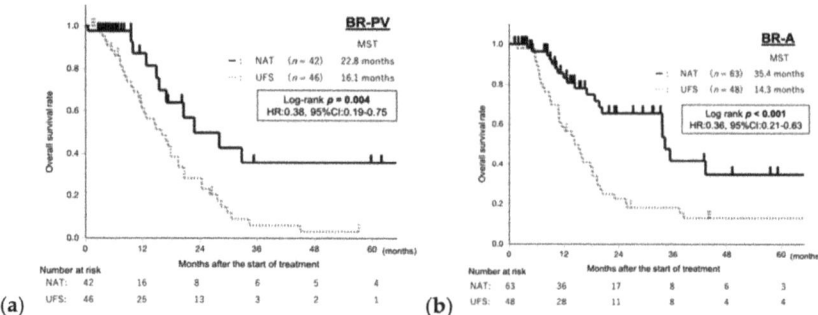

Figure 2. The overall survival in comparison between patients treated with and without NAT in the (**a**) BR-PV and (**b**) BR-A groups. The prognosis of patients treated with NAT was significantly better than that of patients treated without NAT in the BR-PV and BR-A groups ($p = 0.004$ and $p < 0.001$). NAT, neoadjuvant treatment; UFS, upfront surgery; MST, median survival time; HR, hazard ratio; CI, confidence interval.

The 36-month (3-year) OS rates with upfront surgery and NAT were 5.8% versus 35.5% in BR-PV patients and 15.5% versus 41.7% in BR-A patients, respectively.

2.4. Comparison of Regimens in Neoadjuvant Treatment Induction Cases

We compared the regimens of neoadjuvant treatment in each group (Table 4).

In BR-PV patients who underwent FFX/GnP ($n = 26$) vs. gemcitabine (GEM)/S-1 ($n = 2$) vs. GEM/S-1 with radiotherapy (RT) ($n = 14$), the median survival times (MSTs) were 32.9, 10.0 and 20.6 months, respectively, and the prognosis tended to be better in the FFX/GnP group. The number of resected cases was 36 (86%).

In BR-A patients who underwent FFX/GnP ($n = 29$) vs. FFX/GnP with RT ($n = 7$) vs. GEM/S-1 ($n = 10$) vs. GEM/S-1 with RT ($n = 17$), the MSTs were 35.4, 18.7, 43.2 and 19.7 months, respectively, with a better prognosis in the FFX/GnP group. The number of resected cases was 39 (62%).

The R0 rate tended to be higher in regimens with RT.

Table 4. Comparison of regimens in patients who underwent NAT.

	BR-PV ($n = 42$)						BR-A ($n = 63$)					
	n	MST (Months)	CA19-9 Normalized	Resection	R0 Rate	Evans Grade $\geq$IIb	n	MST (Months)	CA19-9 Normalized	Resection	R0 Rate	Evans Grade $\geq$IIb
FFX/GnP	26	32.9	47%	22 (85%)	86%	24%	29	35.4	40%	17 (59%)	71%	21%
FFX/GnP with RT	0						7	18.7	75%	4 (57%)	100%	0%
Old NAC	2	10	0%	2 (100%)	50%	0%	10	43.2	38%	9 (90%)	67%	0%
Old NAC with RT	14	20.6	50%	12 (86%)	100%	36%	17	19.7	20%	9 (53%)	100%	33%

Old NAC means neoadjuvant chemotherapy including gemcitabine, S-1, and GEM with S-1; FFX, FOLFIRINOX; GnP, gemcitabine along with nab-paclitaxel; RT, radiotherapy; NAC, neoadjuvant chemotherapy; MST, median survival time.

2.5. Prognostic Factors in Patients Who Underwent Resection after NAT

2.5.1. Definition of Cutoff Values for PNI

Receiver operating characteristic (ROC) curve analysis was performed with data from 36 BR-PV PDAC patients who underwent surgical resection between January 2002 and December 2018 to examine the association between PNI and 2-year survival. The area under the curve (AUC) was 0.728, and the best cutoff value was calculated as 42.65 (Figure 3a). Moreover, ROC curve analysis was performed with data from 39 BR-A PDAC patients. The AUC curve was 0.820, and the best cutoff value was calculated as 42.50 (Figure 3b). We eventually determined that the cutoff value for PNI was 42.5.

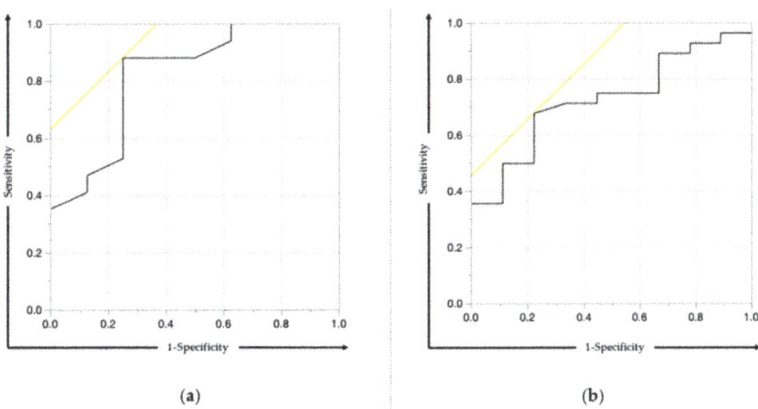

Figure 3. ROC analysis for the prediction of 2-year survival according to the preoperative PNI. (**a**) The AUC was 0.820 in BR-PV patients. (**b**) The AUC was 0.728 in BR-A patients. AUC, area under the curve; PNI, prognostic nutritional index.

2.5.2. Univariate and Multivariate Analyses of Prognostic Factors in BR-PDAC Patients Who Underwent Resection after Neoadjuvant Treatment

Table 5 shows the results of univariate analysis of prognostic factors in BR-PDAC patients who underwent resection after NAT. The cutoff values for continuous variables except preoperative PNI were determined using median values of all BR-PDAC patients who underwent resection after NAT.

In 36 BR-PV patients who underwent surgery after NAT, univariate analysis of overall survival revealed that normalization of TM levels ($p = 0.028$), preoperative GPS = 0 ($p = 0.025$), and preoperative high PNI ($p = 0.022$) were significantly associated with better prognosis. There was no significant difference in the multivariate analysis.

In 39 BR-A patients who underwent surgery after NAT, univariate analysis revealed that normalization of TM levels ($p = 0.033$), preoperative high PNI ($p = 0.013$), and intraoperative blood loss $\leq$ 830 mL ($p = 0.013$) were significantly associated with better prognosis. Multivariate analysis showed that preoperative PNI > 42.5 was an independent prognostic factor (HR: 0.15, $p = 0.014$). There was no correlation between the length of NAT and additional RT in survival in either BR-PV or BR-A.

Table 5. Univariate and multivariate analyses of the clinical features of BR-PDAC patients who underwent resection after NAT.

Clinical Factor	BR-PV Univariate			BR-PV Multivariate		BR-A Univariate			BR-A Multivariate	
	No. Patients ($n = 36$)	HR (95% CI)	p	HR (95% CI)	p	No. Patients ($n = 39$)	HR (95% CI)	p	HR (95% CI)	p
Radiation in NAT	12	0.96 (0.23–4.04)	0.955			12	1.37 (0.38–4.87)	0.63		
CA19-9 Before NAT >192 U/mL	17	2.37 (0.58–9.64)	0.23			19	0.41 (0.22–1.48)	0.175		
Preoperative CA19-9 >34 U/mL	17	1.05 (0.26–4.27)	0.945			19	3.90 (0.97–15.72)	0.056		
Tumor marker normalization	20	0.16 (0.031–0.82)	0.028 *	0.28 (0.05–1.71)	0.168	16	0.10 (0.01–0.83)	0.033 *	0.15 (0.01–1.57)	0.064
Preoperative Alb >3.8 g/dL	14	0.55 (0.14–2.24)	0.404			17	0.30 (0.06–1.46)	0.137		
Preoperative CONUT score, >4	5	3.78 (0.92–15.56)	0.065			9	2.48 (0.66–9.34)	0.179		
Preoperative GPS 0	16	0.15 (0.03–0.79)	0.025 *	0.50 (0.05–4.68)	0.547	10	0.52 (0.07–3.78)	0.52		
Preoperative mGPS 0	14	0.25 (0.05–1.28)	0.095			22	0.26 (0.06–1.08)	0.064		
Preoperative NLR >2.52	16	3.17 (0.39–25.86)	0.281			18	1.47 (0.39–5.51)	0.571		
Preoperative PLR >184	11	0.97 (0.23–4.10)	0.972			19	4.15 (0.85–20.26)	0.079		
Preoperative PNI >42.5	16	0.15 (0.03–0.76)	0.022 *	0.32 (0.03–2.98)	0.316	21	0.13 (0.03–0.65)	0.013 *	0.15 (0.02–0.85)	0.014 *
Preoperative LMR >3.50	9	0.19 (0.02–1.72)	0.141			14	0.42 (0.11–1.64)	0.214		
Preoperative SII >512	15	0.89 (0.21–3.74)	0.873			19	4.34 (0.84–22.49)	0.08		
Preoperative CRP/Alb >0.062	12	2.20 (0.43–11.16)	0.341			10	1.75 (0.43–7.08)	0.431		
Preoperative diabetes	11	0.78 (0.18–3.33)	0.739			13	0.91 (0.23–3.55)	0.9		
Preoperative treatment period >60 day	19	1.23 (0.15–10.09)	0.844			29	0.46 (0.12–1.67)	0.237		

Table 5. Cont.

Clinical Factor	BR-PV Univariate			BR-PV Multivariate		BR-A Univariate			BR-A Multivariate	
	No. Patients (n = 36)	HR (95% CI)	p	HR (95% CI)	p	No. Patients (n = 39)	HR (95% CI)	p	HR (95% CI)	p
Preoperative treatment period >90 day	7	1.72 (0.34–8.67)	0.509			14	1.07 (0.28–4.18)	0.918		
Operative time >560 min	7	3.12 (0.74–13.14)	0.121			20	1.73 (0.49–6.09)	0.396		
Intraoperative blood loss >830 ml	21	1.06 (0.25–4.45)	0.941			20	7.42 (1.53–36.1)	0.013 *	2.23 (0.37–13.35)	0.358

CA19-9, carbohydrate antigen 19-9; NAT, neoadjuvant treatment; Alb, albumin; CONUT, controlling nutritional status; GPS, Glasgow prognostic score; mGPS, modified Glasgow prognostic score; NLR, neutrophil/lymphocyte ratio; PLR, platelet/lymphocyte ratio; PNI, prognostic nutritional index; LMR, lymphocyte/monocyte ratio; SII, systemic immune inflammation index; CRP, C-reactive protein; Alb, albumin; * $p < 0.05$.

2.5.3. Prognosis of BR-PDAC Patients Who Underwent Resection after Neoadjuvant Treatment Based on PNI

In BR-PV patients who underwent resection after NAT (n = 36), survival was significantly better in the high PNI (preoperative PNI > 42.50) group (p = 0.029, HR:0.16, 95%CI:0.03–0.83) (Figure 4a). In BR-A patients who underwent resection after NAT (n = 39), survival was significantly better in the high PNI (preoperative PNI > 42.50) group (p = 0.012, HR:0.13, 95%CI:0.03–0.64) (Figure 4b).

Moreover, comparing the high preoperative PNI and low preoperative PNI, there was no statistically significant difference regarding postoperative complications (Clavien–Dindo grade III or more) in both BR-PV and BR-A patients (p = 0.644 and p = 0.580, respectively).

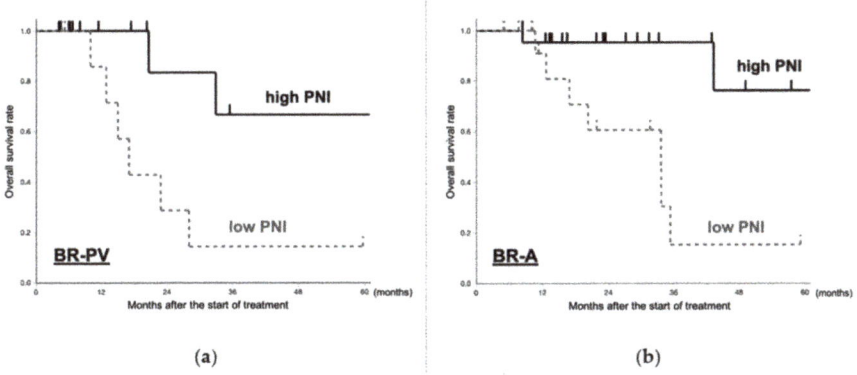

Figure 4. Comparison of the overall survival between high preoperative PNI and low preoperative PNI in the (a) BR-PV and (b) BR-A groups. The prognosis of patients with high preoperative PNI was significantly better than that of patients with low preoperative PNI in the BR-PV and BR-A patients (p = 0.029 and p = 0.012). PNI, prognostic nutritional index.

3. Discussion

There have been many analytical studies on R-PDAC and UR-PDAC, but few have focused on BR-PDAC. The usefulness of NAT for BR-PDAC has been highlighted in several articles [8–11]. Unfortunately, previous reports often analyzed mixed cohorts of patients, including those with BR and locally advanced UR-PDAC, those with BR-PDAC due to the infiltration of celiac and/or superior mesentery arteries (BR-A) and those with only infiltration of the portal system (BR-PV) [12,13]. The surgical strategy and outcome definitely differ between PDAC abutted to the major arteries and PDAC exclusively involving the PV system [14]. Murakami et al. reported that the BR-PV group had a significantly more favorable overall survival than the BR-A group in an analysis of BR patients who underwent upfront surgery [15]. Thus, it seems inappropriate to discuss the efficacy of the treatment strategy using such admixture.

In the present study, we differentiated between BR-A and BR-PV and analyzed the optimal preoperative multidisciplinary treatment and nutritional status before and after NAT for each type. There have been no comprehensive analyses focusing on surgical strategy for this cohort.

3.1. BR-PV

We retrospectively reviewed 88 patients with BR-PV PDAC. The results showed that the prognosis of BR-PV patients who underwent resection after NAT was significantly better than that of patients who underwent upfront surgery without NAT.

Fujii et al. reported that neoadjuvant chemoradiotherapy (NACRT) with S-1 rather than upfront surgery improves R0 rates and increases the survival of patients with BR-PV adenocarcinoma of the pancreatic head but not that of patients with R-PDAC [6]. However, the prognosis tended to be better in the FFX/GnP group than in the NACRT with old chemotherapy group in the present study. Although only 14 BR-PV patients underwent NACRT in this study, chemotherapeutic regimens such as FFX/GnP are expected to be a promising option.

3.2. BR-A

We retrospectively reviewed 111 patients with BR-A PDAC. Similar to that of BR-PV patients, the prognosis of BR-A patients who underwent resection after NAT was significantly better than that of those who underwent upfront surgery without NAT. Moreover, in patients with BR-A, the use of NAT with FFX/GnP significantly prolonged the prognosis.

Nagakawa et al. reported that NACRT, which combines chemotherapy with GEM/S-1, with intensity modified radiotherapy (IMRT) had fewer adverse events and improved the prognosis of BR-A [16]. In addition, they also reported that the R0 resection rate after NACRT was 94.7%. In the present study, the R0 resection rate also tended to be higher in patients who underwent additional RT, although additional RT failed to contribute to patient survival.

Hackert et al. reported that resection rates following FFX were 61% compared with 46% after GEM and RT in patients with locally advanced PDAC [17]. This study did not investigate NACRT, which combines new chemotherapy and RT; thus, it cannot be affirmed. However, the combination of radiation with more effective chemotherapy, such as FFX or GnP, is expected to improve the surgical consequences of BR-A patients. On the other hand, effective chemotherapy may lead to more adverse events. There is a report that NAT with FFX followed by IMRT concurrent with fixed-dose-rate GEM in BR-PDAC is feasible and tolerated [18]. Therefore, the IMRT technique may enable the application of NACRT in combination with more effective chemotherapy.

Over the past decade, newer chemotherapeutic regimens, including FFX and GnP, have emerged as new standard therapies for PDAC, which was formerly a lethal disease, and many studies have demonstrated promising survival rates [8–10,12,13]. However, there are few prospective randomized controlled studies to confirm the efficacy of NAT for patients with BR-PV and BR-A [16]. Evaluation of NAT is required for patients with BR-PV and BR-A in the setting of prospective trials.

3.3. BR-PV and BR-A

From previous reports as well as the results of this study, surgery after NAT is arguably more beneficial than upfront surgery in patients with BR-PDAC; therefore, we focused only on the patients who underwent NAT in the analysis after Section 2.4.

We demonstrated that the long-term survival of patients who underwent resection after NAT was significantly associated with good nutritional status, such as a PNI of more than 42.5 at the time of operation but not at diagnosis. Several studies have reported that preoperative nutrition indices, such as CONUT, mGPS, and PNI, are linked to the prognosis of various malignancies [19–21]. In pancreatic cancer, some indices have also been reported to have an independent association with survival in patients with resectable or BR-PDAC after pancreatectomy [22,23]. Moreover, there was a report that NAT for PDAC could aggravate nutritional status and hamper its postoperative recovery and that malnutrition might decrease the tolerance of NAT [24]. While definitive conclusions cannot be drawn from this retrospective study, these results strongly suggest the need for nutritional care during NAT in patients with PDAC. Systemic chemotherapy generally tends to worsen the patient's nutritional status as a side effect, including loss of appetite or dysgeusia [25]. Active nutritional care during NAC may minimize malnutrition, possibly improving the survival of BR-PDAC patients.

Furthermore, both the BR-PV and BR-A groups had lower median CA19-9 levels at operation in patients who underwent surgery after NAT than those who underwent upfront surgery. Although no significant difference was found in the multivariate analysis, normalization of TM levels was significantly associated with better prognosis in both BR-PV and BR-A patients. Chen et al. reported that long-term (approximately 6 months) chemotherapy after preoperative chemoradiotherapy may improve the prognosis in patients with potentially resectable/BR/UR-PDAC [26]. Satoi et al. also reported that the prognosis was prolonged by giving chemotherapy for 240 days or more in patients with UR-PDAC [27]. Conversely, the results of this study showed that the duration of NAT did not correlate with prognosis for BR-PDAC. It is suggested that the prognosis may be prolonged by surgery after the TM level is greatly reduced, not the length of NAT. Some patients with BR-PDAC became unresectable due to the progression of disease, such as distant metastasis during NAT. Therefore, assessment of TMs may be a more sensitive measure of the indications for resection than the length of treatment. Further exploration will be required for the optimal NAT duration and timing of surgery.

There are several limitations to our study. First, this study was retrospective in design with a relatively small number of patients. Second, the distribution of patients in the different treatment arms was unbalanced. Third, the number of patients receiving NAT has increased since around 2010. The proportion of patients receiving NAT and upfront surgery has changed significantly between 2002 and 2018. Fourth, indications for CRT were biased because CRT was recommended at the physicians' discretion. Finally, we have not started nutritional support for patients with NAT. We plan to explore the effect of nutritional support during NAT for patients with BR-PDAC to confirm the clinical relevance of this study. Further studies with more patients and longer observation periods are needed to evaluate the optimal and detailed strategy of multidisciplinary treatment for BR-PDAC.

In conclusion, these findings suggest that NAT followed by surgery rather than upfront surgery offers clinical benefits to patients with BR-A PDAC. Moreover, nutritional management during NAT may lead to a better prognosis.

4. Materials and Methods

4.1. Study Design

A prospectively maintained pancreatic resection database at two regional high-volume centers, Toyama University Hospital (Toyama, Japan) and Nagoya University Hospital (Nagoya, Japan), was queried to identify patients with BR PDAC who started the initial treatment between January 2002 and December 2018. This study conforms to the ethical guidelines of the World Medical Association Declaration of Helsinki-Ethical Principles for Medical Research Involving Human Subject. Written informed consent for inclusion in the study, as required by the institutional review board of both institutions, was obtained from all patients.

We retrospectively examined 199 patients with BR pancreatic cancer (88 patients with BR-PV and 111 patients with BR-A). For BR-PV and BR-A, the following points were investigated:

1. Comparison of prognosis of upfront surgery vs. NAT by intention to treat analysis;
2. Comparison of regimens in patients who underwent NAT;
3. Prognostic factors in patients who underwent resection after NAT.

4.2. Definitions of BR-PV PDAC and BR-A PDAC Patients

The preoperative resectability status was categorized into R (resectable), BR-PV, BR-A, UR (unresectable)-LA, and UR-M (metastatic) according to the 7th edition of the JPS classification (Table 6) [4].

Table 6. Resectability criteria proposed by the JPS.

Resectability	SubClass	Detail
1. Resectable (R)		No contact of the tumor with the SMV/PV. Abutment/encasement of the SMV/PV of <180° circumference without occlusion (termed R-PV). No contact with any major artery (CA, SMA, or CHA).
2. Borderline resectable (BR)	BR-PV	Tumor abutment/encasement or occlusion of the SMV/PV of ≥180°. No arterial tumor abutment/encasement (CA, SMA, or CHA).
	BR-A	Tumor abutment/encasement of the SMA or CA of <180° without irregularity in the contour of the artery. Tumor abutment/encasement of the CHA without irregularity in the contour of the PHA or CA.
3. Unresectable (UR)	UR-LA (Locally advance)	Tumor abutment/encasement of the SMA or CA of ≥180°. Tumor abutment/encasement of the CHA and extension of abutment/encasement to the PHA or CA. Tumor abutment/encasement of the aorta.
	UR-M (Metastasis)	Distant metastases, including metastases to lymph nodes beyond regional lymph nodes.

JPS, Japan Pancreas Society; SMV, superior mesenteric vein; PV, portal vein; CA, celiac artery; SMA, superior mesenteric artery; CHA, common hepatic artery; PHA, proper hepatic artery.

Patient eligibility was rigorously defined using thin-slice multidetector-row computed tomography. All images were reviewed by two or more experienced radiologists to reaffirm the preoperative staging. Consequently, 199 patients with BR-PDAC (88 patients with BR-PV and 111 patients with BR-A) were enrolled in this study.

4.3. Neoadjuvant Treatment

Some patients received NAT from diagnosis with the following regimens: GnP, FFX, modified FFX (mFFX), or GEM with oral S-1 (the oral 5-fluorouracil prodrug tegafur with oteracil and gimeracil). These chemotherapeutic regimens were selected depending on the patient's background and the period of enrollment. We performed NAT in 105 patients (42 patients with BR-PV and 63 patients with BR-A) from which informed consent was obtained depending on their condition and tumor status. CRT consisted of a photon/proton external beam with 50.4 Gy delivered in 28 fractions combined with systemic chemotherapy involving oral S-1, which was administered twice daily (80 mg/m^2/day) from days 1 to 14 and from days 22 to 35.

4.4. Postoperative Adjuvant Therapy

Postoperative adjuvant chemotherapy was applied unless contraindicated by the patient's condition. In short, the patients received GEM or S-1 for 6 months according to the protocol that was available at the time of treatment [28,29]. GEM at a dose of 1000 mg/m^2 was administered weekly for 3 weeks followed by 1 week of rest; oral S-1 (80 mg/m^2/day) was administered from days 1 to 28 followed by a 2-week rest period. Chemotherapy was initiated at <2 months after the operation in all patients who were considered eligible for the treatment. Computed tomography was routinely performed every 6 months as a postoperative follow-up imaging examination, and a blood test, including evaluation of TMs, was performed every 2 months to evaluate the recurrent disease.

4.5. Data Collection

We collected patient data from the medical records. Pretreatment factors included age, sex, body mass index, tumor size, and blood test results, including serum CA19-9 level. Preoperative factors included chemotherapeutic regimen, length of NAT, and change in CA19-9 level. Perioperative factors included surgical procedures, region of tumor, operative time, blood loss volume, blood transfusion, incidence of postoperative complications according to the Clavien–Dindo classification [30], length of hospital stay, and 90-day mortality.

The tumor-node-metastasis staging system for pancreatic tumors of the seventh edition of the Union for International Cancer Control was applied [31]. The pathological data collected included tumor grade, number of positive lymph nodes, resection margins, perineural invasion, PV invasion, and artery invasion. The surgical margin in this study denoted either the stump of the pancreas or the bile duct or the dissected plane around the pancreas as described by Staley et al. [32]. If viable cancer cells were detected microscopically at the tip of any of these sites, the surgical margin was noted as positive. If the tumor was located at a distance of >1 mm from the surgical margin, the margin was noted as negative.

4.6. Nutritional Status

In the current study, we also investigated several nutritional parameters at diagnosis and at operation, such as the GPS [33], mGPS [33], CONUT [19], PNI [22,33], NLR [33,34], PLR [33], LMR [34], and SII [35], to verify their impact on the operative outcome and the prognosis.

4.7. Statistical Analysis

A biostatistician (K.M.) was responsible for the statistical analysis. The Kaplan–Meier method was used to calculate survival rates, and the difference in survival curves was analyzed by the log-rank test. To detect prognostic factors for survival, we performed Cox proportional hazard analysis, and hazard ratios and 95% confidence intervals (CIs) were calculated. Goodness-of-fit for preoperative PNI was assessed by calculating the AUC of the ROC curve, and the optimal cutoff value was determined using the Youden index. Other cutoff values in Table 3 used their median values. Differences in nominal data between the two groups were examined using the chi-square test or Fisher's exact test when the expected value was <5. Differences in quantitative variables were evaluated using Student's *t*-test or the Mann–Whitney *U* test if the distribution was abnormal. A *p* value < 0.05 was considered statistically significant. All statistical analyses were performed using JMP statistical software (version 14.2; SAS Institute, Cary, NC, USA).

5. Conclusions

NAT using chemotherapy such as FFX or GnP is essential for improving the prognosis of BR pancreatic cancer. This suggests that prognosis may be improved by maintaining good nutritional status during preoperative treatment, not by the length of preoperative treatment. In addition, normalization of TMs by preoperative treatment contributes to the prolongation of survival.

Author Contributions: Conceptualization, N.K., S.Y. and T.F.; methodology, H.T., I.Y. and K.S.; formal analysis, K.M.; investigation F.S., Y.H., K.H., T.W. and K.M. (Kosuke Mori); data curation, H.B., T.M., M.K., M.H., K.M. (Koshi Matsui) and T.O.; writing—original draft preparation, N.K., Y.H. and H.B.; writing—review and editing, N.K., S.Y. and T.F.; supervision, Y.K. and T.F.; project administration, Y.K.; funding acquisition, T.F. All authors have read and agreed to the published version of the manuscript.

Funding: This research was funded by JSPS KAKENHI, grant number 18H02878.

Institutional Review Board Statement: The study was conducted according to the guidelines of the Declaration of Helsinki, and approved by the Institutional Ethics Committee of University of Toyama (protocol code: R2019141 and date of approval: 2 December 2019).

Informed Consent Statement: Patient consent was not required based on the use of anonymized data.

Conflicts of Interest: The authors declare no conflict of interest.

References

1. McGuigan, A.; Kelly, P.; Turkington, R.C.; Jones, C.; Coleman, H.G.; McCain, R.S. Pancreatic cancer: A review of clinical diagnosis, epidemiology, treatment and outcomes. *World J. Gastroenterol.* **2018**, *24*, 4846–4861. [CrossRef] [PubMed]
2. Traverso, L.W. Pancreatic cancer: Surgery alone is not sufficient. *Surg. Endosc.* **2006**, *20*, S446–S449. [CrossRef] [PubMed]
3. NCCN. Clinical Practice Guidelines in Oncology (NCCN Guidelines): NCCN, Pancreatic Adenocarcinoma, Version 1. 2020. Available online: https://www.nccn.org/professionals/physician_gls/pdf/pancreatic.pdf (accessed on 27 September 2020).
4. Japan Pancreas Society. *Classification of Pancreatic Carcinoma*, 4th ed.; Kanehara & Co., Ltd.: Tokyo, Japan, 2017.
5. Varadhachary, G.R.; Tamm, E.P.; Abbruzzese, J.L.; Xiong, H.Q.; Crane, C.H.; Wang, H.; Lee, J.E.; Pisters, P.W.; Evans, D.B.; Wolff, R.A. Borderline resectable pancreatic cancer: Definitions, management, and role of preoperative therapy. *Ann. Surg. Oncol.* **2006**, *13*, 1035–1046. [CrossRef] [PubMed]
6. Fujii, T.; Satoi, S.; Yamada, S.; Murotani, K.; Yanagimoto, H.; Takami, H.; Yamamoto, T.; Kanda, M.; Yamaki, S.; Hirooka, S.; et al. Clinical benefits of neoadjuvant chemoradiotherapy for adenocarcinoma of the pancreatic head: an observational study using inverse probability of treatment weighting. *J. Gastroenterol.* **2016**, *52*, 81–93. [CrossRef]
7. Takahashi, S.; Kinoshita, T.; Konishi, M.; Gotohda, N.; Kato, Y.; Kinoshita, T.; Kobayashi, T.; Mitsunaga, S.; Nakachi, K.; Ikeda, M. Borderline resectable pancreatic cancer: Rationale for multidisciplinary treatment. *J. Hepatobiliary Pancreat. Sci.* **2011**, *18*, 567–574. [CrossRef]
8. Versteijne, E.; Vogel, J.A.; Besselink, M.G.; Busch, O.R.C.; Wilmink, J.W.; Daams, J.G.; van Eijck, C.H.J.; Groot Koerkamp, B.; Rasch, C.R.N.; van Tienhoven, G.; et al. Meta-analysis comparing upfront surgery with neoadjuvant treatment in patients with resectable or borderline resectable pancreatic cancer. *Br. J. Surg.* **2018**, *105*, 946–958. [CrossRef]
9. Miyasaka, Y.; Ohtsuka, T.; Kimura, R.; Matsuda, R.; Mori, Y.; Nakata, K.; Kakihara, D.; Fujimori, N.; Ohno, T.; Oda, Y.; et al. Neoadjuvant Chemotherapy with Gemcitabine Plus Nab-Paclitaxel for Borderline Resectable Pancreatic Cancer Potentially Improves Survival and Facilitates Surgery. *Ann. Surg. Oncol.* **2019**, *26*, 1528–1534. [CrossRef]
10. Janssen, Q.P.; Buettner, S.; Suker, M.; Beumer, B.R.; Addeo, P.; Bachellier, P.; Bahary, N.; Bekaii-Saab, T.; Bali, M.A.; Besselink, M.G.; et al. Neoadjuvant FOLFIRINOX in Patients With Borderline Resectable Pancreatic Cancer: A Systematic Review and Patient-Level Meta-Analysis. *J. Natl. Cancer Inst.* **2019**, *111*, 782–794. [CrossRef]
11. Motoi, F.; Satoi, S.; Honda, G.; Wada, K.; Shinchi, H.; Matsumoto, I.; Sho, M.; Tsuchida, A.; Unno, M.; Study Group of Preoperative Therapy for Pancreatic Cancer (PREP). A single-arm, phase II trial of neoadjuvant gemcitabine and S1 in patients with resectable and borderline resectable pancreatic adenocarcinoma: PREP-01 study. *J. Gastroenterol.* **2019**, *54*, 194–203. [CrossRef]

12. Ferrone, C.R.; Marchegiani, G.; Hong, T.S.; Ryan, D.P.; Deshpande, V.; McDonnell, E.I.; Sabbatino, F.; Santos, D.D.; Allen, J.N.; Blaszkowsky, L.S.; et al. Radiological and surgical implications of neoadjuvant treatment with FOLFIRINOX for locally advanced and borderline resectable pancreatic cancer. *Ann. Surg.* **2015**, *261*, 12–17. [CrossRef]
13. Jang, J.Y.; Han, Y.; Lee, H.; Kim, S.W.; Kwon, W.; Lee, K.H.; Oh, D.Y.; Chie, E.K.; Lee, J.M.; Heo, J.S.; et al. Oncological Benefits of Neoadjuvant Chemoradiation With Gemcitabine Versus Upfront Surgery in Patients With Borderline Resectable Pancreatic Cancer: A Prospective, Randomized, Open-label, Multicenter Phase 2/3 Trial. *Ann. Surg.* **2018**, *268*, 215–222. [CrossRef] [PubMed]
14. Fujii, T.; Yamada, S.; Murotani, K.; Kanda, M.; Sugimoto, H.; Nakao, A.; Kodera, Y. Inverse Probability of Treatment Weighting Analysis of Upfront Surgery Versus Neoadjuvant Chemoradiotherapy Followed by Surgery for Pancreatic Adenocarcinoma with Arterial Abutment. *Medicine (Baltimore)* **2015**, *94*, e1647. [CrossRef] [PubMed]
15. Murakami, Y.; Satoi, S.; Sho, M.; Motoi, F.; Matsumoto, I.; Kawai, M.; Honda, G.; Uemura, K.; Yanagimoto, H.; Shinzeki, M.; et al. National Comprehensive Cancer Network Resectability Status for Pancreatic Carcinoma Predicts Overall Survival. *World J. Surg.* **2015**, *39*, 2306–2314. [CrossRef] [PubMed]
16. Nagakawa, Y.; Hosokawa, Y.; Nakayama, H.; Sahara, Y.; Takishita, C.; Nakajima, T.; Hijikata, Y.; Kasuya, K.; Katsumata, K.; Tokuuye, K.; et al. A phase II trial of neoadjuvant chemoradiotherapy with intensity-modulated radiotherapy combined with gemcitabine and S-1 for borderline-resectable pancreatic cancer with arterial involvement. *Cancer Chemother. Pharmacol.* **2017**, *79*, 951–957. [CrossRef] [PubMed]
17. Hackert, T.; Sachsenmaier, M.; Hinz, U.; Schneider, L.; Michalski, C.W.; Springfeld, C.; Strobel, O.; Jäger, D.; Ulrich, A.; Büchler, M.W. Locally Advanced Pancreatic Cancer: Neoadjuvant Therapy With Folfirinox Results in Resectability in 60% of the Patients. *Ann. Surg.* **2016**, *264*, 457–463. [CrossRef] [PubMed]
18. Tran, N.H.; Sahai, V.; Griffith, K.A.; Nathan, H.; Kaza, R.; Cuneo, K.C.; Shi, J.; Kim, E.; Sonnenday, C.J.; Cho, C.S.; et al. Phase 2 Trial of Neoadjuvant FOLFIRINOX and Intensity Modulated Radiation Therapy Concurrent With Fixed-Dose Rate-Gemcitabine in Patients With Borderline Resectable Pancreatic Cancer. *Int. J. Radiat. Oncol. Biol. Phys.* **2020**, *106*, 124–133. [CrossRef]
19. Kato, Y.; Yamada, S.; Suenaga, M.; Takami, H.; Niwa, Y.; Hayashi, M.; Iwata, N.; Kanda, M.; Tanaka, C.; Nakayama, G.; et al. Impact of the Controlling Nutritional Status Score on the Prognosis After Curative Resection of Pancreatic Ductal Adenocarcinoma. *Pancreas* **2018**, *47*, 823–829. [CrossRef]
20. Liang, R.-F.; Li, J.-H.; Li, M.; Yang, Y.; Liu, Y. The prognostic role of controlling nutritional status scores in patients with solid tumors. *Clin. Chim. Acta* **2017**, *474*, 155–158. [CrossRef]
21. Baba, H.; Tokai, R.; Hirano, K.; Watanabe, T.; Shibuya, K.; Hashimoto, I.; Hojo, S.; Yoshioka, I.; Okumura, T.; Nagata, T.; et al. Risk factors for postoperative pneumonia after general and digestive surgery: A retrospective single-center study. *Surg. Today* **2020**, *50*, 460–468. [CrossRef]
22. Kanda, M.; Fujii, T.; Kodera, Y.; Nagai, S.; Takeda, S.; Nakao, A. Nutritional predictors of postoperative outcome in pancreatic cancer. *Br. J. Surg.* **2011**, *98*, 268–274. [CrossRef]
23. Kawai, M.; Hirono, S.; Okada, K.-I.; Miyazawa, M.; Shimizu, A.; Kitahata, Y.; Kobayashi, R.; Ueno, M.; Hayami, S.; Tanioka, K.; et al. Low lymphocyte monocyte ratio after neoadjuvant therapy predicts poor survival after pancreatectomy in patients with borderline resectable pancreatic cancer. *Surgery* **2019**, *165*, 1151–1160. [CrossRef] [PubMed]
24. Tashiro, M.; Yamada, S.; Sonohara, F.; Takami, H.; Suenaga, M.; Hayashi, M.; Niwa, Y.; Tanaka, C.; Kobayashi, D.; Nakayama, G.; et al. Clinical Impact of Neoadjuvant Therapy on Nutritional Status in Pancreatic Cancer. *Ann. Surg. Oncol.* **2018**, *25*, 3365–3371. [CrossRef] [PubMed]
25. Ziętarska, M.; Krawczyk-Lipiec, J.; Kraj, L.; Zaucha, R.; Małgorzewicz, S. Nutritional status assessment in colorectal cancer patients qualified to systemic treatment. *Contemp. Oncol. (Pozn.)* **2017**, *21*, 157–161. [CrossRef] [PubMed]
26. Chen, K.T.; Devarajan, K.; Milestone, B.N.; Cooper, H.S.; Denlinger, C.; Cohen, S.J.; Meyer, J.E.; Hoffman, J.P. Neoadjuvant Chemoradiation and Duration of Chemotherapy Before Surgical Resection for Pancreatic Cancer: Does Time Interval Between Radiotherapy and Surgery Matter? *Ann. Surg. Oncol.* **2014**, *21*, 662–669. [CrossRef] [PubMed]
27. Satoi, S.; Yamaue, H.; Kato, K.; Takahashi, S.; Hirono, S.; Takeda, S.; Eguchi, H.; Sho, M.; Wada, K.; Shinchi, H.; et al. Role of adjuvant surgery for patients with initially unresectable pancreatic cancer with a long-term favorable response to non-surgical anti-cancer treatments: Results of a project study for pancreatic surgery by the Japanese Society of Hepato-Biliary-Pancreatic Surgery. *J. Hepatobiliary Pancreat. Sci.* **2013**, *20*, 590–600. [PubMed]
28. Oettle, H.; Neuhaus, P.; Hochhaus, A.; Hartmann, J.T.; Gellert, K.; Ridwelski, K.; Niedergethmann, M.; Zülke, C.; Fahlke, J.; Arning, M.B.; et al. Adjuvant chemotherapy with gemcitabine and long-term outcomes among patients with resected pancreatic cancer: The CONKO-001 randomized trial. *JAMA* **2013**, *310*, 1473–1481. [CrossRef] [PubMed]
29. Uesaka, K.; Boku, N.; Fukutomi, A.; Okamura, Y.; Konishi, M.; Matsumoto, I.; Kaneoka, Y.; Shimizu, Y.; Nakamori, S.; Sakamoto, H.; et al. Adjuvant chemotherapy of S-1 versus gemcitabine for resected pancreatic cancer: A phase 3, open-label, randomised, non-inferiority trial (JASPAC 01). *Lancet* **2016**, *388*, 248–257. [CrossRef]
30. Dindo, D.; Demartines, N.; Clavien, P.A. Classification of surgical complications: A new proposal with evaluation in a cohort of 6336 patients and results of a survey. *Ann. Surg.* **2004**, *240*, 205–213. [CrossRef] [PubMed]
31. Cong, L.; Liu, Q.; Zhang, R.; Cui, M.; Zhang, X.; Gao, X.; Guo, J.; Dai, M.; Zhang, T.; Liao, Q.; et al. Tumor size classification of the 8th edition of TNM staging system is superior to that of the 7th edition in predicting the survival outcome of pancreatic cancer patients after radical resection and adjuvant chemotherapy. *Sci. Rep.* **2018**, *8*, 10383. [CrossRef]

32. Staley, C.A.; Cleary, K.R.; Abbruzzese, J.L.; Lee, J.E.; Ames, F.C.; Fenoglio, C.J.; Evans, D.B. The Need for Standardized Pathologic Staging of Pancreaticoduodenectomy Specimens. *Pancreas* **1996**, *12*, 373–380. [CrossRef]
33. Xiao, Y.; Xie, Z.; Shao, Z.; Chen, W.; Xie, H.; Qin, G.; Zhao, N. Prognostic value of postdiagnostic inflammation-based scores in short-term overall survival of advanced pancreatic ductal adenocarcinoma patients. *Medicine* **2017**, *96*, e9247. [CrossRef] [PubMed]
34. Sierzega, M.; Lenart, M.; Rutkowska, M.; Surman, M.; Mytar, B.; Matyja, A.; Siedlar, M.; Kulig, J. Preoperative Neutrophil-Lymphocyte and Lymphocyte-Monocyte Ratios Reflect Immune Cell Population Rearrangement in Resectable Pancreatic Cancer. *Ann. Surg. Oncol.* **2017**, *24*, 808–815. [CrossRef] [PubMed]
35. Jomrich, G.; Gruber, E.S.; Winkler, D.; Hollenstein, M.; Gnant, M.; Sahora, K.; Schindl, M. Systemic Immune-Inflammation Index (SII) Predicts Poor Survival in Pancreatic Cancer Patients Undergoing Resection. *J. Gastrointest. Surg.* **2020**, *24*, 610–618. [CrossRef] [PubMed]

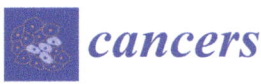

Review
Surgical Treatment of Pancreatic Ductal Adenocarcinoma

Kongyuan Wei and Thilo Hackert *

Department of General, Visceral and Transplantation Surgery, University of Heidelberg, Im Neuenheimer Feld 420, 69120 Heidelberg, Germany; jasonwky@163.com
* Correspondence: thilo_hackert@med.uni-heidelberg.de; Tel.: +49-6221-565150

Simple Summary: Surgery is the only potential cure for pancreatic ductal adenocarcinoma and should always be combined with adjuvant chemotherapy or other multimodal treatment. Besides the advances in such multimodal approaches, there has been substantial progress in surgical techniques to especially address advanced resections. These techniques include specific operative steps, such as 'artery first' or 'uncinate first' approaches as well as techniques that allow safe vascular resection and reconstruction to achieve radical tumor removal. Most recently, also minimally-invasive and robotic approaches have been adopted for pancreatic cancer surgery; however, there is no high-level evidence on these evolving techniques especially with regards to long-term results compared to conventional surgical techniques.

Abstract: Pancreatic ductal adenocarcinoma (PDAC) represents an aggressive tumor of the digestive system with still low five-year survival of less than 10%. Although there are improvements for multimodal therapy of PDAC, surgery still remains the effective way to treat the disease. Combined with adjuvant and/or neoadjuvant treatment, pancreatic surgery is able to enhance the five-year survival up to around 20%. However, pancreatic resection is always associated with a high risk of complications and regarded as one of the most complex fields in abdominal surgery. This review gives a summary on the surgical treatment for PDAC based on the current literature with a special focus on resection techniques.

Keywords: pancreatic ductal adenocarcinoma; surgical treatment; technical advances

1. Introduction

Pancreatic ductal adenocarcinoma (PDAC) still remains a big therapeutic challenge for its poor prognosis and will likely becomes the second cause of cancer death within the next decade [1,2]. Although there are mounts of advanced treatments including adjuvant chemotherapy, surgical therapy is always regarded as the most effective one to attain the long-term survival for the patients with PDAC [3]. Unfortunately, less than 20% of patients with pancreatic cancer are considered as the surgically resectable cases until now [2]. Additionally, most of the patients with metastatic disease are not suitable for resection according to the safety and efficacy affected by the historical concerns [4]. However, owing to the development of systematic chemotherapy and improvement of surgery, extended indications of the pancreatic resection are applied in clinical practice, including technical advancements as well as patient criteria such as advanced age [5].

1.1. Definition of Resectability

There are various classifications reported for the differentiation of resectable, borderline-resectable, and unresectable pancreatic cancers [6–11]. The definition of resectability is made mainly based on scientific associations as well as the MD Anderson Classification [8,10]. The AHPBA/SSO/SSAT Classification was modified by the National Comprehensive Cancer Network (NCCN) further as well as the International Study Group of Pancreatic Surgery (ISGPS) [11,12]. Therefore, resectability now is classified by the invasion of important adjacent vessels, especially referring to the celiac trunk, superior mesenteric artery (SMA), and the portal (PV) or superior mesenteric vein (SMV). Pancreatic cancer is regarded as resectable if there are no major vessels involved. Borderline resectable pancreatic cancer is defined as a pancreatic cancer with involvement of the portal vein and/or superior mesenteric vein and the involved segments of vessels allow resection and reconstruction (Figure 1).

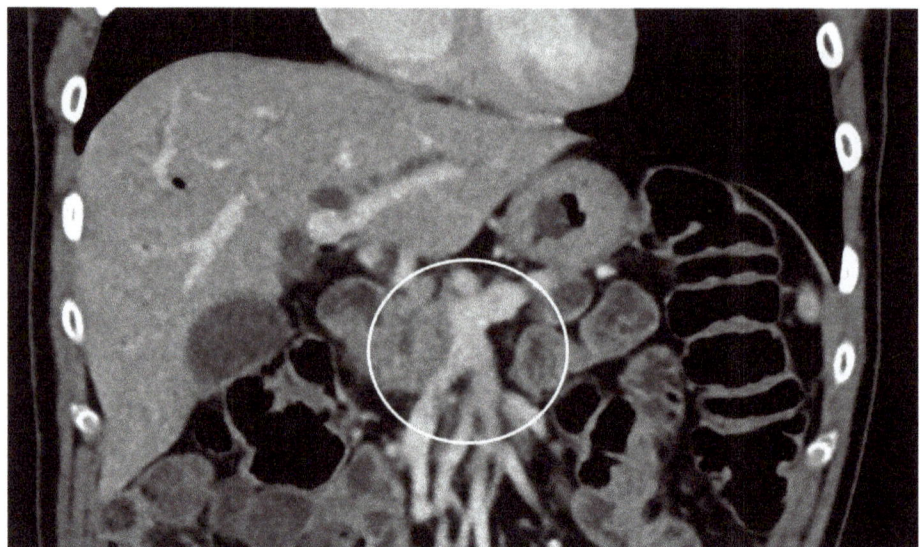

Figure 1. Anatomical borderline resectability, contrast enhanced CT scan, and coronary reformatting. Pancreatic head cancer with contact to superior mesenteric vein/portal vein confluence (white circle), vascular reconstruction technically possible.

Furthermore, if the superior mesenteric artery or the celiac trunk are invaded, pancreatic tumors are considered as locally advanced and unresectable, however arterial resections and reconstructions can be performed by experienced surgeons. Actually, for determination of resectability, the relationship between the tumor and mesenteric/hepatic vessels is the critical topic to obtain R0 resection [13–15]. Hence, through preoperative staging and imaging, pancreatic tumors are divided into four types: resectable, borderline resectable, locally advanced and metastatic. Currently, upfront surgery is recommended in resectable pancreatic cancer [7,11,12]. In contrary to the surgical and anatomical considerations to evaluate resectability, the International Association of Pancreatology developed a more comprehensive definition of resectability using three different factors: 1. anatomical; 2. biological; 3. conditional [7]. For anatomical criteria it basically includes the above mentioned factors and basically a serum carbohydrate antigen (CA) 19-9 level more than 500 U/mL or regional lymph node metastases diagnosed by biopsy or positron emission tomography-computed tomography. Potentially resectable disease based on anatomic criteria is transferred to borderline resectability if these factors are present. Conditional factors include the ECOG classification of patients and may also shift potentially resectable disease based on anatomic and biologic criteria towards a borderline resectable status if classification equals or exceeds ECOG 2 [7]. The detailed definition of anatomical resectability is displayed in Table 1. Recently, the BACAP Consortium published a BACAP Score to predict the resectability of pancreatic adenocarcinoma based on anatomical considerations (vascular thrombosis, tumor localization, tumor size) as well as conditional evaluation (WHO performance status) and symptoms (pain, weight loss) [16]. Based on the analysis of a prospectively collected 814-patient cohort, this score will be evaluated in further clinical trials.

Table 1. International consensus of classification of BR PDAC based on anatomical definition using CT imaging including coronal and sagittal sections [7].

Category	Anatomical Feature
Resectable: R	SMV/PV: no tumor contact or unilateral narrowing
	SMA, CA, CHA: no tumor contact
Borderline resectable: BR	Subclassified according to SMV/PV involvement alone or arterial invasion
BR-PV (SMV/PV involvement alone)	SMV/PV: tumor contact 180 or greater or bilateral narrowing/occlusion, not exceeding the inferior border of the duodenum.
	SMA, CA, CHA: no tumor contact/invasion
BR-A (arterial involvement)	SMA, CA: tumor contact of less than 180 without showing deformity/stenosis
	CHA: tumor contact without showing tumor contact of the PHA and/or CA.
Unresectable: UR	Subclassified according to the status of distant metastasis
Locally advanced: LA	SMV/PV: bilateral narrowing/occlusion, exceeding the inferior border of the duodenum
	SMA, CA: tumor contact/invasion of 180 or more degree #.
	CHA: tumor contact/invasion showing tumor contact/invasion of the PHA and/or CA.
	AO: tumor contact or invasion.
Metastatic: M	Distant metastasis $.

#: In cases with CA invasion of 180 or more without involvement of the aorta and with intact and uninvolved gastroduodenal artery thereby permitting a distal pancreatectomy with en bloc celiac axis resection (DP-CAR), some members prefer this criteria to be in the BR-A category. $: including macroscopic para aortic and extra abdominal lymph node metastasis.

Nowadays, CT, MRI, and PET are applied in the imaging detection and staging for patients with pancreatic cancer as well as endoscopic ultrasound (EUS). Contrast-enhanced CT is regarded as primary approach for the diagnosis and resectability evaluation. MRI is an alternative choice and is superior to CT when evaluating ductal anatomy with MRCP [17]. Besides, MRI is superior to detect the liver metastases compared to CT with higher sensitivity [18]. Recently, PET-MRI has been reported to have equal efficacy in resectability evaluation for the patients with PDAC [19]. Yamada et al. showed that EUS combined with elastography (EG) had better diagnostic performance in evaluating vascular invasion for PDAC compared to CT [20]. In addition, Ehrlich et al. also demonstrated that for patients with borderline resectable pancreatic cancer and locally advanced pancreatic cancer, EUS-FNA (fine-needle aspiration) has the potential to ensure the diagnose as well as local resectability accurately and suggested it as a routine approach for PDAC patients [21]. However, a recent meta-analysis indicated that CT might be superior to EUS in resectability evaluation; so a controversy about EUS application still remains and more high-quality clinical trials need to be conducted in the future to achieve more high-level evidence [22–24].

1.2. Neoadjuvant and Adjuvant Therapy

The impact of adjuvant chemotherapy to improve survival after resection of pancreatic cancer has been undoubtedly be proven during the last two decades, namely by the ESPAC study group as well as the PRODIGE consortium who continuously developed standards for adjuvant treatment by conducting large multicenter RCTs [25–28].

The latest of these studies reported median survival times of 30 and 54 months, respectively, as well as a 5-year survival of 30% which shows the essential need for adjuvant systemic treatment after pancreatic cancer resection [26,28]. This has ultimately been adopted in national and international guidelines [29].

Today there is a worldwide trend to increase the proportion of patients receiving neoadjuvant therapy. While neoadjuvant therapy is inevitable in locally advanced pancreatic cancers to achieve a chance of conversion surgery afterwards, its use in borderline-resectable and especially resectable pancreatic cancer is currently still based on weak evidence, although observational and a limited number of randomized controlled trials suggest its benefit when borderline resectable disease is considered.

Yet, the main dilemma remains the selection of patients for neoadjuvant treatment and the selection of the specific treatment protocol. Neoadjuvant chemotherapy alone or in combination with radiotherapy is widely used in numerous varying protocols on one hand, on the other hand these protocols are often based on institutional or national preferences and—in contrast to adjuvant protocols—no standards are set on the basis of high-quality evidence [30,31].

Briefly, the debate on upfront surgery versus neoadjuvant treatment still remains. The Dutch Randomized Phase III PREOPANC Trial demonstrated that there was no significant difference in overall survival benefit between the preoperative chemoradiotherapy and upfront surgery for resectable and borderline resectable pancreatic cancer [32]. Given the observation that upfront surgery combined with adjuvant therapy can attain an average 19% five-year overall survival which increases up to 50% in prognostically favorable subgroups neoadjuvant therapy is still far from being the standard based on high-level evidence [33]. If neoadjuvant therapy is chosen, another unsolved question is the need for additional adjuvant therapy after resection. A recently published study pooling observational data of 520 patient after induction FOLFIRINOX treatment and consecutive resection showed that an additional adjuvant protocol did not generally show any benefit but may be recommended for pathologically lymph-node positive patients [34]. A phase 2 Randomized Clinical Trial discovered that perioperative chemotherapy did not significantly improve two-year overall survival for resectable PDAC whereas may increase actual resectability rates—an observation which is certainly explained by a selection effect during neoadjuvant treatment [35]. All in all, adjuvant and especially neoadjuvant treatment are currently in a dynamic state and numerous studies are ongoing.

2. Surgery

2.1. Standard Resection

Pancreaticoduodenectomy (PD) has been widely applied since in 1940, Whipple reported the classical procedure including distal gastrectomy and total duodenectomy and although this approach has been modified in some steps it is still basically similar to what is performed today [36].

PD includes a standardized lymphadenectomy along the right side of the vascular structures (porto-mesenteric veins, superior mesenteric artery, celiac axis) and the hepatoduodenal ligament. Nowadays, PD is routinely performed under preservation of the pylorus as recent studies have confirmed that pylorus preservation does not have any disadvantages compared to pylorus resection or classical Whipple procedures in terms of functional (especially regarding delayed gastric emptying) and oncological outcomes unless the tumor extends towards the pylorus, which then—unquestionably—requires resection of the distal stomach.

For tumors of the body and tail of the pancreas, a distal pancreatectomy and splenectomy with respective lymphadenectomy from the left side of the vascular structures is mandatory.

In case of unfavorable location of the tumor in the center of the pancreas or synchronous multiple PDAC, a total pancreatectomy and splenectomy may be required. Regarding all resection techniques, it is of the utmost importance to achieve a radical (R0) resection status. This can best be achieved by a complete dissection of all lymphatic and soft tissue along the arterial structures to reduce the risk of remaining microscopic tumor persistence and early recurrence.

2.2. Specific Techniques

2.2.1. Artery First Approach

The core principle of this procedure is to identify the SMA early at the origin of the aorta and the approach has been described for different ways of access to the artery [37,38].

The idea of the approach to evaluate any potential tumor adherence to the SMA at the beginning of the operation and either stop resection or plan an arterial resection if required and indicated. After exposing the SMA from the left-sided access (opening Treitz ligament) a Kocher maneuver is required to expose the anterior surface of the inferior vena cava and the aorta with an early identification of the left renal vein and the origin of the SMA. After the accurate dissection along the SMA is finished, the soft tissue between the SMA and the celiac trunk should also be removed. By this procedure, a very controlled and radical resection on the right side of the arterial axis (SMA/celiac trunk) is achieved, while the autonomous nerves on the left side of the arteries are spared to reduce the incidence of postoperative diarrhea. For the radical resection of pancreatic head tumors which involve the posterior and right side of the SMA, the artery first technique is beneficial and recommended. A recent meta-analysis indicated that the SMA artery first approach can decrease the overall complication rate (OR 0.62, 95% 17 CI 0.47 to 0.81, $p = 0.001$) and reduce blood loss (WMD -264.84, 95% CI -336.1 to 18 -193.58, $p < 0.001$) compared to the normal procedure in pancreaticoduodenectomy and attain an increased R0 resection rate (OR 2.92, 95% CI 1.72 to 4.96, $p < 0.001$) and three-year OS (OR 2.15, 95% CI 1.34 to 3.43, $p = 0.001$) showing that the artery first approach can have superior clinical outcomes [39]. Until now, many different artery first approaches have been developed, such as the posterior approach, the right/medial uncinate approach, the inferior infracolic or mesenteric approach or the hanging maneuver [40]. This underlines the importance of paying attention to the status of the SMA and achieving an increased R0 rate through the meticulous dissection of the right margin of the SMA.

2.2.2. Uncinate Process First

The Uncinate first approach describes a modified technique of resection along of the right margin of the SMV and SMA through a special method. This approach includes the division of the proximal jejunum and translocation of the first jejunal loop before other steps of dissection. Afterwards, the pancreatic head is dissected retrogradely and finally leading to the transection of the pancreas at its neck [41]. The first step of the approach is to open Treitz ligament from the left side of the mesenteric root after the Kocher maneuver with wide mobilization of the duodenum. After division and skeletonizing the first jejunal loop, this is then pulled through to the right side of the mesenteric root and resection can be continued as described above. When using this method, there is no need to use tunneling to transect the pancreas above the portal vein for the specimen is usually already mobilized extensively. Through the retrograde approach, the resection may be more radical due to a clear visualization of the medial resection margin throughout the entire preparation and both superior mesenteric vessels, arteries and veins are clearly seen which may reduce blood loss. Hence, it is recommended as an additional technique in modern pancreatic surgery. Recently, it was demonstrated that also laparoscopic uncinate first approach is a feasible method for pancreatic head neoplasms with high lymph node harvests (19.3 vs. 13.9 ($p = 0.03$)) and no significant difference in R0 resection, operative time and median length of stay compared to laparoscopic classical approach [42]. Zhang et al. reported that laparoscopic pancreaticoduodenectomy (LPD) combined with the uncinate process first approach improved the laparoscopic resection technique with low risk of postoperative complications and high rate of curative resection [43]. Wang et al. described that LPD with uncinate process first reduced the operative time, decreased the bleeding amount during the operation and protected the variant hepatic artery suggesting that it is safe and feasible to conduct LPD together with uncinate first approach [44]. Additionally, a recent comparative study displayed that LPD with the uncinate process-first approach was feasible compared to traditional pancreatic surgery for this new technique can achieve less blood loss and a shorter first flatus time together with diet start time [45].

2.2.3. The TRIANGLE Operation

The TRIANGLE operation aims to develop a novel method for the patients with locally advanced pancreatic cancer after the neoadjuvant therapy and was described in 2017 [46]. The rationale of this procedure is the observation that after neoadjuvant therapy conventional imaging fails to differentiate between actual tumor encasement or abutment and only fibrotic residual tissue mainly to the arterial structures. Therefore, the technique comprises dissection of all soft tissue along the CA, SMA, SMV, and PV in association with a radical tumor removal. During the resection process, if must be proven that the specific periarterial tissue does not include viable tumor by frozen section; afterwards a radical artery-sparing approach can be conducted. This results in an anatomic triangle bordered by the SMA, CA, and portal vein revealed by the dissection and finally resection indicating the comprehensive removal of all soft tissue contained within these borders—usually fibrotic, neural, and lymphatic tissue (Figure 2). It is essential for the artery to be reached on the adventitial layer which opens longitudinally and allows to carry out the lymphadenectomy and soft tissue removal of the respective area. Above all, this technique allows patients after neoadjuvant therapy have the chance to attain a comprehensive tumor removal. Furthermore, the major advantage is the avoidance of arterial resection and reconstruction.

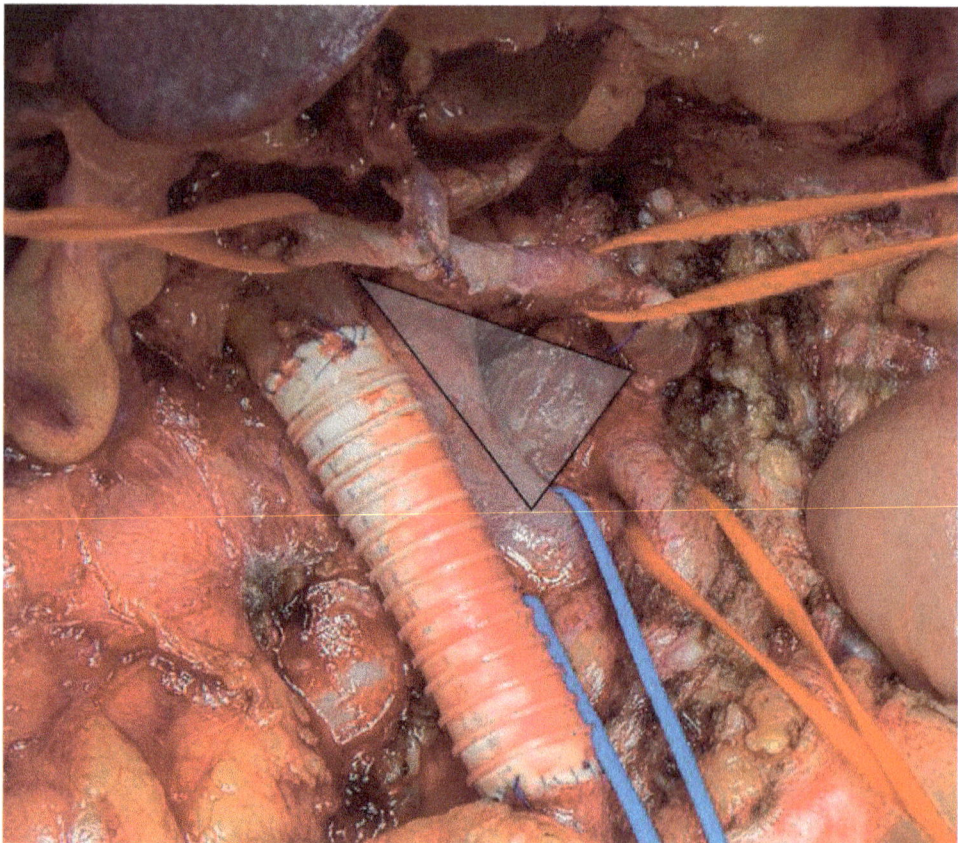

Figure 2. Intraoperative view after radical resection in pancreatic cancer (TRIANGLE operation). Porto-mesenteric vein resection and reconstruction with ringed allograft, dissection of all soft tissue (grey triangle) between celiac axis and superior mesenteric artery (red tapes) as well as the replaced mesenterico-portal vein. Blue tape: left kidney vein.

Furthermore, the major advantage is the avoidance of arterial resection and reconstruction. However, when required, the TRIANGLE operation can be combined with and arterial resection and reconstruction, a venous resection is frequently required in this situation. Rosso et al. described that the "triangle operation" for borderline resectable pancreatic head cancer was safe and efficient [47].

2.2.4. Venous Bypass First

One of the most challenging procedures during pancreatectomy can arise when venous infiltration of the portal/superior mesenteric vein axis is basically possible but hampered by large collateral vessels which implies that preparation may take a rather long time with the consecutive need for a long clamping time towards the small bowel with venous congestion [48]. In such situations, including cavernous transformation of the portal vein, a new surgical technique called "venous bypass graft first" is the procedure of choice [49,50]. The idea of this procedure is to create an initial venous bypass graft placement between the superior mesenteric vein or its tributaries and the portal vein in order to avoid bleeding as well as venous congestion of the small bowel. If the portal vein is not accessible in the hepatoduodenal ligament or liver hilum, this bypass can be performed between superior mesenteric vein and inferior cava vein after the Kocher/Cattel-Braasch maneuver is completed before proceeding with the resection of the pancreatic head. As cavernous transformation of the portal vein is caused by a complete portal/superior mesenteric vein occlusion; otherwise, it is an unsolved obstacle for resection, the step-by-step pancreatic head resections with a 'venous bypass graft first' approach should be carried out to overcome this problem. The approach includes preoperative assessment of the superior mesenteric and portal vein, exploration, and identification of venous vessels suitable for a graft placement. By this technique, a continuous porto-venous inflow to the liver during the resection phase is ensured if performed as a mesenterico-portal bypass. If this is not directly possible, at least a severe venous congestion of the small bowel can be avoided. in cases of temporary mesenterico-caval shunting and final restoration of the portal vein inflow reconstruction to the portal vein after completed tumor resection.

2.2.5. Periarterial Divestment

Due to the increasing application of neoadjuvant therapy in PDAC, especially in locally advanced disease, surgical strategies and concepts have gradually changed as well as resection techniques, especially for cases which have been down-staged or shown a stable disease. It still remains controversial whether it is mandatory to perform arterial resection for arterial involvement in pancreatic cancer. An alternative approach has been described as the "periarterial divestment" technique [51,52]. This technique comprises a radical tumor clearance without arterial resection instead. Because of the inaccuracy of detection of true arterial involvement and true arterial invasion through current imaging methods, operative exploration should be performed.

The technique of periarterial divestment describes the sub-adventitial dissection in the layer between the arterial wall and remnant tumor/fibrous tissue which allows a radical removal without an arterial replacement. All in all, 'artery first' approach, 'uncinate process first', 'triangle operation', 'venous bypass first', and 'periarterial divestment' are complementary techniques in pancreatic cancer surgery. These mainly vessel-oriented technical approaches of pancreatic head resection allow removal of all putatively tumor-infiltrated soft tissue with the utmost aim for an improved R0 resection rate [53].

2.3. Vascular (Venous and Arterial) Resection

2.3.1. Venous Resection

Vascular resection, especially for venous resection has now been widely applied with pancreaticoduodenectomy in selected patients. The earliest surgery focusing on the superior mesenteric vein (SMV) was reported by Moore in 1951 during pancreatic surgery [54]. Afterwards, en bloc pancreatoduodenectomy with vein resection was described by Fortner and indicated that the technique is safe and favorable [55]. Venous resections have been modified and refined to be a routine surgical procedure in high volume centers [56,57]. It is possible to perform vein resection in patients with PDAC during all types of pancreatic surgery including pancreaticoduodenectomy, distal, or total pancreatectomies. The ISGPS classified mesentericoportal vein resections into four groups which was mainly considered by the approaches of resection and reconstruction [12]. Regarding outcomes of these techniques, vascular resection along with multiple treatments is beneficial for the patients with pancreatic cancer especially in the long-term overall survival. [58]. Several observational studies [59,60] demonstrated that neoadjuvant systematic chemotherapy can lead to increased radical resection chances for patients with complex tumor-vessel anatomy. The 2019 French Recommendations for the Vascular Resection for Pancreatic Cancer [60] has suggested that neoadjuvant treatment should be applied in case of venous tumor involvement followed by pancreatectomy with venous resection and can potentially be curative for the respective patients. It is unquestionable that venous resection during PD must also aim to obtain negative resection margins, while the reported effects on survival remain controversial [61]. A meta-analysis showed that pancreatectomy combined with venous resection needed longer operative time and had increased perioperative blood loss compared to the group of pancreatectomy without venous resection [62]. Patients with venous resection attained reduced R0 rates. There was no significant difference in postoperative complications between the two groups. In terms of survival, patients with venous resection had lower one-, three-, and five-year survival. The most recent meta-analysis [63] described that patients with pancreaticoduodenectomy plus venous resection seemed to attain a larger tumor size, positive lymph nodes and R1 resection rates and higher 30 day mortality. However, there was no significant difference in rates of total complications. In terms of long-term outcomes, patients with venous resection had lower one-year overall survival (OS), three-year OS, and five-year OS. A retrospective study [64] revealed that patients during pancreatic resection with venous vascular resection attained higher morbidity, lower five-year disease-free survival (7% and 20%, $p = 0.018$) and five-year disease-specific survival (19% and 35%, $p = 0.42$). Controversially to the reported impaired survival after venous resection, a recent propensity score-matched analysis [65] showed similar survival in pancreaticoduodenectomy with venous resection and pancreaticoduodenectomy alone groups after adjustment for baseline characteristics. A Japanese study [66] described the feasibility of venous resection and—in combination with adjuvant therapy—favorable outcomes reaching a 30-month median survival time in borderline resectable patients. This underlines the need to perform a venous resection whenever required to achieve negative resection margins and not to compromise radicality by avoidance of vascular resection and reconstruction. However, the effects of the various treatment options—including neoadjuvant therapy—in this setting require further evaluation and more high-level studies need to be conducted in the future.

2.3.2. Artery Resection

In the 1950s, arterial resection was initially described during abdominal surgery by Appleby on resection of the celiac axis during extended gastrectomy including distal pancreatectomy [67]. In contrast to vein resection, artery resection is more debatable for its increased morbidity and mortality and mostly considered as an individual decision in selected patients [68]. However, the modified Appleby procedure which implies distal pancreatectomy, splenectomy, and celiac axis resection under preservation of the stomach has been shown to be beneficial for the patients with advanced tumors of the pancreatic body and tail [69]. This procedure can achieve median survival times of at least 18 months when combined with a multimodal treatment concept and is gaining increasing acceptance today [70]. Furthermore, during recent years, the techniques of replacement applied for the hepatic artery or the superior mesenteric artery have been improved and procedures such as splenic artery use have been described for restoration of hepatic or small-intestine perfusion (Figures 3 and 4) [71]. Oba et al. confirmed that arterial resection it is more likely to attain preferable long-term outcome after the application of preoperative neoadjuvant treatments [72]. A Japanese study reported that patients with distal pancreatectomy plus celiac axis resection who underwent preoperative therapy achieved better one-, two-, and five-year overall survivals (100%, 90%, and 78.8%) than those who underwent upfront surgery (77.9%, 51.5%, and 26.7%; $p < 0.0001$) [73]. A recent meta-analysis showed that patients undergoing pancreatic surgery with artery resection had a greater risk of postoperative mortality (RR: 4.09, $p < 0.001$), morbidity (RR: 1.4, $p = 0.01$) and worse three-year survival [74]. Regarding specific complications and outcomes, the postoperative complications and the length of hospital stay and non-R0 rate were not significantly different compared to those without artery resection. A single-center cohort study reported that pancreatectomy with artery resection can attain better one-, three-, and five-year survival rates compared to palliation for patients with LAPC [75]. Another recent study covering nearly 40 years of experience showed that any type of arterial resection was performed at a frequency of 6% (44/730 patients) and confirmed the safety and efficacy of these operations for patients with locally advanced pancreatic cancer, additionally suggesting preoperative therapy with artery resection as a useful concept for locally advanced pancreatic cancer [76]. An important aspect in selecting patients properly and gaining sufficient surgical experience to safely perform such procedure which has recently been shown in two large series that demonstrated the impact of the surgical learning curve in two single center collectives of 111 and 195 patients, respectively [77,78].

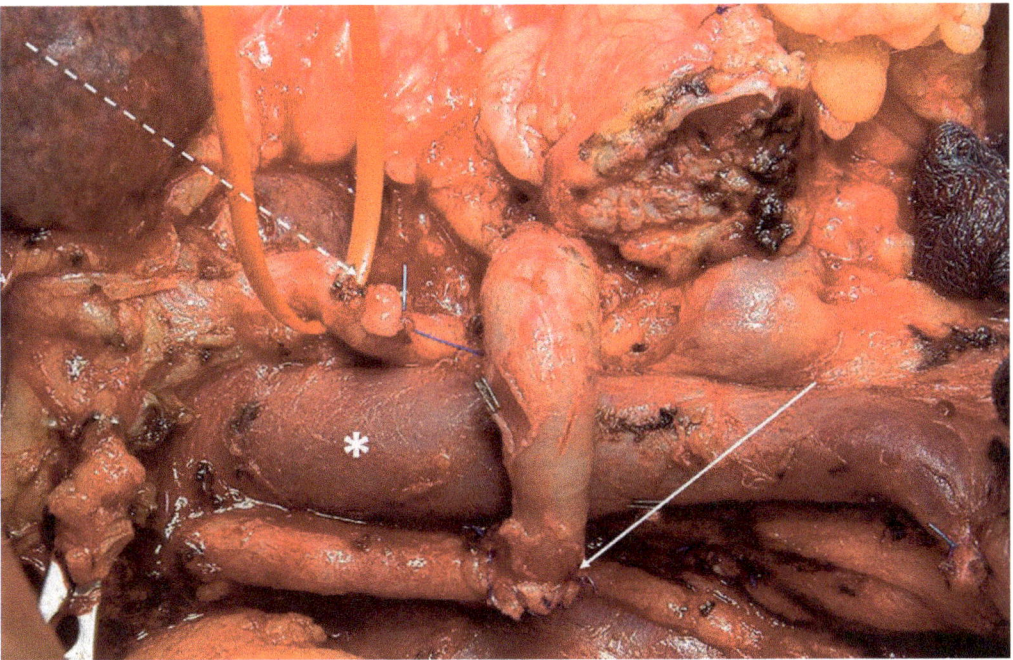

Figure 3. Example of splenic artery transposition on an aberrant right hepatic artery after resection of the aberrant hepatic artery due to tumor infiltration. Proper left hepatic artery with red tape and stump of the gastroduodenal artery (broken white arrow); portal vein (white asterisk); transposed splenic artery with end-to-end anastomosis on the aberrant right hepatic artery.

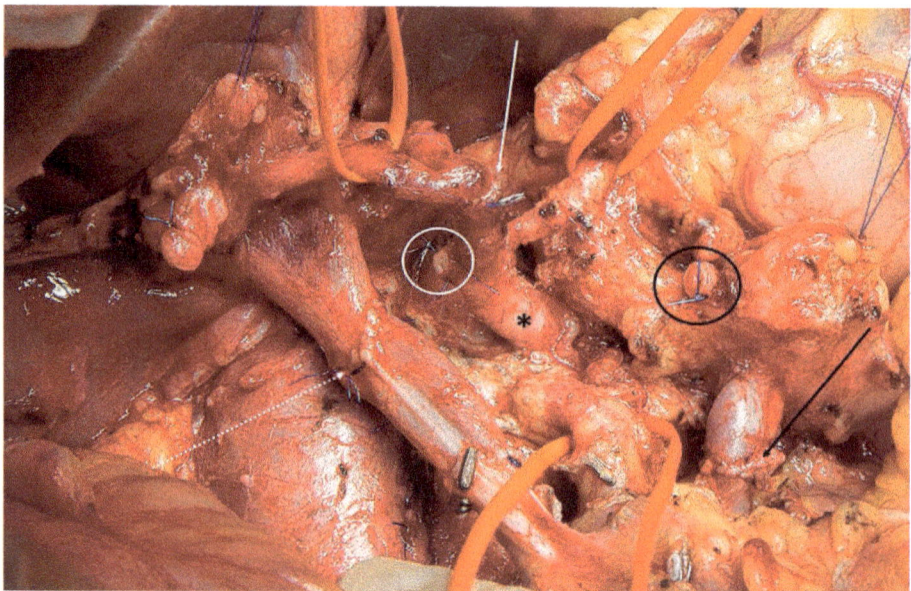

Figure 4. Intraoperative view after combined arterial and venous resection during partial pancreato-duodenectomy. Resection of the common hepatic artery (white circle) and reconstruction by splenic artery transposition with end-to-end anastomosis (white arrow) on the proper hepatic artery (upper left red tape). Distal splenic artery stump (black circle) below the pancreatic cut margin; black asterisk: celiac axis; end-to-end reconstruction of the superior mesenteric/portal vein (dotted white arrow) and splenic vein on inferior mesenteric vein (black circle); upper right red tape: left gastric artery; lower middle red tape: superior mesenteric artery.

2.4. Multivisceral Resection

In addition to vascular resections, also multivisceral resections have been applied increasingly nowadays to attempt to achieve margin-negative resection. Previous studies indicate that pancreaticoduodenectomy with multivisceral resection is associated with increased morbidity and potentially mortality with conflicting results in terms of oncologic outcomes [79–81]. A systematic review suggested that multivisceral pancreatectomies was safe and feasible in selected patients [82]. A case-matched study showed that multivisceral distal pancreatectomy was able to achieve radical tumor removal providing beneficial survival outcomes [83]. Furthermore, a single center analysis demonstrated that multivisceral resection in pancreatic surgery was suitable for locally advanced pancreatic carcinoma of the body and/or tail [84], comparable results were achieved in a current multi-center publication, proving that distal pancreatectomy with multivisceral resection is viable in order to obtain free margins which is the key to achieve long-term survival [85].

2.5. MIS/Robotic Surgery

With the rapid development of technology, minimal invasive pancreatic surgery has been popularly applied worldwide. The first laparoscopic pancreatectomy was reported in 1996 while the first robotic pancreatic resections were described in 2003 [86,87]. A recent international evidence-based guideline on minimally-invasive pancreatic surgery demonstrated that open, laparoscopic and robotic pancreatic surgery all have their own aspects in treating patients with pancreatic diseases and it is quite possible to achieve promising clinical outcomes by applying these advanced technologies [88]. An international consensus statement on robotic pancreatic surgery showed that robotic pancreatic surgery is safe and feasible compared to open pancreatic surgery [89]. Another international expert consensus on laparoscopic pancreaticoduodenectomy (PD) also showed that laparoscopic pancreaticoduodenectomy was safe and effective for experienced surgeons [90]. Furthermore, a current network meta-analysis indicated that laparoscopic PD and robotic PD had a reduced length of hospital stay, operative bleeding and overall complications while on the other hand achieving a similar number of retrieved lymph nodes, tumor-free resection margins, clinically relevant postoperative pancreatic fistula, severe postoperative complications [91]. Besselink et al. demonstrated that minimally invasive distal pancreatectomy (DP) is technically safe, whereas oncological feasibility needs to be evaluated carefully. With respect to minimally invasive PD, some advantages have been shown in comparison to open PD [92]. However, due to a limited level of evidence, this has to be regarded with care, but minimally-invasive PD could be beneficial for selected patients with better short-term clinical outcomes. Without doubt, there is a strong need for more high-quality trials to confirm potential advantages of minimally invasive pancreatic surgery.

2.5.1. Laparoscopic and Robotic Distal Pancreatectomy

The latest study indicated a shorter length of hospital, less delayed gastric emptying, higher rates of postoperative pancreatic fistula in minimally invasive distal pancreatectomy in contrast to open distal pancreatectomy [93]. The DIPLOMA study indicated that minimally invasive distal pancreatectomy attained less median blood loss, shorter hospital stay and less lymph node retrieval [94]. Furthermore, the LEOPARD randomized controlled trial proved that the less operative blood loss and the rate of delayed gastric emptying. However, longer operation times (217 vs. 179 min, $p = 0.005$) were observed in minimally invasive distal pancreatectomy [95]. A multicenter study described no significant differences in the incidence of clinically relevant postoperative pancreatic fistula in robotic distal pancreatectomy in contrast with open pancreatectomy [96].

2.5.2. Laparoscopic and Robotic Pancreatoduodenectomy

A recent study showed that laparoscopic pancreaticoduodenectomy had lower blood loss, longer operative time. However, there were no obvious differences among 90-day overall mortality, Clavien-Dindo 3 complications and postoperative length of hospital stay in contrast to open surgery [97]. This meta-analysis included—among two other studies—the LEOPARD-2 randomized controlled phase 2/3 trial which reported more complication-related deaths in the laparoscopic group compared to open pancreaticoduodenectomy with no obvious difference in time to functional recovery between the two groups and thereby weakened the conclusion that laparoscopic pancreaticoduodenectomy is potentially harmful [98]. Yet, this procedure is probably only feasible in highly-specialized centers with a respective high case load. However, the level of the current evidence focusing on minimal invasive pancreaticoduodenectomy may be too low, hence, more high-quality studies need to be carried out to enhance the future evidence, as especially for robotic procedures no randomized controlled trials are available to date.

3. Conclusions and Future Perspective

Over the past decades, surgical therapy for pancreatic cancer has been changing and developing rapidly allowing extended resections and improved complication. Given the advanced technology and comprehensive strategies, approaches of curative resections have improved as well as the quality of perioperative management. As a result, the mortality rate after pancreatic surgery has reduced obviously to a current rate of less than 5% in specialized centers. Although centralization has not become reality in all countries around the world, this should be the benchmark and especially advanced pancreatic surgery should be clearly limited to high-volume centers. Combined with multimodal treatment, pancreatic surgery allows to improve the quality of life and long-term survival for patients in different stages of pancreatic cancer. In terms of surgical techniques, open, laparoscopic and robotic procedures all will exert their own merit in their particular field to achieve benefit for the patients at the greatest extent.

Author Contributions: K.W.: study concept and design, drafting of the manuscript. T.H.: idea, study supervision, tables and figures preparation, critical revision of the manuscript. All authors have read and agreed to the published version of the manuscript.

Funding: This research received no external funding.

Institutional Review Board Statement: Not applicable as no humans or animals were involved in this study.

Informed Consent Statement: Not applicable.

Data Availability Statement: Not applicable.

Conflicts of Interest: The authors declare no conflict of interest.

Abbreviations

AHPBA	American Hepato-Pancreato-Biliary Association
SSO	Society of Surgical Oncology
SSAT	Society for Surgery of the Alimentary Tract
ECOG	Eastern Cooperative Oncology Group
BACAP	The National Anatomo-Clinical Database on Pancreatic Adenocarcinoma
SMV	superior mesenteric vein
PV	portal vein
SMA	superior mesenteric artery
CA	celiac artery
CHA	common hepatic artery
PHA	proper hepatic artery
LAPC	locally advanced pancreatic cancer
WMD	weighted mean difference
OR	odds ratio
CI	confidence interval

References

1. Hackert, T.; Sachsenmaier, M.; Hinz, U.; Schneider, L.; Michalski, C.W.; Springfeld, C.; Strobel, O.; Jager, D.; Ulrich, A.; Buchler, M.W. Locally advanced pancreatic cancer: Neoadjuvant therapy with folfirinox results in resectability in 60% of the patients. *Ann. Surg.* **2016**, *264*, 457–463. [CrossRef]
2. Kleeff, J.; Korc, M.; Apte, M.; La Vecchia, C.; Johnson, C.D.; Biankin, A.V.; Neale, R.E.; Tempero, M.; Tuveson, D.A.; Hruban, R.H.; et al. Pancreatic cancer. *Nat. Rev. Dis. Primers* **2016**, *2*, 16022. [CrossRef] [PubMed]
3. Vincent, A.; Herman, J.; Schulick, R.; Hruban, R.; Goggins, M. Pancreatic cancer. *Lancet* **2011**, *378*, 607–620. [CrossRef]
4. De Dosso, S.; Siebenhuner, A.R.; Winder, T.; Meisel, A.; Fritsch, R.; Astaras, C.; Szturz, P.; Borner, M. Treatment landscape of metastatic pancreatic cancer. *Cancer Treat Rev.* **2021**, *96*, 102180. [CrossRef]
5. Satoi, S.; Yamamoto, T.; Uchida, K.; Fujii, T.; Kin, T.; Hirano, S.; Hanada, K.; Itoi, T.; Murakami, Y.; Igarashi, H.; et al. Optimal treatment for octogenarians with resectable and borderline resectable pancreatic ductal adenocarcinoma: A multicenter retrospective study. *Pancreas* **2020**, *49*, 837–844. [CrossRef] [PubMed]
6. Windsor, J.A.; Barreto, S.G. The concept of 'borderline resectable' pancreatic cancer: Limited foundations and limited future? *J. Gastrointest. Oncol.* **2017**, *8*, 189–193. [CrossRef]
7. Isaji, S.; Mizuno, S.; Windsor, J.A.; Bassi, C.; Fernández-Del Castillo, C.; Hackert, T.; Hayasaki, A.; Katz, M.H.G.; Kim, S.-W.; Kishiwada, M.; et al. International consensus on definition and criteria of borderline resectable pancreatic ductal adenocarcinoma 2017. *Pancreatology* **2018**, *18*, 2–11. [CrossRef] [PubMed]
8. Callery, M.P.; Chang, K.J.; Fishman, E.K.; Talamonti, M.S.; William Traverso, L.; Linehan, D.C. Pretreatment assessment of resectable and borderline resectable pancreatic cancer: Expert consensus statement. *Ann. Surg. Oncol.* **2009**, *16*, 1727–1733. [CrossRef]
9. Varadhachary, G.R.; Tamm, E.P.; Abbruzzese, J.L.; Xiong, H.Q.; Crane, C.H.; Wang, H.; Lee, J.E.; Pisters, P.W.; Evans, D.B.; Wolff, R.A. Borderline resectable pancreatic cancer: Definitions, management, and role of preoperative therapy. *Ann. Surg. Oncol.* **2006**, *13*, 1035–1046. [CrossRef] [PubMed]
10. Katz, M.H.; Pisters, P.W.; Evans, D.B.; Sun, C.C.; Lee, J.E.; Fleming, J.B.; Vauthey, J.N.; Abdalla, E.K.; Crane, C.H.; Wolff, R.A.; et al. Borderline resectable pancreatic cancer: The importance of this emerging stage of disease. *J. Am. Coll. Surg.* **2008**, *206*, 833–846. [CrossRef]
11. Tempero, M.A.; Malafa, M.P.; Chiorean, E.G.; Czito, B.; Scaife, C.; Narang, A.K.; Fountzilas, C.; Wolpin, B.M.; Al-Hawary, M.; Asbun, H.; et al. Pancreatic adenocarcinoma, version 1.2019. *J. Natl. Compr. Cancer Netw.* **2019**, *17*, 202–210. [CrossRef]

12. Bockhorn, M.; Uzunoglu, F.G.; Adham, M.; Imrie, C.; Milicevic, M.; Sandberg, A.A.; Asbun, H.J.; Bassi, C.; Büchler, M.; Charnley, R.M.; et al. Borderline resectable pancreatic cancer: A consensus statement by the International Study Group of Pancreatic Surgery (ISGPS). *Surgery* **2014**, *155*, 977–988. [CrossRef] [PubMed]
13. Helmink, B.A.; Snyder, R.A.; Idrees, K.; Merchant, N.B.; Parikh, A.A. Advances in the surgical management of resectable and borderline resectable pancreas cancer. *Surg. Oncol. Clin. N. Am.* **2016**, *25*, 287–310. [CrossRef]
14. Satoi, S.; Yamamoto, T.; Yamaki, S.; Sakaguchi, T.; Sekimoto, M. Surgical indication for and desirable outcomes of conversion surgery in patients with initially unresectable pancreatic ductal adenocarcinoma. *Ann. Gastroenterol. Surg.* **2019**, *4*, 6–13. [CrossRef] [PubMed]
15. Nakamura, T.; Asano, T.; Okamura, K.; Tsuchikawa, T.; Murakami, S.; Kurashima, Y.; Ebihara, Y.; Noji, T.; Nakanishi, Y.; Tanaka, K.; et al. A preoperative prognostic scoring system to predict prognosis for resectable pancreatic cancer: Who will benefit from upfront surgery? *J. Gastrointest. Surg.* **2019**, *23*, 990–996. [CrossRef]
16. Maulat, C.; Canivet, C.; Touraine, C.; Gourgou, S.; Napoleon, B.; Palazzo, L.; Flori, N.; Piessen, G.; Guibert, P.; Truant, S.; et al. A new score to predict the resectability of pancreatic adenocarcinoma: The BACAP Score. *Cancers* **2020**, *12*, 783. [CrossRef]
17. Nguyen, A.H.; Melstrom, L.G. Use of imaging as staging and surgical planning for pancreatic surgery. *Hepatobiliary Surg. Nutr.* **2020**, *9*, 603–614. [CrossRef] [PubMed]
18. Motosugi, U.; Ichikawa, T.; Morisaka, H.; Sou, H.; Muhi, A.; Kimura, K.; Sano, K.; Araki, T. Detection of pancreatic carcinoma and liver metastases with gadoxetic acid-enhanced MR imaging: Comparison with contrast-enhanced multi-detector row CT. *Radiology* **2011**, *260*, 446–453. [CrossRef]
19. Joo, I.; Lee, J.M.; Lee, D.H.; Lee, E.S.; Paeng, J.C.; Lee, S.J.; Jang, J.Y.; Kim, S.W.; Ryu, J.K.; Lee, K.B. Assessment of pancreatic cancer with FDG PET/MR imaging versus FDG PET/CT plus contrast-enhanced multidetector CT: A prospective preliminary study. *Radiology* **2017**, *282*, 149–159. [CrossRef]
20. Yamada, K.; Kawashima, H.; Ohno, E.; Ishikawa, T.; Tanaka, H.; Nakamura, M.; Miyahara, R.; Ishigami, M.; Hirooka, Y.; Fujishiro, M. Diagnosis of vascular invasion in pancreatic ductal adenocarcinoma using endoscopic ultrasound elastography. *BMC Gastroenterol.* **2020**, *20*, 81. [CrossRef]
21. Ehrlich, D.; Ather, N.; Rahal, H.; Donahue, T.R.; Hines, O.J.; Kim, S.; Sedarat, A.; Muthusamy, V.R.; Watson, R. The utility of EUS-FNA to determine surgical candidacy in patients with pancreatic cancer after neoadjuvant therapy. *J. Gastrointest. Sur.* **2020**, *24*, 2807–2813. [CrossRef] [PubMed]
22. Muhammad, I.O.R.; Chan, B.P.H.; Far, P.M.; Mbuagbaw, L.; Thabane, L.; Taghoobi, M. Endoscopic ultrasound versus computed tomography in determining the resectability of pancreatic cancer: A diagnostic test accuracy meta-analysis. *Saudi J. Gastroenterol.* **2020**, *26*, 113–119.
23. Hyungjin, R.; Park, M.S. The role of imaging in current treatment strategies for pancreatic adenocarcinoma. *Korean J. Radiol.* **2021**, *22*, 23–40.
24. Larghi, A.; Rimbaş, M.; Rizzatti, G.; Quero, G.; Gasbarrini, A.; Costamagna, G.; Alfieri, S. Resectable pancreatic solid lesions: Time to move from surgical diagnosis? *Endosc. Ultrasound* **2020**, *9*, 76–82. [CrossRef] [PubMed]
25. Neoptolemos, J.P.; Dunn, J.A.; Stocken, D.D.; Almond, J.; Link, K.; Beger, H.; Bassi, C.; Falconi, M.; Pederzoli, P.; Dervenis, C.; et al. Adjuvant chemoradiotherapy and chemotherapy in resectable pancreatic cancer: A randomised controlled trial. *Lancet* **2001**, *358*, 1576–1585. [CrossRef]
26. Neoptolemos, J.P.; Moore, M.J.; Cox, T.F.; Valle, J.W.; Palmer, D.H.; McDonald, A.C.; Carter, R.; Tebbutt, N.C.; Dervenis, C.; Smith, D.; et al. Effect of adjuvant chemotherapy with fluorouracil plus folinic acid or gemcitabine vs observation on survival in patients with resected ampullary adenocarcinoma: The ESPAC-3 periampullary cancer randomized trial. *JAMA* **2012**, *308*, 147–156. [CrossRef] [PubMed]
27. Neoptolemos, J.P.; Palmer, D.H.; Ghaneh, P.; Psarelli, E.E.; Valle, J.W.; Halloran, C.M.; Faluyi, O.; O'Reilly, D.A.; Cunningham, D.; Wadsley, J.; et al. Comparison of adjuvant gemcitabine and capecitabine with gemcitabine monotherapy in patients with resected pancreatic cancer (ESPAC-4): A multicentre, open-label, randomised, phase 3 trial. *Lancet* **2017**, *389*, 1011–1024. [CrossRef]
28. Conroy, T.; Hammel, P.; Hebbar, M.; Abdelghani, B.M.; Wie, A.C.; Raoul, J.L.; Chone, L.; Francois, E.; Artru, P.; Biagi, J.J.; et al. FOLFIRINOX or gemcitabine as adjuvant therapy for pancreatic cancer. *N. Engl. J. Med.* **2018**, *379*, 2395–2406. [CrossRef]
29. Sohal, D.P.S.; Kennedy, E.B.; Cinar, P.; Conroy, T.; Copur, M.S.; Crane, C.H.; Garrido-Laguna, I.; Lau, M.W.; Johnson, T.; Krishnamurthi, S.; et al. Metastatic pancreatic cancer: ASCO guideline update. *J. Clin. Oncol.* **2020**. [CrossRef]
30. Xiang, M.; Heestand, G.M.; Chang, D.T.; Pollom, E.L. Neoadjuvant treatment strategies for resectable pancreas cancer: A propensity-matched analysis of the National Cancer Database. *Radiother. Oncol.* **2020**, *143*, 101–107. [CrossRef]
31. Murphy, J.E.; Wo, J.Y.; Ryan, D.P.; Jiang, W.; Yeap, B.Y.; Drapek, L.C.; Blaszkowsky, L.S.; Kwak, E.L.; Allen, J.N.; Clark, J.W.; et al. Total neoadjuvant therapy with FOLFIRINOX followed by individualized chemoradiotherapy for borderline resectable pancreatic adenocarcinoma: A phase 2 clinical trial. *JAMA Oncol.* **2018**, *4*, 963–969. [CrossRef] [PubMed]
32. Versteijne, E.; Suker, M.; Groothuis, K.; Akkermans-Vogelaar, J.M.; Besselink, M.G.; Bonsing, B.A.; Buijsen, J.; Busch, O.R.; Creemers, G.J.M.; van Dam, R.M.; et al. Preoperative chemoradiotherapy versus immediate surgery for resectable and borderline resectable pancreatic cancer: Results of the Dutch randomized phase III PREOPANC trial. *J. Clin. Oncol.* **2020**, *38*, 1763–1773. [CrossRef] [PubMed]

33. Strobel, O.; Lorenz, P.; Hinz, U.; Gaida, M.; Konig, A.K.; Hank, T.; Niesen, W.; Kaiser, J.; Al-Saeedi, M.; Bergmann, F.; et al. Actual five-year survival after upfront resection for pancreatic ductal adenocarcinoma: Who beats the odds? *Ann. Surg.* **2020**. [CrossRef] [PubMed]
34. Van Roessel, S.; van Veldhuisen, E.; Klompmaker, S.; Janssen, Q.P.; Hilal, M.A.; Alseidi, A.; Balduzzi, A.; Balzano, G.; Bassi, C.; Berrevoet, F.; et al. Evaluation of adjuvant chemotherapy in patients with resected pancreatic cancer after neoadjuvant FOLFIRINOX treatment. *JAMA Oncol.* **2020**, *6*, 1–8. [CrossRef] [PubMed]
35. Sohal, D.P.S.; Duong, M.; Ahmad, S.A.; Gandhi, N.S.; Beg, M.S.; Wang-Gillam, A.; Wade, J.L.; Chiorean, E.G.; Guthrie, K.A.; Lowy, A.M. Efficacy of perioperative chemotherapy for resectable pancreatic adenocarcinoma: A phase 2 randomized clinical trial. *JAMA Oncol.* **2021**, *7*, 421–427. [CrossRef]
36. Whipple, A.O. Pancreaticoduodenectomy for islet carcinoma: A five-year follow-up. *Ann. Surg.* **1945**, *121*, 847–852. [CrossRef] [PubMed]
37. Weitz, J.; Rahbari, N.; Koch, M.; Büchler, M.W. The "artery first" approach for resection of pancreatic head cancer. *J. Am. Coll. Surg.* **2010**, *210*, e1–e4. [CrossRef]
38. Sanjay, P.; Takaori, K.; Govil, S.; Shrikhande, S.V.; Windsor, J.A. 'Artery-first' approaches to pancreatoduodenectomy. *Br. J. Surg.* **2012**, *99*, 1027–1035. [CrossRef]
39. Jiang, X.; Yu, Z.; Ma, Z.; Deng, H.; Ren, W.; Shi, W.; Jiao, Z. Superior mesenteric artery first approach can improve the clinical outcomes of pancreaticoduodenectomy: A meta-analysis. *Int. J. Surg.* **2020**, *73*, 14–24. [CrossRef]
40. Mora-Oliver, I.; Garcés-Albir, M.; Dorcaratto, D.; Muñoz-Forner, E.; Izquierdo Moreno, A.; Carbonell-Aliaga, M.P.; Sabater, L. Pancreatoduodenectomy with artery-first approach. *Minerva Chir.* **2019**, *74*, 226–236. [CrossRef]
41. Hackert, T.; Werner, J.; Weitz, J.; Schmidt, J.; Büchler, M.W. Uncinate process first—a novel approach for pancreatic head resection. *Langenbecks Arch. Surg.* **2010**, *395*, 1161–1164. [CrossRef]
42. Pędziwiatr, M.; Pisarska, M.; Małczak, P.; Major, P.; Wierdak, M.; Radkowiak, D.; Kulawik, J.; Dembiński, M.; Budzyński, A. Laparoscopic uncinate process first pancreatoduodenectomy-feasibility study of a modified 'artery first' approach to pancreatic head cancer. *Langenbecks Arch. Surg.* **2017**, *402*, 917–923. [CrossRef]
43. Zhang, Y.; Sun, D.L.; Chen, X.M. The uncinate process first approach in laparoscopic pancreaticoduodenectomy: A single-institution experience. *Surg. Laparosc. Endosc. Percutan. Tech.* **2017**, *27*, e141–e144. [CrossRef]
44. Wang, S.P.; Liu, S.Y.; Zhang, W.; Wang, Y.C.; Ji, B.; Meng, L.Y.; Liu, Y.H. The value of "posterior approach, uncinate process priority, artery first" in laparoscopic pancreatoduodenectomy. *Chin. Med. J.* **2020**, *100*, 3328–3331.
45. Chen, X.M.; Sun, D.L.; Zhang, Y. Laparoscopic versus open pancreaticoduodenectomy combined with uncinated process approach: A comparative study evaluating perioperative outcomes (Retrospective cohort study). *Int. J. Surg.* **2018**, *51*, 170–173. [CrossRef]
46. Hackert, T.; Strobel, O.; Michalski, C.W.; Mihaljevic, A.L.; Mehrabi, A.; Müller-Stich, B.; Berchtold, C.; Ulrich, A.; Buchler, M.W. The TRIANGLE operation–Radical surgery after neoadjuvant treatment for advanced pancreatic cancer: A single arm observational study. *HPB* **2017**, *19*, 1001–1007. [CrossRef]
47. Rosso, E.; Zimmitto, G.; Ianelli, A.; Garatti, M. The 'TRIANGLE operation' by laparoscopy: Radical pancreaticoduodenectomy with major vascular resection for borderline resectable pancreatic head cancer. *Ann. Surg. Oncol.* **2020**, *27*, 1613–1614. [CrossRef] [PubMed]
48. Terasaki, F.; Fukami, Y.; Maeda, A.; Takayama, Y.; Takahashi, T.; Uji, M.; Kaneoka, Y. Comparison of end-to-end anastomosis and interposition graft during pancreatoduodenectomy with portal vein reconstruction for pancreatic ductal adenocarcinoma. *Langenbecks Arch. Surg.* **2019**, *404*, 191–201. [CrossRef] [PubMed]
49. Schmidt, T.; Strobel, O.; Schneider, M.; Diener, M.K.; Berchtold, C.; Mihaljevic, A.L.; Mehrabi, A.; Müller-Stich, B.P.; Hackert, T.; Büchler, M.W. Cavernous transformation of the portal vein in pancreatic cancer surgery-venous bypass graft first. *Langenbecks Arch. Surg.* **2020**, *405*, 1045–1050. [CrossRef]
50. Kinny-Köster, B.; van Oosten, F.; Habib, J.R.; Javed, A.A.; Cameron, J.L.; Lafaro, K.J.; Burkhart, R.A.; Burns, W.R.; He, J.; Fishman, E.K.; et al. Mesoportal bypass, interposition graft, and mesocaval shunt: Surgical strategies to overcome superior mesenteric vein involvement in pancreatic cancer. *Surgery* **2020**, *168*, 1048–1055. [CrossRef]
51. Diener, M.K.; Mihaljevic, A.L.; Strobel, O.; Loos, M.; Schmidt, T.; Schneider, M.; Berchtold, C.; Mehrabi, A.; Müller-Stich, B.P.; Jiang, K.; et al. Periarterial divestment in pancreatic cancer surgery. *Surgery* **2020**, in press. [CrossRef]
52. Cai, B.; Lu, Z.; Neoptolemos, J.P.; Diener, M.K.; Li, M.; Yin, L.; Gao, Y.; Wei, J.; Chen, J.; Guo, F.; et al. Sub-adventitial divestment technique for resecting artery-involved pancreatic cancer: A retrospective cohort study. *Langenbecks Arch. Surg.* **2021**. [CrossRef]
53. Schneider, M.; Strobel, O.; Hackert, T.; Büchler, M.W. Pancreatic resection for cancer-the Heidelberg technique. *Langenbecks Arch. Surg.* **2019**, *404*, 1017–1022. [CrossRef] [PubMed]
54. Moore, G.E.; Sako, Y.; Thomas, L.B. Radical pancreatoduodenectomy with resection and reanastomosis of the superior mesenteric vein. *Surgery* **1951**, *30*, 550–553. [PubMed]
55. Fortner, J.G. Regional resection of cancer of the pancreas: A new surgical approach. *Surgery* **1973**, *73*, 307–320. [PubMed]
56. Hackert, T.; Schneider, L.; Büchler, M.W. Current state of vascular resections in pancreatic cancer surgery. *Gastroenterol. Res. Pract.* **2015**, *2015*, 120207. [CrossRef]
57. Turrini, O.; Ewald, J.; Barbier, L.; Mokart, D.; Blache, J.L.; Delpero, J.R. Should the portal vein be routinely resected during pancreaticoduodenectomy for adenocarcinoma? *Ann. Surg.* **2013**, *257*, 726–730. [CrossRef]

58. Katz, M.H.; Wang, H.; Fleming, J.B.; Sun, C.C.; Hwang, R.F.; Wolff, R.A.; Varadhachary, G.; Abbruzzese, J.L.; Crane, C.H.; Krishnan, S.; et al. Long-term survival after multidisciplinary management of resected pancreatic adenocarcinoma. *Ann. Surg. Oncol.* **2009**, *16*, 836–847. [CrossRef] [PubMed]
59. Younan, G.; Tsai, S.; Evans, D.B.; Christians, K.K. Techniques of vascular resection and reconstruction in pancreatic cancer. *Surg. Clin. N. Am.* **2016**, *96*, 1351–1370. [CrossRef]
60. Delpero, J.R.; Suvanet, A. Vascular resection for pancreatic cancer: 2019 French recommendations based on a literature review from 2008 to 6–2019. *Front. Oncol.* **2020**, *10*, 40. [CrossRef]
61. Kasumova, G.G.; Conway, W.C.; Tseng, J.F. The role of venous and arterial resection in pancreatic cancer surgery. *Ann. Surg. Oncol.* **2018**, *25*, 51–58. [CrossRef] [PubMed]
62. Wang, X.; Demir, I.E.; Schorn, S.; Jäger, C.; Scheufele, F.; Friess, H.; Ceyhan, G.O. Venous resection during pancreatectomy for pancreatic cancer: A systematic review. *Transl. Gastroenterol. Hepatol.* **2019**, *4*, 46. [CrossRef]
63. Fancellu, A.; Petrucciani, N.; Porcu, A.; Deiana, G.; Sanna, V.; Ninniri, C.; Perra, T.; Celoria, V.; Nigri, G. The impact on survival and morbidity of portal-mesenteric resection during pancreaticoduodenectomy for pancreatic head adenocarcinoma: A systematic review and meta-analysis of comparative studies. *Cancers* **2020**, *12*, 1976. [CrossRef] [PubMed]
64. Belfiori, G.; Fiorentini, G.; Tamburrino, D.; Partelli, S.; Pagnanelli, M.; Gasparini, G.; Castoldi, R.; Balzano, G.; Rubini, C.; Zamboni, G.; et al. Vascular resection during pancreatectomy for pancreatic head cancer: A technical issue or a prognostic sign? *Surgery* **2021**, *169*, 403–410. [CrossRef] [PubMed]
65. Xie, Z.B.; Li, J.; Gu, J.C.; Jin, C.; Zou, C.F.; Fu, D.L. Pancreatoduodenectomy with portal vein resection favors the survival time of patients with pancreatic ductal adenocarcinoma: A propensity score matching analysis. *Oncol. Lett.* **2019**, *18*, 4563–4572. [CrossRef]
66. Murakami, Y.; Satoi, S.; Motoi, F.; Sho, M.; Kawai, M.; Matsumoto, I.; Honda, G.; Multicentre Study Group of Pancreatobiliary Surgery (MSG-PBS). Portal or superior mesenteric vein resection in pancreatoduodenectomy for pancreatic head carcinoma. *Br. J. Surg.* **2015**, *102*, 837–846. [CrossRef]
67. Appleby, L.H. The coeliac axis in the expansion of the operation for gastric carcinoma. *Cancer* **1953**, *6*, 704–707. [CrossRef]
68. Klaiber, U.; Mihaljevic, A.; Hackert, T. Radical pancreatic cancer surgery—with arterial resection. *Transl. Gastroenterol. Hepatol.* **2019**, *4*, 8. [CrossRef]
69. Yamamoto, T.; Satoi, S.; Kawai, M.; Motoi, F.; Sho, M.; Uemura, K.I.; Matsumoto, I.; Honda, G.; Okada, K.I.; Akahori, T.; et al. Is distal pancreatectomy with en-bloc celiac axis resection effective for patients with locally advanced pancreatic ductal adenocarcinoma? -Multicenter surgical group study. *Pancreatology* **2018**, *18*, 106–113. [CrossRef]
70. Klompmaker, S.; de Roii, T.; Korteweg, J.J.; van Dieren, S.; van Lienden, K.P.; van Gulik, T.M.; Busch, O.R.; Besselink, M.G. Systematic review of outcomes after distal pancreatectomy with coeliac axis resection for locally advanced pancreatic cancer. *Br. J. Surg.* **2016**, *103*, 941–949. [CrossRef]
71. Hackert, T.; Weitz, J.; Buchler, M.W. Splenic artery use for arterial reconstruction in pancreatic surgery. *Langenbecks Arch. Surg.* **2014**, *399*, 667–671. [CrossRef]
72. Oba, A.; Bao, Q.R.; Barnett, C.C.; Al-Musawi, M.H.; Croce, C.; Schulick, R.D.; Del Chiaro, M. Vascular resections for pancreatic ductal adenocarcinoma: Vascular resections for PDAC. *Scand. J. Surg.* **2020**, *109*, 18–28. [CrossRef]
73. Nakamura, T.; Hirano, S.; Noji, T.; Asano, T.; Okamura, K.; Tsuchikawa, T.; Murakami, S.; Kurashima, Y.; Ebihara, Y.; Nakanishi, Y. Distal pancreatectomy with en bloc celiac axis resection (modified appleby procedure) for locally advanced pancreatic body cancer: A single-center review of 80 consecutive patients. *Ann. Surg. Oncol.* **2016**, *23*, 969–975. [CrossRef]
74. Małczak, P.; Sierżęga, M.; Stefura, T.; Kacprzyk, A.; Droś, J.; Skomarovska, O.; Krzysztofik, M.; Major, P.; Pędziwiatr, M. Arterial resections in pancreatic cancer–Systematic review and meta-analysis. *HPB* **2020**, *22*, 961–968. [CrossRef]
75. Del Chiaro, M.; Rangelova, E.; Halimi, A.; Ateeb, Z.; Scandavini, C.; Valente, R.; Segersvärd, R.; Arnelo, U.; Verbeke, C.S. Pancreatectomy with arterial resection is superior to palliation in patients with borderline resectable or locally advanced pancreatic cancer. *HPB* **2019**, *21*, 219–225. [CrossRef] [PubMed]
76. Sonohara, F.; Yamada, S.; Takami, H.; Hayashi, M.; Kanda, M.; Tanaka, C.; Kobayashi, D.; Nakayama, G.; Koike, M.; Fujiwara, M.; et al. Novel implications of combined arterial resection for locally advanced pancreatic cancer in the era of newer chemo-regimens. *Eur. J. Surg. Oncol.* **2019**, *45*, 1895–1900. [CrossRef]
77. Tee, M.C.; Krajewski, A.C.; Groeschl, R.T.; Farnell, M.B.; Nagorney, D.M.; Kendrick, M.L.; Cleary, S.P.; Smoot, R.L.; Croome, K.P.; Truty, M.J. Indications and perioperative outcomes for pancreatectomy with arterial resection. *J. Am. Coll. Surg.* **2018**, *227*, 255–269. [CrossRef] [PubMed]
78. Loos, M.; Kester, T.; Klaiber, U.; Mihaljevic, A.L.; Mehrabi, A.; Müller-Stich, B.M.; Diener, M.K.; Schneider, M.A.; Berchtold, C.; Hinz, U.; et al. Arterial resection in pancreatic cancer surgery: Effective after a learning curve. *Ann. Surg.* **2020**. [CrossRef]
79. Bhayani, N.H.; Enomoto, L.M.; James, B.C.; Ortenzi, G.; Kaifi, J.T.; Kimchi, E.T.; Staveley-O'Carroll, K.F.; Gusani, N.J. Multivisceral and extended resections during pancreatoduodenectomy increase morbidity and mortality. *Surgery* **2014**, *155*, 567–574. [CrossRef] [PubMed]
80. Kulemann, B.; Hoeppner, J.; Wittel, U.; Glatz, T.; Keck, T.; Wellner, U.F.; Bronsert, P.; Sick, O.; Hopt, U.T.; Makowiec, F.; et al. Perioperative and long-term outcome after standard pancreaticoduodenectomy, additional portal vein and multivisceral resection for pancreatic head cancer. *J. Gastrointest. Surg.* **2015**, *19*, 438–444. [CrossRef]

81. Hartwig, W.; Gluth, A.; Hinz, U.; Koliogiannis, D.; Strobel, O.; Hackert, T.; Werner, J.; Büchler, M.W. Outcomes after extended pancreatectomy in patients with borderline resectable and locally advanced pancreatic cancer. *Br. J. Surg.* **2016**, *103*, 1683–1694. [CrossRef]
82. Petrucciani, N.; Debs, T.; Nigri, G.; Giannini, G.; Sborlini, E.; Kassir, R.; Ben Amor, I.; Iannelli, A.; Valabrega, S.; D'Angelo, F.; et al. Pancreatectomy combined with multivisceral resection for pancreatic malignancies: Is it justified? Results of a systematic review. *HPB* **2018**, *20*, 3–10. [CrossRef]
83. Malinka, T.; Klein, F.; Andreou, A.; Pratschke, J.; Bahra, M. Distal pancreatectomy combined with multivisceral resection is associated with postoperative complication rates and survival comparable to those after standard procedures. *J. Gastrointest. Surg.* **2018**, *22*, 1549–1556. [CrossRef] [PubMed]
84. Beetz, O.; Sarisin, A.; Kaltenborn, A.; Klempnauer, J.; Winkler, M.; Grannas, G. Multivisceral resection for adenocarcinoma of the pancreatic body and tail-a retrospective single-center analysis. *World J. Surg. Oncol.* **2020**, *18*, 218. [CrossRef] [PubMed]
85. Ramia, J.M.; Del Río-Martín, J.V.; Blanco-Fernández, G.; Cantalejo-Díaz, M.; Rotellar-Sastre, F.; Sabater-Orti, L.; Carabias-Hernandez, A.; Manuel-Vázquez, A.; Hernández-Rivera, P.J.; Jaén-Torrejimeno, I.; et al. Distal pancreatectomy with multivisceral resection: A retrospective multicenter study–Case series. *Int. J. Surg.* **2020**, *82*, 123–129. [CrossRef] [PubMed]
86. Salky, B.A.; Edye, M. Laparoscopic pancreatectomy. *Surg. Clin. N. Am.* **1996**, *76*, 539–545. [CrossRef]
87. Melvin, W.S.; Needleman, B.J.; Krause, K.R.; Ellison, E.C. Robotic resection of pancreatic neuroendocrine tumor. *J. Laparoendosc. Adv. Surg. Tech.* **2003**, *13*, 33–36. [CrossRef]
88. Asbun, H.J.; Moekotte, A.L.; Vissers, F.L.; Kunzler, F.; Cipriani, F.; Alseidi, A.; D'Angelica, M.I.; Balduzzi, A.; Bassi, C.; Björnsson, B.; et al. The Miami international evidence-based guidelines on minimally invasive pancreas resection. *Ann. Surg.* **2020**, *271*, 1–14. [CrossRef]
89. Liu, R.; Wakabayashi, G.; Palanivelu, C.; Tsung, A.; Yang, K.; Goh, B.K.P.; Chong, C.C.; Kang, C.M.; Peng, C.; Kakiashvili, E.; et al. International consensus statement on robotic pancreatic surgery. *Hepatobiliary Surg. Nutr.* **2019**, *8*, 345–360. [CrossRef]
90. Qin, R.; Kendrick, M.L.; Wolfgang, C.L.; Edil, B.H.; Palanivelu, C.; Parks, R.W.; Yang, Y.; He, J.; Zhang, T.; Mou, Y.; et al. International expert consensus on laparoscopic pancreaticoduodenectomy. *Hepatobiliary Surg. Nutr.* **2020**, *9*, 464–483. [CrossRef]
91. Aiolfi, A.; Lombardo, F.; Bonitta, G.; Danelli, P.; Bona, D. Systematic review and updated network meta-analysis comparing open, laparoscopic, and robotic pancreaticoduodenectomy. *Updates Surg.* **2020**. [CrossRef]
92. Van Hilst, J.; de Graaf, N.; Hilal, M.A.; Besselink, M.G. The landmark series: Minimally invasive pancreatic resection. *Ann. Surg. Oncol.* **2021**, *28*, 1447–1456. [CrossRef]
93. Korrel, M.; Vissers, F.L.; van Hilst, J.; de Rooij, T.; Dijkgraaf, M.G.; Festen, S.; Groot Koerkamp, B.; Busch, O.R.; Luyer, M.D.; Sandström, P.; et al. Minimally invasive versus open distal pancreatectomy: An individual patient data meta-analysis of two randomized controlled trials. *HPB* **2020**, *23*, 323–330. [CrossRef] [PubMed]
94. van Hilst, J.; de Rooij, T.; Klompmaker, S.; Rawashdeh, M.; Aleotti, F.; Al-Sarireh, B.; Alseidi, A.; Ateeb, Z.; Balzano, G.; Berrevoet, F.; et al. Minimally invasive versus open distal pancreatectomy for ductal adenocarcinoma (DIPLOMA): A pan-european propensity score matched study. *Ann. Surg.* **2019**, *269*, 10–17. [CrossRef]
95. de Rooij, T.; van Hilst, J.; van Santvoort, H.; Boerma, D.; van den Boezem, P.; Daams, F.; van Dam, R.; Dejong, C.; van Duyn, E.; Dijkgraaf, M.; et al. Minimally invasive versus open distal pancreatectomy (LEOPARD): A multicenter patient-blinded randomized controlled trial. *Ann. Surg.* **2019**, *269*, 2–9. [CrossRef]
96. Magistri, P.; Boggi, U.; Esposito, A.; Carrano, F.M.; Pesi, B.; Ballarin, R.; De Pastena, M.; Menonna, F.; Moraldi, L.; Melis, M.; et al. Robotic vs open distal pancreatectomy: A multi-institutional matched comparison analysis. *J. Hepatobiliary Pancreat. Sci.* **2020**. [CrossRef]
97. Nickel, F.; Haney, C.M.; Kowalewski, K.F.; Probst, P.; Limen, E.F.; Kalkum, E.; Diener, M.K.; Strobel, O.; Müller-Stich, B.P.; Hackert, T. Laparoscopic versus open pancreaticoduodenectomy: A systematic review and meta-analysis of randomized controlled trials. *Ann. Surg.* **2020**, *271*, 54–66. [CrossRef] [PubMed]
98. van Hilst, J.; de Rooij, T.; Bosscha, K.; Brinkman, D.J.; van Dieren, S.; Dijkgraaf, M.G.; Gerhards, M.F.; de Hingh, I.H.; Karsten, T.M.; Lips, D.J.; et al. Laparoscopic versus open pancreatoduodenectomy for pancreatic or periampullary tumours (LEOPARD-2): A multicentre, patient-blinded, randomised controlled phase 2/3 trial. *Lancet Gastroenterol. Hepatol.* **2019**, *4*, 199–207. [CrossRef]

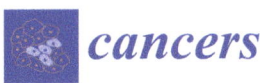

Review

Radical Resection for Locally Advanced Pancreatic Cancers in the Era of New Neoadjuvant Therapy—Arterial Resection, Arterial Divestment and Total Pancreatectomy

Yosuke Inoue *[ ], Atushi Oba, Yoshihiro Ono, Takafumi Sato, Hiromichi Ito and Yu Takahashi

Division of Hepatobiliary and Pancreatic Surgery, Cancer Institute Hospital, Japanese Foundation for Cancer Research, Tokyo 135-8550, Japan; atsushi.oba@jfcr.or.jp (A.O.); yoshihiro.ono@jfcr.or.jp (Y.O.); takafumi.sato@jfcr.or.jp (T.S.); hiromichi.ito@jfcr.or.jp (H.I.); yu.takahashi@jfcr.or.jp (Y.T.)
* Correspondence: yosuke.inoue@jfcr.or.jp; Tel.: +81-3-3520-0111; Fax: +81-3-3570-0343

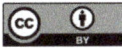

Citation: Inoue, Y.; Oba, A.; Ono, Y.; Sato, T.; Ito, H.; Takahashi, Y. Radical Resection for Locally Advanced Pancreatic Cancers in the Era of New Neoadjuvant Therapy—Arterial Resection, Arterial Divestment and Total Pancreatectomy. *Cancers* **2021**, *13*, 1818. https://doi.org/10.3390/cancers13081818

Academic Editor: Sohei Satoi

Received: 10 February 2021
Accepted: 7 April 2021
Published: 10 April 2021

Publisher's Note: MDPI stays neutral with regard to jurisdictional claims in published maps and institutional affiliations.

Copyright: © 2021 by the authors. Licensee MDPI, Basel, Switzerland. This article is an open access article distributed under the terms and conditions of the Creative Commons Attribution (CC BY) license (https://creativecommons.org/licenses/by/4.0/).

Simple Summary: Aggressive arterial resection or total pancreatectomy in surgical treatment for locally advanced pancreatic cancer (LAPC) has gradually been encouraged thanks to new chemotherapy regimens such as FOLFIRINOX or Gemcitabine and nab-paclitaxel, which have provided more adequate patient selection and local tumor suppression, justifying aggressive local resection. The development of surgical techniques provides the safety of arterial resection (AR) for even major visceral arteries, such as the celiac axis or superior mesenteric artery. Total pancreatectomy has been re-evaluated as an effective option to balance both the local control and postoperative safety. In this review, we investigate the recent reports focusing on arterial resection and total pancreatectomy for locally advanced pancreatic cancer (LAPC) and discuss the rationale of such an aggressive approach in the treatment of PC.

Abstract: Aggressive arterial resection (AR) or total pancreatectomy (TP) in surgical treatment for locally advanced pancreatic cancer (LAPC) had long been discouraged because of their high mortality rate and unsatisfactory long-term outcomes. Recently, new chemotherapy regimens such as FOLFIRINOX or Gemcitabine and nab-paclitaxel have provided more adequate patient selection and local tumor suppression, justifying aggressive local resection. In this review, we investigate the recent reports focusing on arterial resection and total pancreatectomy for LAPC and discuss the rationale of such an aggressive approach in the treatment of PC. AR for LAPCs is divided into three, according to the target vessel. The hepatic artery resection is the simplest one, and the reconstruction methods comprise end-to-end, graft or transposition, and no reconstruction. Celiac axis resection is mainly done with distal pancreatectomy, which allows collateral arterial supply to the liver via the pancreas head. Resection of the superior mesenteric artery is increasingly reported, though its rationale is still controversial. Total pancreatectomy has been re-evaluated as an effective option to balance both the local control and postoperative safety. In conclusion, more and more aggressive pancreatectomy has become justified by the principle of total neoadjuvant therapy. Further technical standardization and optimal neoadjuvant strategy are mandatory for the global dissemination of aggressive pancreatectomies.

Keywords: pancreatic cancer; arterial resection; total pancreatectomy; neoadjuvant therapy

1. Introduction

Pancreatic cancer (PC) is a dismal clinical entity [1]. For localized PCs, resection is the only chance for cure. Theoretically, R0 resection is one essential philosophy for cancer treatment even if the local tumor has invaded major visceral arteries. However, the aggressive biology of PC accompanied with occult metastasis has precluded simply extending the resection. Pancreatectomy is accompanied by high morbidity, and extended resection, including arterial resection (AR) or multi-organ resection, has been a challenge because of its substantial mortality [2,3]. Total pancreatectomy (TP) is an option to achieve R0 resection in locally advanced PCs. The rationale of TP for PC, however, has long been in controversy due to complicated short-time outcomes, including malnutrition or brittle diabetes, along with unsatisfactory long-term survival [4].

New-generation chemotherapies, i.e., FOLFIRINOX [5] or gemcitabine (GEM) + nab-paclitaxel (GNP) [6], have changed the paradigm of the treatment strategy for unresectable locally advanced (LA) PCs. In this review, we investigate the recent innovation of aggressive resection for LAPCs including AR or TP and discuss the future perspective of extended resections for advanced PCs.

2. Arterial Resections

2.1. Overview

Pancreatic ductal adenocarcinoma has an invasive nature, and our predecessor surgeons have tried to improve the prognosis by achieving R0 resection by extending resection. Fortner et al. reported the first series of extended resections named regional pancreatectomy [7]. This report described a novel approach of pancreatectomy for PCs, including TP and routine portomesentericosplenic confluence resection en bloc with the surrounding soft tissue. AR was concomitantly performed if needed. However, their results showed severe short-term outcomes and insufficient long-term survivals and was not accepted as a reasonable method to improve the treatment outcomes of LAPCs [2,7]. Since then, advances in surgical techniques and perioperative management have made venous resection and reconstruction during pancreatectomy safe [8,9]. Recent reports have documented favorable short-term outcomes of venous resection in patients with localized PCs [10,11]; however, the R0 resection rate, as well as long-term survival, remained unsatisfactory, because the most frequent site of cancer-positive margin was located at the superior mesenteric artery (SMA) margin [12,13], which could not be overcome by venous resection alone. Therefore, the necessity of more radical dissection, including arterial resection, remained and has become more prominent in the past two decades, although recent meta-analyses concluded that pancreatectomy with ARs remained a challenge, because it increased the complexity of the procedure and was associated with increased morbidity and mortality in comparison to non-AR pancreatectomies [14,15].

2.2. Management for the Involvement of the Superior Mesenteric Artery

In advanced pancreatic uncinate cancers, the superior mesenteric artery (SMA) is the most common artery that is invaded and becomes a reason for unresectable or pathologically noncurative resection [12,13,16]. Until recent years, a large series of SMA resections for PCs was quite limited, and mortality after SMA resection had reportedly been higher than ordinal pancreatectomies, which discouraged the aggressive resection of LAPCs involving the SMA [17–20] (Table 1). As an alternative, periadventitial dissection (PAD) of the SMA had been proposed to pursue the local control of the peri-SMA region. Inoue et al. presented a standardized technique of SMA-PAD using the supracolic anterior artery-first approach, which resulted in no mortality over 158 patients, with a R0 rate of 74% [16,21]. Extended resection of the peri-SMA nerve plexus was assumed to cause neurogenic diarrhea, which would lead to insufficient patient recovery or adjuvant therapy. Inoue et al. documented that the incremental administration of an opium tincture according to the frequency of watery diarrhea was effective and easy to adjust to, with satisfactory diarrhea control, leading to sufficient adjuvant therapy introduction (83%) [16]. For more advanced tumors that cause encasement of the artery, SMA resection would be required. Recently, some high-volume centers with outstanding expertise in pancreatic resections have reported large series of arterial resections for PCs, including more than 30 cases of SMA resections [22,23]. Bachellier et al. [22] reported a large single-center series, including 34 SMA resections. They achieved the lowest mortality ever (5.1% of all patients with AR), which represented the improved safety of SMA resection and reconstruction. They mainly employed an end-to-end anastomosis using autografts such as a great saphenous vein and noted that reconstruction with an artificial graft caused thrombosis, leading to in-hospital mortality. Loos et al. [23] reported another large series involving 30 SMA resections with an acceptable mortality of 6.7%. They also performed a learning curve analysis and concluded that even an experienced pancreatic surgeon needed more than 12 cases of AR to minimize the mortality. An optimal reconstruction technique has never been established and likely depends on the length of a resected segment. Previous reports on SMA reconstruction employed end-to-end anastomosis or anastomosis to the aorta with or without graft interposition (Figure 1A,B,D,E) and a rotation of the splenic artery (SpA) (Figure 1C) [10,17,20,22–34]. Westermark et al. [35] proposed a safe technique of end-to-end anastomosis of the SMA. They recommended the Cattel-Braasch maneuver, wherein the total mesentery is detached from the retroperitoneum to facilitate a tension-free anastomosis. Sterile ice in a surgical towel was placed in the lower sub-mesocolic abdomen to reduce the warm ischemia of the small intestine. The Cattel-Braasch maneuver enabled tension-free anastomosis even after SMA resection of 4 cm in length. Accordingly, SMA resection is now no more an anecdotal tool but one possible option for LA pancreatic head cancers. Reports focusing on the long-term outcomes after SMA resection are still limited.

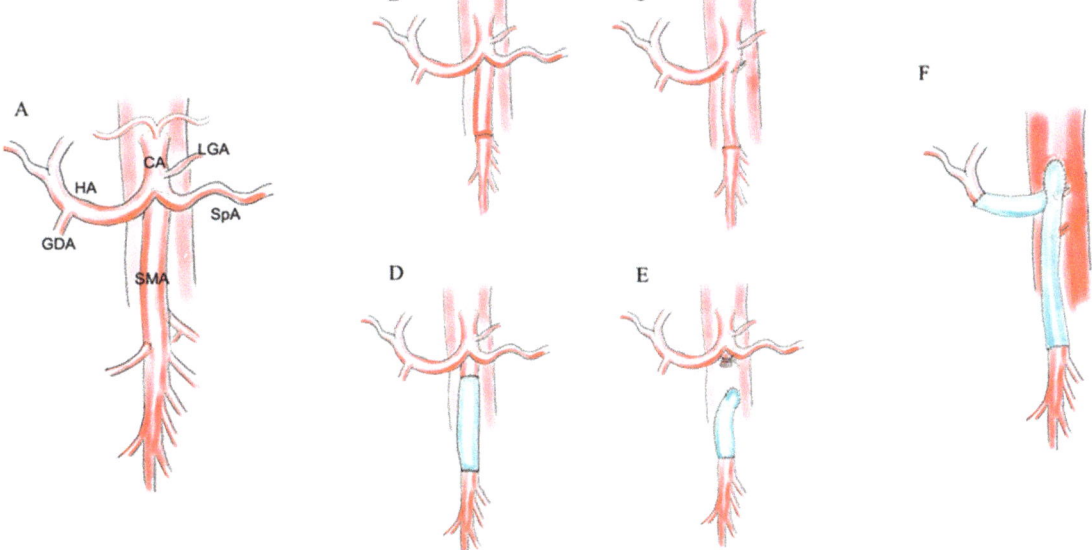

Figure 1. Reconstruction of the superior mesenteric artery. (**A**) Basic anatomy of relevant vessels in SMA resection. (**B**) Direct end-to-end anastomosis. (**C**) Transposition of SpA to be anastomosed with the distal stump of the SMA. (**D**) End-to-end anastomosis with graft interposition. (**E**) Graft interposition from the aorta to the distal stump of the SMA. (**F**) Combined resection and reconstruction of the HA and SMA using interposition grafts. HA, hepatic artery, SpA, splenic artery, GDA, gastroduodenal artery, SMA, superior mesenteric artery, MCA, middle colic artery and LGA, left gastric artery.

Table 1. Previous reports about resection of the superior mesenteric artery.

Author	Year	Country	N	NAT (%)	Procedures	Reconstruction Method	Study Period	Mortality (%)
Li [24]	2004	China	11	ND	PD	Graft 8, interposition from the aorta 3	1994–2003	ND
Nakao [10]	2006	Japan	3	ND	PD, TP	ND	1981–2005	35.7 **
Yekebas [20]	2008	Germany	3	ND	PD, DP	EEA 1, graft 2	1994–2005	33
Amano [17]	2009	Japan	12	13 **	PD, TP	EEA 3, SpA transposition 7 *, graft 2	2005–2009	17
Boggi [25]	2009	Italy	6	ND	PD	EEA 1, graft 5	1987–2004	4.0 **
Martin [26]	2009	USA	2	100	PD, TP	Graft 2	1999–2007	0
Kitagawa [19]	2011	Japan	17	ND	PD	EEA 1, graft 16	2002–2011	12
Bockhorn [27]	2011	Germany	3	ND	PD, TP	Graft 3	1994–2004	14 **
Rehders [28]	2012	Germany	4	ND	PD	EEA 3, graft 1	2004–2010	ND
Gong [29]	2013	China	10	ND	PD	ND	2006–2011	6.7 **
Sgroi [30]	2015	USA	4	38 **	PD	EEA 4	2003–2013	ND
Glebova [31]	2016	USA	2	28 **	PD	EEA 1, graft 1	1989–2014	ND
Perinel [32]	2016	France	6	67	TP	SpA transposition 6	2008–2014	0
Tee [33]	2018	USA	15	75 **	PD, DP, TP	EEA, graft, or reconstruction †	1990–2017	7.0
Loveday [34]	2019	Canada	10	94 **	PD, DP, TP	EEA, interposition from the aorta †	2009–2016	3.2 **
Bachellier [22]	2020	France	34	75 **	PD, DP, TP	EEA or graft 34 †	1990–2017	5.7
Loos [23]	2020	Germany	30	49 **	PD, DP, TP	EEA, graft, transposition †	2003–2019	6.7

NAT, neoadjuvant therapy, ND, not described, PD, pancreaticoduodenectomy, TP, total pancreatectomy, DP, distal pancreatectomy, EEA, end-to-end anastomosis and SpA, splenic artery. * The hepatic artery was anastomosed to the SpA with total pancreatectomy; ** Incidence among all patients with arterial resection. † Each number was not documented.

2.3. Resection of the Hepatic Artery

Advanced cancers located at the pancreatic neck often invade the common and proper hepatic artery (HA), as well as the gastroduodenal artery (GDA). In such cases, segmental resection of the HA, including the root of the GDA, is suggested. If cancer invasion is limited and resected segment is short, end-to-end anastomosis is often possible. Recent guidelines have also described the combined HA or celiac axis (CA) resection as one of the putative options for LAPC [36]. Although a large series that specifically focuses on HA resection is limited, there are many small case series, including five to 20 patients who mainly underwent pancreaticoduodenectomy (PD) with concomitant resection of the HA until recently [10,17,20,24–27,29–32,37–39] (Table 2). Amano H et al. first reported a medium series of HA resections in which they described the details of techniques and outcomes about HA reconstruction. The in-hospital mortality rate was 7%, accompanied by an R0 rate of 80% and a median survival time (MST) of 12 months. The authors concluded that HA resection is justified only when surgery of R0 has taken place for selected patients with PC. Regarding the reconstruction technique of the HA, several reports described HA reconstruction, which was dominantly done by end-to-end anastomosis (Figure 2A,B) [24–27,30–32,37]. Short-segment resection of the HA was simple and safe and could be recommended as an entry procedure of AR for pancreatic surgeons who perform pancreatic head resection. In a case where the HA is resected in a long segment, arterial transposition (Figure 2C,D) [17,32] or interposition using the autograft to bridge between the celiac axis or aorta and proper HA is required (Figure 2E) [24,25,27,31]. To simplify and reduce the number of anastomoses, transposition of the SpA or colic artery should first be considered. The right inferior phrenic artery is an alternative option for a small orifice of the left HA. Although SpA transposition is usually performed with TP to gain enough length of the SpA pedicle, preservation of the pancreas tail would be possible if the left gastric artery (LGA) and great pancreatic artery are preserved. Desaki et al. reported a case series of SpA resection during PD mainly for PCs and documented that no clinically relevant splenic infarction was observed [40]. On the other hand, the omittance of HA reconstruction would be possible if we performed a specific preparation for HA resection. Miyazaki et al. proposed the novel management of HA resection with preoperative HA embolization to enhance the collateral hepatic arterial inflow [38]. After HA resection, backflow from the proper HA stump was observed. If the backflow was strong enough, they omitted HA reconstruction. In a 21-patient series, they reconstructed HA in only one patient, and eventually, 33% of the patients suffered postoperative liver infarction, but there was no in-hospital mortality.

Table 2. Previous reports about resection of the hepatic artery.

Author	Year	Country	N	NAT (%)	Procedures	Reconstruction Method	Study Period	Mortality (%)
Li [24]	2004	China	8	ND	PD	EEA 5, graft 3	1994–2003	ND
Nakao [10]	2006	Japan	9	ND	PD, TP	ND	1981–2005	ND
Yekebas [20]	2008	Germany	10	ND	PD, TP, DP	EEA 10	1994–2005	0
Amano H [17]	2009	Japan	15	13 [†]	PD, TP	EEA 3, GDA 4 *, SpA 6 **, Others 3	2005–2009	6.7
Boggi [25]	2009	Italy	12	ND	PD	EEA 6, graft 5, no reconstruction 1	1987–2004	4 [†]
Martin [26]	2009	USA	3	33	PD, TP	EEA 3	1999–2007	0
Bockhorn [27]	2011	Germany	18	ND	PD, TP	EEA 10, graft 8	1994–2004	14 [†]
Gong [29]	2013	China	5	ND	PD	ND	2006–2011	6.7 [†]
Amano R [37]	2015	Japan	7	100	PD, TP	EEA 6, no reconstruction 1	2012–2013	0
Sgroi [30]	2015	USA	7	38 [†]	PD	EEA 7	2003–2013	ND
Glebova [31]	2016	USA	18	28 [†]	PD	EEA 15, graft 2, no reconstruction 1	1989–2014	ND
Perinel [32]	2016	France	6	0	TP	SpA 3, no reconstruction 3 [‡]	2008–2014	0
Miyazaki [38]	2017	Japan	21	43	PD, TP	EEA1, no reconstruction 20	2019–2015	0
Tee [33]	2018	USA	60	75 [†]	PD, DP, TP	EEA or graft or reconstruction [§]	1990–2017	13
Loveday [34]	2019	Canada	10	94 [†]	PD, DP, TP	EEA, interposition from the aorta [†]	2009–2016	3.2 [†]
Bachellier [22]	2020	France	29	75 [†]	PD, DP, TP	EEA or graft 20 [§], no reconstruction 9 [§]	1990–2017	5.1 [†]
Loos [23]	2020	Germany	85	49 [†]	PD, DP, TP	EEA, graft, transposition [§]	2003–2019	16.7

EEA, end-to-end anastomosis, ND, not described, PD, pancreaticoduodenectomy, TP, total pancreatectomy, DP, distal pancreatectomy, GDA, gastroduodenal artery and SpA, splenic artery. * The replaced hepatic artery was anastomosed to the GDA. ** The hepatic artery was anastomosed to the SpA with total pancreatectomy. [†] Incidences among all patients with arterial resection. [‡] Includes patients who had replaced HA. [§] Each number was not documented.

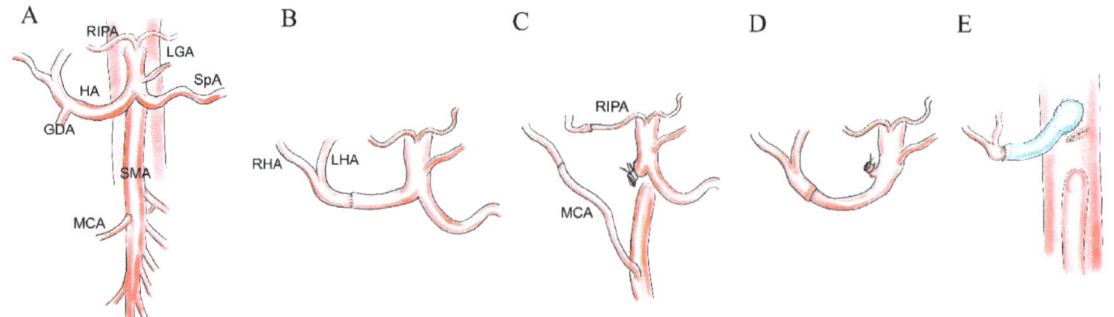

Figure 2. Reconstruction of the hepatic artery. (**A**) Basic anatomy of the relevant vessels in HA resection. (**B**) Direct end-to-end anastomosis. (**C**) Transposition of the MCA and RIPA to be anastomosed with the RHA and LHA. (**D**) Transposition of the SpA to be anastomosed with the proper HA. (**E**) Graft interposition from the aorta to the stump of the proper HA. HA, hepatic artery, RIPA, right inferior phrenic artery, SpA, splenic artery, GDA, gastroduodenal artery, SMA, superior mesenteric artery, MCA, middle colic artery, LGA left gastric artery, RHA, right hepatic artery and LHA, left hepatic artery.

2.4. Resection of the Celiac Axis

CA resection for advanced pancreatic body cancer was an exceptional situation of arterial resection, wherein reconstruction of the hepatic artery was considered to be unnecessary because of the peripancreatic collateral arterial flow that originated from the SMA [41]. Pancreatic body cancers frequently involve the celiac–hepatic artery system, and distal pancreatectomy with celiac axis resection (DP-CAR) was a reasonable choice to achieve an en-bloc eradication of the tumor and its invasion. The concept of DP-CAR was a modification of the Appleby procedure originally for advanced gastric cancers [41]. The first report about DP-CAR was written by Hishinuma et al. in 1991, and they documented the preservation of the whole stomach during CAR and distinguished DP-CAR from the Appleby procedure in that the stomach was preserved [42]. Afterward, several small series of DP-CARs were reported [43–47], and in 2007, Hirano et al. first described the short- and long-term outcomes of the standardized DP-CAR [48]. They reported 23 patients who underwent DP-CARs with no mortality and had acceptable overall survival (five-year survival rate, 42% and median survival time, 21 months). This pivotal report encouraged pancreatic surgeons worldwide to perform DP-CAR as a promising option to balance surgical and oncological safety. However, as the cases accumulated, ischemic complications involving the stomach or liver became prominent, as well as post-pancreatectomy hemorrhage, caused by the insufficient drainage of postoperative pancreatic fistula, leading to non-negligible mortality [49–54] (Table 3). Ischemic gastropathy or stomach perforation were complications specific to DP-CARs, which often included resection of the LGA, as well as the left gastroepiploic artery. Moreover, radical retroperitoneal dissection during DP-CAR includes resection of the left inferior phrenic artery. These sacrifices of critical gastric inflows potentially lead to life-threatening gastropathy [55]. As for liver infarction, collateral hepatic flow via the GDA was theoretically sufficient for liver perfusion. However, excessive dissection of the GDA sometimes leads to arterial stenosis, which causes depression of the hepatic arterial flow [56]. Depression of the proper hepatic artery induces recurrent cholangitis, liver abscess or cholecystitis. Cholecystitis was reported to be one possible cause of postoperative major intervention [50,55]. Therefore, the gallbladder should be resected routinely during DP-CAR. In the early years, preoperative arterial embolization of the HA or LGA to enhance the collateral flow was encouraged to avoid ischemic complications. However, recent reports found no positive impact of arterial embolization on the prevention of postoperative ischemic complications [55–58]. Another possible resolution is an intraoperative reconstruction of the LGA. Sato et al. first described reconstruction of the LGA to avoid ischemic gastropathy after DP-CAR [59]. The authors used a pedicle of the middle colic artery as an origin of the arterial supply. The right branch of the middle colic artery is usually away from the pancreatic body cancer and used as a suitable counterpart of the LGA. The efficacy of the anastomosis should be confirmed promptly and objectively after anastomosis. Oba et al. reported the intraoperative evaluation of the patency of LGA anastomosis using indocyanine green fluorescence imaging [60]. By these managements, the safety of DP-CARs would be improved.

Table 3. Previous reports of distal pancreatectomy with celiac axis resections (DP-CARs).

Author	Year	Country	N	Study Period	Preoperative Embolization (%)	LGA Flow Preservation (%)	Ischemic Complication (%) Stomach	Ischemic Complication (%) Liver	Mortality (%)
Klompmaker [49]	2019	Europa	191	2000–2016	38	12	11	23	9.5
Nakamura [50]	2016	Japan	80	1998–2015	100	6.3	29	6	5
Yamamoto [53]	2017	Japan	72	2001–2011	ND	ND	ND	ND	4.2
Okada [55]	2018	Japan	50	2004–2017	92	46	10	56	8
Yoshitomi [58]	2019	Japan	38	2010–2016	74	0	10	3	3
Ocuin [48]	2016	USA	30	2007–2015	ND	0	7	ND	14
Yoshiya [49]	2019	Japan	20	2008–2018	80	0	0	ND	0
Beane [51]	2015	USA	20	2011–2012	ND	0	0	0	10
Oba [57]	2019	Japan	18	2014–2017	0	89	11	ND	0

LGA, left gastric artery and ND, not described.

3. Total Pancreatectomy

TP was reported by Rockey et al. for the first time [61]. Although TP was attempted to improve the survival of patients with PC with the rationale to avoid anastomosis-related morbidity and mortality in early years [62,63], Warren et al. documented that TP led to pancreatic endocrine and exocrine insufficiency, resulting in brittle diabetes due to a lack of endocrine and malabsorption caused by exocrine deficiency [64]. Later, TP was indicated with the intention to improve the local control in extensive pancreatic cancers [7]. However, as was described by Fortner et al., a simple extension of resection resulted in poor short-term outcomes accompanied by unsatisfactory survival [2]. In the 1980s, TP was attempted to eradicate multicentric carcinogenesis in the whole pancreas, but it failed to improve the survival of patients with PS, because the incidence of tumor multicentricity proved to be low [4,65]. Therefore, TP has been discouraged for the curative treatment of PCs [66]. After 2000, the introduction of long-acting insulin formulations facilitated the easy control of blood sugar levels after TP. As a result, endocrine-related mortality has been rarely reported ever since. As for exocrine insufficiency, diarrhea was the most frequent sequelae after TP, and 23.5% of patients who underwent TP still had symptoms, despite pancreatic enzyme administration [67]. Moreover, malabsorption causes postoperative steatohepatitis, which potentially leads to life-threatening hepatic decompensation [68]. Hata et al. identified female gender, malnutrition and insufficient pancreatic enzyme substitution as significant prognostic factors of post-TP steatohepatitis and suggested that high-dose pancreatic enzyme replacement therapy might have preventive effects on hepatic steatosis occurring after a pancreatectomy [69]. Anyway, the development and standardization of the surgical technique fostered by the case accumulation and centralization of complicated procedures has gradually made the surgical outcomes of TP an acceptable level, like partial pancreatectomy [70–73]. Long-term survivals have gradually become better and better. Until the middle of the 2000s, the MST of patients who underwent TP for PCs was about one year or less [4,74,75]. Schmidt et al. reported a substantial improvement in survival after TP for pancreatic neck cancers, documenting an MST of 18 months [76]. After 2010, a large series comprising 289 patients with TP for PCs documented an MST of 18.1 months [72]. Accordingly, TP was gradually reappraised as a reasonable option to achieve a cure for selective patients with PC [70,72,77–83] (Table 4). If TP was applied to LAPCs to obtain a cure or long-term survival, we would have to consider the quality of life after TP, as well as the absolute surgical safety or survival time.

Recently, several reports documented a significant reduction of physical functioning [84] or both the physical and emotional composite scores [85,86]. Stoop et al. stated in the latest report that the quality of life after TP was reduced in comparison to the general population but remained stable compared with the preoperative situation [84]. They demonstrated the challenges of endocrine (96% of patients involved) and exocrine insufficiency (64% of patients involved) after TP and claimed that the management of both insufficiencies should be improved further to overcome the quality of life reduction after TP.

Table 4. Previous reports about total pancreatectomy for pancreatic cancers.

Author	Year	Country	N	Study Period	Mortality (%)	R0 Resection Rate (%)	Median Survival Time (Months)
Brooks [74]	1989	USA	48	1970–1986	8.3	ND	12
Launois [75]	1993	France	47	1968–1986	15	ND	8
Karpoff [4]	2001	USA	35	1983–1998	5.7	82	7.9
Schmit [76]	2007	USA	33	1992–2006	6	100	18
Reddy [70]	2009	USA	100	1970–2007	8	78	12
Nathan [77]	2009	USA	376	1998–2004	8.6	ND	15
Hartwig [71]	2015	Germany	289	2001–2012	7.8	ND	18
Satoi [78]	2016	Japan	45	2001–2011	0	76	17
Johnston [79]	2016	USA	2582	1998–2004	5.5	76	15
Xiong [80]	2017	China	50	2009–2015	6	90	18
Passeri [81]	2019	USA	807	1998–2006	5.6	76	17
Hashimoto [82]	2020	Japan	1393	2013–2016	1.1	ND	ND
Stoop [83]	2020	Sweden	90	2008–2017	3.4	ND	ND

ND, not described.

4. Recent Evolution of Radical Pancreatectomies in the Era of New Regimens and Future Perspective

4.1. Recent Reports of Extremely Radical Pancreatectomy

The respective techniques of arterial resection or total pancreatectomy have gradually matured and become common among experienced pancreatic surgeons; however, extremely radical pancreatectomy involving major arterial resection with or without total pancreatectomy is still controversial in that long-term survival is not considered worth carrying the surgical risks for patients with LAPC [3,17,70–72]. However, the introduction of new-generation chemotherapy regimens such as FOLFIRINOX [5] or GNP [6] has gradually changed the paradigm of indication for these surgical challenges. In recent years, multiple high-volume pancreatic centers have reported extremely radical pancreatectomy after intensive neoadjuvant therapy (NAT) using FOLFIRINOX or GNP.

Tee et al. first reported a large series of AR combined with new-generation NAT for advanced PCs [33]. In this study, 111 patients underwent pancreatectomy with AR, including any hepatic (54%), any celiac (44%), any superior mesenteric (14%) or multiple ARs (14%), with revascularization in 55% (Figure 1F). TP was performed on 20 (18%) patients. The majority of cases underwent planned AR (77%), and most of the procedures were performed post-2010 (78%). The most common indication for pancreatectomy was for PC in 87 (78%) patients. Of these patients, 65 (75%) were treated with neoadjuvant systemic chemotherapy that included FOLFIRINOX, GNP or both, with the majority (88%) also receiving sequential chemoradiation with a total dose of 50.4Gy with various radiation sensitizers. Ninety-day major morbidity (≥grade III) and mortality was 54% and 13% mainly due to post-pancreatectomy hemorrhage, postoperative pancreatic fistula or ischemia. They emphasized that a significant decrease in mortality was achieved in patients who underwent ARs post-2010 (9% compared with 29% in patients before 2010, $p = 0.02$). From the same group, Truty et al. reported a systematic classification of CAR, which included three levels according to the extent of the resection: class 1, celiac only; class 2, celiac and PHA and class 3, SMA additional to class 1 or 2 [57]. Ninety-day mortality was 10%, with a significant improvement in the last 50 consecutive cases (4%).

The R0 resection rate (88%) was associated with chemoradiation ($p = 0.004$). The MST was 36.2 months, superior from the neoadjuvant chemotherapy (8.0 vs. 43.5 months). Truty et al. also reported a large series comprising 194 borderline resectable or LAPC [87]. En-bloc venous and/or arterial resection was required in 125 (65%) patients, with 94% of patients achieving R0 margins. TP was performed in 25 (13%) patients. The 90-day mortality was 6.7%. Among patients without mortality, epochally favorable survival outcomes were obtained (the median, one-year, two-year and three-year overall survivival (OS) rates were 58.8 months, 96%, 78% and 62%, respectively). They emphasized the efficacy of total neoadjuvant therapy (TNT) with favorable prognostic factors: extended duration (six cycles) of neoadjuvant chemotherapy, optimal post-chemotherapy CA19-9 response and major pathological response. Bachellier et al. reported a large AR series for PCs with excellent postoperative outcomes [22]. The most impactful point was that this study included 35 SMA resections, which was the largest ever. The overall mortality and morbidity were 5.1% and 41.5%, respectively. Preoperative radiation was not employed, assumably to secure the safety of complicated AR of the major visceral arteries. TP was performed in 18 (15%) patients. Some patients (75.4%) underwent NAT. The median, one-year, three-year and five-year OS rates after resection were 13.7 months, 59%, 13% and 12%, respectively. They identified that R0 resection (hazard ratio: 0.60, $p = 0.01$) and pathological venous invasion (hazard ratio: 1.67, $p = 0.04$) were independent prognostic factors. Loos et al. reported the largest AR series (195 patients) for LAPCs recently [23]. They compared AR with periadventitial dissection (PAD; $n = 190$), which was an optional technique to achieve R0 resection in borderline resectable or LAPCs, and revealed higher rates of postoperative pancreatic fistula (4.2% after PAD vs. 10.3% after AR; $p = 0.022$), post-pancreatectomy hemorrhage (4.7% vs. 14.9%; $p = 0.001$), ischemia (4.2% vs. 15.9%; $p < 0.0001$) and relaparotomy (12.6% vs. 26.9%; $p = 0.001$) after AR. The overall mortality rate of AR was higher than that of PAD (12.8% vs. 4.7%; $p = 0.005$). Although the mortality rate became lower and lower through the study period, AR remained more dangerous than PAD. The authors concluded even experienced pancreatic surgeons needed a learning curve of 15 ARs to safely perform the procedure. These results indicated the difficulty of AR to be disseminated globally. The median and five-year OS rates were 21.5 months and 15%, respectively, after PAD and 17.7 months and 9% after AR ($p = 0.099$). These results were attributed to more advanced stages and less incidences of NAT in the AR group.

4.2. En-Bloc Arterial Resection or Arterial Divestment?

There still remains controversy over the issue of whether we choose AR for major vessels or not, especially for the SMA. Even in highly selected patients, the SMA resection is regarded as difficult to be generalized. To balance surgical and oncological safety, the arterial divestment technique has been proposed as an alternative for SMA resection. "Divestment" means "undressing" or "circumferential dissection". The detailed technique and outcomes of arterial divestment were described in recent reports from the Heidelberg group [88,89]. The SMA was dissected using an artery-first approach through a wide Kocher maneuver, and if needed, a Cattel-Braasch maneuver was added. The authors recommend intraoperative sampling of the periadventitial tissue around the SMA, and if the cancer was positive, divestment was first attempted. Cai et al. recommended in their report that peri-adventitial dissection should be done with cold dissection using the tip of a right-angled clamp or the nonworking tip of energy devices [89]. Burn injury on the arterial wall would be a risk of postoperative aneurysm. If the dissection was difficult due to direct encasement, finally, AR was employed. To select among the three choices: divestment, AR or aborting resection before the point of no return, an artery-first approach is mandatory. The safety of the divestment technique was reported by a recent article from the same group of Heidelberg [23]. Inoue et al. [16] described the details of periadventitial dissection around the SMA, which resulted in no mortality by the use of an artery-first approach. It did not preclude postoperative recovery or adjuvant therapy if the neurogenic diarrhea was adequately controlled. However, the safe utilization of this technique has never been generalized. Sabater et al. [90] conducted the first randomized trial to compare the oncological and surgical outcomes between artery-first PD and standard PD. The authors concluded that they found no difference either in the R0 resection rates (67.9 % vs. 77.3 %, $p = 0.194$) or in the postoperative complications (overall morbidity rate; 67.9% vs. 73.3%, $p = 0.484$) in patients undergoing artery-first PD versus standard PD. Although this trial included only resectable PCs and other periampullary malignancies, and their conclusions could not be applied directly to the management of LAPCs, this technique should be carefully applied by an expert pancreatic surgeon at a high-volume center. Another important matter is when and how we decide the approach to the SMA. Habib et al. [91] also encouraged SMA divestment for selected patients after new-generation NAT. They also indicated the usefulness of the preoperative radiological finding of circumferential SMA encasement. Halo sign, wherein the SMA was surrounded by hypodense tissue without narrowing, was potentially a candidate for resection using arterial divestment. On the other hand, string sign, wherein the SMA was surrounded by periadventitial tissue forming an irregular narrowing (like a string), was not a candidate for R0 resection, even with arterial divestment. Habib et al. and the John's Hopkins group did not regard a patient with string sign as an adequate candidate for resection, because they could not justify SMA resection due to the high morbidity and mortality. However, the radiological change after NAT did not represent a pathological regression of the tumor cells, and decision-making by the preoperative findings alone would include the risk of overdiagnosis and loss of chance for a cure. Del Chiaro also advocated intraoperative decision-making of the divestment or AR [92]. The author also recommended performing the divestment technique by the surgical team experienced in AR, because we have to prepare for unexpected arterial injury during SMA dissection, which requires complex vascular reconstruction.

On the other hand, Truty et al. [87] strongly recommended a planned en-bloc resection, even for the SMA. Their recent report still included a high mortality rate (9 out of 71 LAPC patients) after aggressive AR, but they stated that the safety of AR has become more robust recently and documented a surprisingly high R0 rate and long-term survival. Actually, the intraoperative judgement of periadventitial cancer invasion requires a test dissection, which potentially cuts into the cancer tissue. The superiority of planned en-bloc portal vein resection in obtaining R0 to unplanned venous resection after a test dissection was recently documented [93]. The en-bloc approach is exactly the principle of regional pancreatectomy suggested by Fortner et al. [7], and the reappraisal of regional en-bloc resection has been reported, such as for portal vein resection [94]. If the safety of AR is guaranteed, the same theory should be justified in SMA resection as well. For pancreatectomy with complicated AR, the efficacy of concomitant TP has been reappraised. The total removal of the pancreatic gland makes the procedure safer by eliminating the problem of pancreas fistula and its potentially fatal effect on arterial anastomosis [95,96]. This strategy, which was originally suggested at the dawn of the radical resection of PCs, has become justified after the improvement of the perioperative management of TP patients through several decades.

4.3. Rationale of Total Neoadjuvant Therapy

Another recent topic relevant to extremely radical pancreatectomy for PCs is the rationale of TNT. TNT has been advocated for LA gastrointestinal cancers, i.e., esophageal cancers [97] or rectal cancers [98,99], wherein the surgical burden of resection likely hampers prompt postoperative recovery and adequate adjuvant systemic chemotherapy. For LAPCs, due to a lack of effective regimens, TNT has long been out of the question, and the efficacy of TNT was suggested only recently. Murphy et al. reported a prospective single-arm phase II trial evaluating the efficacy of TNT using FOLFIRINOX for LAPCs with the primary endpoint of the R0 resection rate [100]. This report was the first concrete evidence of TNT for PCs. Forty-nine LAPC patients were enrolled. Eight cycles of FOLFIRINOX were administered, followed by short- or long-course chemoradiotherapy, depending on the radiological findings after FOLFIRINOX. Thirty-nine (80%) patients completed eight cycles. One patient (2%) had a radiographic complete response. Twenty-three patients

(49%) had a partial response, while 21 (45%) had a stable disease. Two patients (4%) had a progressive disease by the response evaluation criteria in solid tumours (RECIST) criteria. Thirty-four patients (69%) underwent surgical resection. Finally, 30 (61%) patients achieved R0 resection. TNT with FOLFIRINOX was feasible and provided a favorable long-term survival (median progression-free survival was 17.5 months (95% CI: 13.9–22.7), and median MST was 31.4 months (95% CI, 18.1–38.5)). For LAPCs, intensive neoadjuvant therapy has already become a consensus, and the next issue is how we can standardize the optimal contents, dose and duration of NAT. Moreover, scientifically reliable evidence for neoadjuvant therapy for PCs [101,102] is still sparse compared to adjuvant therapy [103–106] so far. Whether or not we should really omit adjuvant therapy remains unclear.

5. Conclusions

In this review, the recent development of radical pancreatectomy, including arterial resection, arterial divestment or total pancreatectomy, was discussed. Thanks to the recent improvement of chemotherapy using multiple agents, both tumor suppression and patient selection have become pragmatic. Simple resection of the HA or CA and TP has likely become a matured technique. To implement ERP including SMA resection or combined major arterial resections, the further accumulation of cases, the establishment of a standardized technique and optimal neoadjuvant therapy should be pursued.

Author Contributions: Conceptualization, Y.I. and Y.T.; methodology, Y.I.; writing—original draft preparation, Y.I.; writing—review and editing, A.O., Y.O., T.S. and H.I. and supervision, Y.T. All authors have read and agreed to the published version of the manuscript.

Funding: This research received no external funding.

Conflicts of Interest: The authors declare no conflict of interest.

References

1. Siegel, R.L.; Miller, K.D.; Jemal, A. Cancer statistics, 2019. *CA Cancer J. Clin.* **2019**, *69*, 7–34. [CrossRef] [PubMed]
2. Fortner, J.G. Regional pancreatectomy for cancer of the pancreas, ampulla, and other related sites. Tumor staging and results. *Ann. Surg.* **1984**, *199*, 418–425. [CrossRef]
3. Mollberg, N.; Rahbari, N.N.; Koch, M.; Hartwig, W.; Hoeger, Y.; Büchler, M.W.; Weitz, J. Arterial resection during pancreatectomy for pancreatic cancer: A systematic review and meta-analysis. *Ann. Surg.* **2011**, *254*, 882–893. [CrossRef] [PubMed]
4. Karpoff, H.M.; Klimstra, D.S.; Brennan, M.F.; Conlon, K.C. Results of total pancreatectomy for adenocarcinoma of the pancreas. *Arch. Surg.* **2001**, *136*, 44–47; discussion 48. [CrossRef]
5. Conroy, T.; Desseigne, F.; Ychou, M.; Bouche, O.; Guimbaud, R.; Becouarn, Y.; Adenis, A.; Raoul, J.L.; Gourgou-Bourgade, S.; de la Fouchardiere, C.; et al. Folfirinox versus gemcitabine for metastatic pancreatic cancer. *N. Engl. J. Med.* **2011**, *364*, 1817–1825. [CrossRef] [PubMed]
6. Von Hoff, D.D.; Ervin, T.; Arena, F.P.; Chiorean, E.G.; Infante, J.; Moore, M.; Seay, T.; Tjulandin, S.A.; Ma, W.W.; Saleh, M.N.; et al. Increased survival in pancreatic cancer with nab-paclitaxel plus gemcitabine. *N. Engl. J. Med.* **2013**, *369*, 1691–1703. [CrossRef] [PubMed]
7. Fortner, J.G.; Kim, D.K.; Cubilla, A.; Turnbull, A.; Pahnke, L.D.; Shils, M.E. Regional pancreatectomy: En bloc pancreatic, portal vein and lymph node resection. *Ann. Surg.* **1977**, *186*, 42–50. [CrossRef] [PubMed]
8. Evans, D.B.; Farnell, M.B.; Lillemoe, K.D.; Vollmer, C., Jr.; Strasberg, S.M.; Schulick, R.D. Surgical treatment of resectable and borderline resectable pancreas cancer: Expert consensus statement. *Ann. Surg. Oncol.* **2009**, *16*, 1736–1744. [CrossRef] [PubMed]
9. Tseng, J.F.; Tamm, E.P.; Lee, J.E.; Pisters, P.W.; Evans, D.B. Venous resection in pancreatic cancer surgery. *Best Pract. Res. Clin. Gastroenterol.* **2006**, *20*, 349–364. [CrossRef]
10. Nakao, A.; Takeda, S.; Inoue, S.; Nomoto, S.; Kanazumi, N.; Sugimoto, H.; Fujii, T. Indications and techniques of extended resection for pancreatic cancer. *World J. Surg.* **2006**, *30*, 976–982. [CrossRef]
11. Tseng, J.F.; Raut, C.P.; Lee, J.E.; Pisters, P.W.; Vauthey, J.N.; Abdalla, E.K.; Gomez, H.F.; Sun, C.C.; Crane, C.H.; Wolff, R.A.; et al. Pancreaticoduodenectomy with vascular resection: Margin status and survival duration. *J. Gastroint. Surg.* **2004**, *8*, 935–949; discussion 949–950. [CrossRef]
12. Esposito, I.; Kleeff, J.; Bergmann, F.; Reiser, C.; Herpel, E.; Friess, H.; Schirmacher, P.; Buchler, M.W. Most pancreatic cancer resections are r1 resections. *Ann. Surg. Oncol.* **2008**, *15*, 1651–1660. [CrossRef]
13. Verbeke, C.S.; Leitch, D.; Menon, K.V.; McMahon, M.J.; Guillou, P.J.; Anthoney, A. Redefining the r1 resection in pancreatic cancer. *Br. J. Surg.* **2006**, *93*, 1232–1237. [CrossRef] [PubMed]

14. Rebelo, A.; Büdeyri, I.; Heckler, M.; Partsakhashvili, J.; Ukkat, J.; Ronellenfitsch, U.; Michalski, C.W.; Kleeff, J. Systematic review and meta-analysis of contemporary pancreas surgery with arterial resection. *Langenbeck's Arch. Surg.* **2020**, *405*, 903–919. [CrossRef]
15. Małczak, P.; Sierżęga, M.; Stefura, T.; Kacprzyk, A.; Droś, J.; Skomarovska, O.; Krzysztofik, M.; Major, P.; Pędziwiatr, M. Arterial resections in pancreatic cancer—Systematic review and meta-analysis. *HPB* **2020**, *22*, 961–968. [CrossRef]
16. Inoue, Y.; Saiura, A.; Oba, A.; Kawakatsu, S.; Ono, Y.; Sato, T.; Mise, Y.; Ishizawa, T.; Takahashi, Y.; Ito, H. Optimal extent of superior mesenteric artery dissection during pancreaticoduodenectomy for pancreatic cancer: Balancing surgical and oncological safety. *J. Gastrointest. Surg.* **2019**, *23*, 1373–1383. [CrossRef] [PubMed]
17. Amano, H.; Miura, F.; Toyota, N.; Wada, K.; Katoh, K.; Hayano, K.; Kadowaki, S.; Shibuya, M.; Maeno, S.; Eguchi, T.; et al. Is pancreatectomy with arterial reconstruction a safe and useful procedure for locally advanced pancreatic cancer? *J. Hepato-Biliary-Pancreat. Surg.* **2009**, *16*, 850–857. [CrossRef] [PubMed]
18. Jegatheeswaran, S.; Baltatzis, M.; Jamdar, S.; Siriwardena, A.K. Superior mesenteric artery (sma) resection during pancreatectomy for malignant disease of the pancreas: A systematic review. *HPB* **2017**, *19*, 483–490. [CrossRef] [PubMed]
19. Kitagawa, H.; Ohta, T.; Tajima, H.; Nakagawara, H.; Makino, I.; Takamura, H.; Tani, T.; Kayahara, M. En bloc resection including the superior mesenteric artery and vein of locally advanced pancreatic carcinomas. *Nihon Geka Gakkai Zasshi* **2011**, *112*, 164–169.
20. Yekebas, E.F.; Bogoevski, D.; Cataldegirmen, G.; Kunze, C.; Marx, A.; Vashist, Y.K.; Schurr, P.G.; Liebl, L.; Thieltges, S.; Gawad, K.A.; et al. En bloc vascular resection for locally advanced pancreatic malignancies infiltrating major blood vessels: Perioperative outcome and long-term survival in 136 patients. *Ann. Surg.* **2008**, *247*, 300–309. [CrossRef]
21. Inoue, Y.; Saiura, A.; Yoshioka, R.; Ono, Y.; Takahashi, M.; Arita, J.; Takahashi, Y.; Koga, R. Pancreatoduodenectomy with systematic mesopancreas dissection using a supracolic anterior artery-first approach. *Ann. Surg.* **2015**, *262*, 1092–1101. [CrossRef]
22. Bachellier, P.; Addeo, P.; Faitot, F.; Nappo, G.; Dufour, P. Pancreatectomy with arterial resection for pancreatic adenocarcinoma: How can it be done safely and with which outcomes?: A single institution's experience with 118 patients. *Ann. Surg.* **2020**, *271*, 932–940. [CrossRef]
23. Loos, M.; Kester, T.; Klaiber, U.; Mihaljevic, A.L.; Mehrabi, A.; Muller-Stich, B.M.; Diener, M.K.; Schneider, M.A.; Berchtold, C.; Hinz, U.; et al. Arterial resection in pancreatic cancer surgery: Effective after a learning curve. *Ann. Surg.* **2020**. Jun 12. [CrossRef] [PubMed]
24. Li, B.; Chen, F.Z.; Ge, X.H.; Cai, M.Z.; Jiang, J.S.; Li, J.P.; Lu, S.H. Pancreatoduodenectomy with vascular reconstruction in treating carcinoma of the pancreatic head. *Hepatobiliary Pancreat. Dis. Int.* **2004**, *3*, 612–615. [PubMed]
25. Boggi, U.; Del Chiaro, M.; Croce, C.; Vistoli, F.; Signori, S.; Moretto, C.; Amorese, G.; Mazzeo, S.; Cappelli, C.; Campani, D.; et al. Prognostic implications of tumor invasion or adhesion to peripancreatic vessels in resected pancreatic cancer. *Surgery* **2009**, *146*, 869–881. [CrossRef]
26. Martin, R.C., 2nd; Scoggins, C.R.; Egnatashvili, V.; Staley, C.A.; McMasters, K.M.; Kooby, D.A. Arterial and venous resection for pancreatic adenocarcinoma: Operative and long-term outcomes. *Arch. Surg.* **2009**, *144*, 154–159. [CrossRef] [PubMed]
27. Bockhorn, M.; Burdelski, C.; Bogoevski, D.; Sgourakis, G.; Yekebas, E.F.; Izbicki, J.R. Arterial en bloc resection for pancreatic carcinoma. *Br. J. Surg.* **2011**, *98*, 86–92. [CrossRef]
28. Rehders, A.; Stoecklein, N.H.; Güray, A.; Riediger, R.; Alexander, A.; Knoefel, W.T. Vascular invasion in pancreatic cancer: Tumor biology or tumor topography? *Surgery* **2012**, *152*, S143–S151. [CrossRef] [PubMed]
29. Gong, Y.; Zhang, L.; He, T.; Ding, J.; Zhang, H.; Chen, G.; Zhang, D.; Wu, Z.; Chen, Q.; Fan, H.; et al. Pancreaticoduodenectomy combined with vascular resection and reconstruction for patients with locally advanced pancreatic cancer: A multicenter, retrospective analysis. *PLoS ONE* **2013**, *8*, e70340.
30. Sgroi, M.D.; Narayan, R.R.; Lane, J.S.; Demirjian, A.; Kabutey, N.K.; Fujitani, R.M.; Imagawa, D.K. Vascular reconstruction plays an important role in the treatment of pancreatic adenocarcinoma. *J. Vasc. Surg.* **2015**, *61*, 475–480. [CrossRef]
31. Glebova, N.O.; Hicks, C.W.; Tosoian, J.J.; Piazza, K.M.; Abularrage, C.J.; Schulick, R.D.; Wolfgang, C.L.; Black, J.H., 3rd. Outcomes of arterial resection during pancreatectomy for tumor. *J. Vasc. Surg.* **2016**, *63*, 722–729.e1. [CrossRef] [PubMed]
32. Perinel, J.; Nappo, G.; El Bechwaty, M.; Walter, T.; Hervieu, V.; Valette, P.J.; Feugier, P.; Adham, M. Locally advanced pancreatic duct adenocarcinoma: Pancreatectomy with planned arterial resection based on axial arterial encasement. *Langenbeck's Arch. Surg.* **2016**, *401*, 1131–1142. [CrossRef] [PubMed]
33. Tee, M.C.; Krajewski, A.C.; Groeschl, R.T.; Farnell, M.B.; Nagorney, D.M.; Kendrick, M.L.; Cleary, S.P.; Smoot, R.L.; Croome, K.P.; Truty, M.J. Indications and perioperative outcomes for pancreatectomy with arterial resection. *J. Am. Coll. Surg.* **2018**, *227*, 255–269. [CrossRef]
34. Loveday, B.P.T.; Zilbert, N.; Serrano, P.E.; Tomiyama, K.; Tremblay, A.; Fox, A.M.; Segedi, M.; O'Malley, M.; Borgida, A.; Bianco, T.; et al. Neoadjuvant therapy and major arterial resection for potentially reconstructable arterial involvement by stage 3 adenocarcinoma of the pancreas. *HPB* **2019**, *21*, 643–652. [CrossRef]
35. Westermark, S.; Rangelova, E.; Ansorge, C.; Lundell, L.; Segersvärd, R.; Del Chiaro, M. Cattell-braasch maneuver combined with local hypothermia during superior mesenteric artery resection in pancreatectomy. *Langenbeck's Arch. Surg.* **2016**, *401*, 1241–1247. [CrossRef] [PubMed]
36. Tempero, M.A.; Malafa, M.P.; Chiorean, E.G.; Czito, B.; Scaife, C.; Narang, A.K.; Fountzilas, C.; Wolpin, B.M.; Al-Hawary, M.; Asbun, H.; et al. Pancreatic adenocarcinoma, version 1. 2019. *J. Natl. Compr. Cancer Netw.* **2019**, *17*, 202–210. [CrossRef] [PubMed]

37. Amano, R.; Kimura, K.; Nakata, B.; Yamazoe, S.; Motomura, H.; Yamamoto, A.; Tanaka, S.; Hirakawa, K. Pancreatectomy with major arterial resection after neoadjuvant chemoradiotherapy gemcitabine and s-1 and concurrent radiotherapy for locally advanced unresectable pancreatic cancer. *Surgery* **2015**, *158*, 191–200. [CrossRef] [PubMed]
38. Miyazaki, M.; Yoshitomi, H.; Takano, S.; Shimizu, H.; Kato, A.; Yoshidome, H.; Furukawa, K.; Takayashiki, T.; Kuboki, S.; Suzuki, D.; et al. Combined hepatic arterial resection in pancreatic resections for locally advanced pancreatic cancer. *Langenbeck's Arch. Surg.* **2017**, *402*, 447–456. [CrossRef]
39. Wang, C.; Wu, H.; Xiong, J.; Zhou, F.; Tao, J.; Liu, T.; Zhao, G.; Gou, S. Pancreaticoduodenectomy with vascular resection for local advanced pancreatic head cancer: A single center retrospective study. *J. Gastrointest. Surg.* **2008**, *12*, 2183–2190. [CrossRef]
40. Desaki, R.; Mizuno, S.; Tanemura, A.; Kishiwada, M.; Murata, Y.; Azumi, Y.; Kuriyama, N.; Usui, M.; Sakurai, H.; Tabata, M.; et al. A new surgical technique of pancreaticoduodenectomy with splenic artery resection for ductal adenocarcinoma of the pancreatic head and/or body invading splenic artery: Impact of the balance between surgical radicality and qol to avoid total pancreatectomy. *Biomed. Res. Int.* **2014**, *2014*, 219038. [CrossRef] [PubMed]
41. Appleby, L.H. The coeliac axis in the expansion of the operation for gastric carcinoma. *Cancer* **1953**, *6*, 704–707. [CrossRef]
42. Hishinuma, S.; Ogata, Y.; Matsui, J.; Ozawa, I.; Inada, T.; Shimizu, H.; Eckhauser, F. Two cases of cancer of the pancreatic body undergoing gastric preservation with distal pancreatectomy combined with resection of the celiac axis. *Jpn. J. Gastroenterol. Surg.* **1991**, *24*, 2782–2786. [CrossRef]
43. Kondo, S.; Katoh, H.; Hirano, S.; Ambo, Y.; Tanaka, E.; Okushiba, S.; Morikawa, T. Results of radical distal pancreatectomy with en bloc resection of the celiac artery for locally advanced cancer of the pancreatic body. *Langenbeck's Arch. Surg.* **2003**, *388*, 101–106.
44. Konishi, M.; Kinoshita, T.; Nakagori, T.; Inoue, K.; Oda, T.; Kimata, T.; Kikuchi, H.; Ryu, M. Distal pancreatectomy with resection of the celiac axis and reconstruction of the hepatic artery for carcinoma of the body and tail of the pancreas. *J. Hepato-Biliary-Pancreat. Surg.* **2000**, *7*, 183–187. [CrossRef] [PubMed]
45. Kimura, W.; Han, I.; Furukawa, Y.; Sunami, E.; Futakawa, N.; Inoue, T.; Shinkai, H.; Zhao, B.; Muto, T.; Makuuchi, M.; et al. Appleby operation for carcinoma of the body and tail of the pancreas. *Hepato-Gastroenterol.* **1997**, *44*, 387–393.
46. Ozaki, H.; Kinoshita, T.; Kosuge, T.; Yamamoto, J.; Shimada, K.; Inoue, K.; Koyama, Y.; Mukai, K. An aggressive therapeutic approach to carcinoma of the body and tail of the pancreas. *Cancer* **1996**, *77*, 2240–2245. [CrossRef]
47. Mayumi, T.; Nimura, Y.; Kamiya, J.; Kondo, S.; Nagino, M.; Kanai, M.; Miyachi, M.; Hamaguchi, K.; Hayakawa, N. Distal pancreatectomy with en bloc resection of the celiac artery for carcinoma of the body and tail of the pancreas. *Int. J. Pancreatol.* **1997**, *22*, 15–21. [CrossRef] [PubMed]
48. Hirano, S.; Kondo, S.; Hara, T.; Ambo, Y.; Tanaka, E.; Shichinohe, T.; Suzuki, O.; Hazama, K. Distal pancreatectomy with en bloc celiac axis resection for locally advanced pancreatic body cancer: Long-term results. *Ann. Surg.* **2007**, *246*, 46–51. [CrossRef] [PubMed]
49. Klompmaker, S.; Peters, N.A.; van Hilst, J.; Bassi, C.; Boggi, U.; Busch, O.R.; Niesen, W.; Van Gulik, T.M.; Javed, A.A.; Kleeff, J.; et al. Outcomes and risk score for distal pancreatectomy with celiac axis resection (dp-car): An international multicenter analysis. *Ann. Surg. Oncol.* **2019**, *26*, 772–781. [CrossRef]
50. Nakamura, T.; Hirano, S.; Noji, T.; Asano, T.; Okamura, K.; Tsuchikawa, T.; Murakami, S.; Kurashima, Y.; Ebihara, Y.; Nakanishi, Y.; et al. Distal pancreatectomy with en bloc celiac axis resection (modified appleby procedure) for locally advanced pancreatic body cancer: A single-center review of 80 consecutive patients. *Ann. Surg. Oncol.* **2016**, *23*, 969–975. [CrossRef] [PubMed]
51. Ocuin, L.M.; Miller-Ocuin, J.L.; Novak, S.M.; Bartlett, D.L.; Marsh, J.W.; Tsung, A.; Lee, K.K.; Hogg, M.E.; Zeh, H.J.; Zureikat, A.H. Robotic and open distal pancreatectomy with celiac axis resection for locally advanced pancreatic body tumors: A single institutional assessment of perioperative outcomes and survival. *HPB* **2016**, *18*, 835–842. [CrossRef] [PubMed]
52. Yoshiya, S.; Fukuzawa, K.; Inokuchi, S.; Kosai-Fujimoto, Y.; Sanefuji, K.; Iwaki, K.; Motohiro, A.; Itoh, S.; Harada, N.; Ikegami, T.; et al. Efficacy of neoadjuvant chemotherapy in distal pancreatectomy with en bloc celiac axis resection (dp-car) for locally advanced pancreatic cancer. *J. Gastrointest. Surg.* **2019**, *24*, 1605–1611. [CrossRef] [PubMed]
53. Yamamoto, T.; Satoi, S.; Kawai, M.; Motoi, F.; Sho, M.; Uemura, K.I.; Matsumoto, I.; Honda, G.; Okada, K.I.; Akahori, T.; et al. Is distal pancreatectomy with en-bloc celiac axis resection effective for patients with locally advanced pancreatic ductal adenocarcinoma? -multicenter surgical group study. *Pancreatology* **2018**, *18*, 106–113. [CrossRef] [PubMed]
54. Beane, J.D.; House, M.G.; Pitt, S.C.; Kilbane, E.M.; Hall, B.L.; Parmar, A.D.; Riall, T.S.; Pitt, H.A. Distal pancreatectomy with celiac axis resection: What are the added risks? *HPB* **2015**, *17*, 777–784. [CrossRef] [PubMed]
55. Okada, K.I.; Kawai, M.; Hirono, S.; Miyazawa, M.; Kitahata, Y.; Ueno, M.; Hayami, S.; Shimokawa, T.; Yamaue, H. Ischemic gastropathy after distal pancreatectomy with en bloc celiac axis resection for pancreatic body cancer. *Langenbeck's Arch. Surg.* **2018**, *403*, 561–571. [CrossRef] [PubMed]
56. Ueda, A.; Sakai, N.; Yoshitomi, H.; Furukawa, K.; Takayashiki, T.; Kuboki, S.; Takano, S.; Suzuki, D.; Kagawa, S.; Mishima, T.; et al. Is hepatic artery coil embolization useful in distal pancreatectomy with en bloc celiac axis resection for locally advanced pancreatic cancer? *World J. Surg. Oncol.* **2019**, *17*, 124. [CrossRef] [PubMed]
57. Truty, M.J.; Colglazier, J.J.; Mendes, B.C.; Nagorney, D.M.; Bower, T.C.; Smoot, R.L.; DeMartino, R.R.; Cleary, S.P.; Oderich, G.S.; Kendrick, M.L. En bloc celiac axis resection for pancreatic cancer: Classification of anatomical variants based on tumor extent. *J. Am. Coll. Surg.* **2020**, *231*, 8–29. [CrossRef] [PubMed]

58. Yoshitomi, H.; Sakai, N.; Kagawa, S.; Takano, S.; Ueda, A.; Kato, A.; Furukawa, K.; Takayashiki, T.; Kuboki, S.; Miyzaki, M.; et al. Feasibility and safety of distal pancreatectomy with en bloc celiac axis resection (dp-car) combined with neoadjuvant therapy for borderline resectable and unresectable pancreatic body/tail cancer. *Langenbeck's Arch. Surg.* **2019**, *404*, 451–458. [CrossRef]
59. Sato, T.; Inoue, Y.; Takahashi, Y.; Mise, Y.; Ishizawa, T.; Tanakura, K.; Ito, H.; Saiura, A. Distal pancreatectomy with celiac axis resection combined with reconstruction of the left gastric artery. *J. Gastrointest. Surg.* **2017**, *21*, 910–917. [CrossRef]
60. Oba, A.; Inoue, Y.; Sato, T.; Ono, Y.; Mise, Y.; Ito, H.; Ishizawa, T.; Takahashi, Y.; Saiura, A. Impact of indocyanine green-fluorescence imaging on distal pancreatectomy with celiac axis resection combined with reconstruction of the left gastric artery. *HPB* **2019**, *21*, 619–625. [CrossRef]
61. Rockey, E.W. Total pancreatectomy for carcinoma: Case report. *Ann. Surg.* **1943**, *118*, 603–611. [CrossRef] [PubMed]
62. ReMine, W.H.; Priestley, J.T.; Judd, E.S.; King, J.N. Total pancreatectomy. *Ann. Surg.* **1970**, *172*, 595–604. [CrossRef] [PubMed]
63. Ross, D.E. Cancer of the pancreas; a plea for total pancreatectomy. *Am. J. Surg.* **1954**, *87*, 20–33. [CrossRef]
64. Warren, K.W.; Poulantzas, J.K.; Kune, G.A. Life after total pancreatectomy for chronic pancreatitis: Clinical study of eight cases. *Ann. Surg.* **1966**, *164*, 830–834. [CrossRef]
65. Nakao, A.; Ichihara, T.; Nonami, T.; Harada, A.; Koshikawa, T.; Nakashima, N.; Nagura, H.; Takagi, H. Clinicohistopathologic and immunohistochemical studies of intrapancreatic development of carcinoma of the head of the pancreas. *Ann. Surg.* **1989**, *209*, 181–187. [CrossRef]
66. Ihse, I.; Anderson, H.; Andrén, S. Total pancreatectomy for cancer of the pancreas: Is it appropriate? *World J. Surg.* **1996**, *20*, 288–293; discussion 294. [CrossRef]
67. Scholten, L.; Stoop, T.F.; Del Chiaro, M.; Busch, O.R.; van Eijck, C.; Molenaar, I.Q.; de Vries, J.H.; Besselink, M.G. Dutch Pancreatic Cancer, G. Systematic review of functional outcome and quality of life after total pancreatectomy. *Br. J. Surg.* **2019**, *106*, 1735–1746. [CrossRef]
68. Dresler, C.M.; Fortner, J.G.; McDermott, K.; Bajorunas, D.R. Metabolic consequences of (regional) total pancreatectomy. *Ann. Surg.* **1991**, *214*, 131–140. [CrossRef]
69. Hata, T.; Ishida, M.; Motoi, F.; Sakata, N.; Yoshimatsu, G.; Naitoh, T.; Katayose, Y.; Egawa, S.; Unno, M. Clinical characteristics and risk factors for the development of postoperative hepatic steatosis after total pancreatectomy. *Pancreas* **2016**, *45*, 362–369. [CrossRef] [PubMed]
70. Reddy, S.; Wolfgang, C.L.; Cameron, J.L.; Eckhauser, F.; Choti, M.A.; Schulick, R.D.; Edil, B.H.; Pawlik, T.M. Total pancreatectomy for pancreatic adenocarcinoma: Evaluation of morbidity and long-term survival. *Ann. Surg.* **2009**, *250*, 282–287. [CrossRef]
71. Hartwig, W.; Gluth, A.; Hinz, U.; Koliogiannis, D.; Strobel, O.; Hackert, T.; Werner, J.; Büchler, M.W. Outcomes after extended pancreatectomy in patients with borderline resectable and locally advanced pancreatic cancer. *Br J Surg.* **2016**, *103*, 1683–1694. [CrossRef]
72. Hartwig, W.; Gluth, A.; Hinz, U.; Bergmann, F.; Spronk, P.E.; Hackert, T.; Werner, J.; Büchler, M.W. Total pancreatectomy for primary pancreatic neoplasms: Renaissance of an unpopular operation. *Ann. Surg.* **2015**, *261*, 537–546. [CrossRef]
73. Müller, M.W.; Friess, H.; Kleeff, J.; Dahmen, R.; Wagner, M.; Hinz, U.; Breisch-Girbig, D.; Ceyhan, G.O.; Büchler, M.W. Is there still a role for total pancreatectomy? *Ann. Surg.* **2007**, *246*, 966–974, discussion 974–965. [CrossRef]
74. Brooks, J.R.; Brooks, D.C.; Levine, J.D. Total pancreatectomy for ductal cell carcinoma of the pancreas. An update. *Ann. Surg.* **1989**, *209*, 405–410. [CrossRef]
75. Launois, B.; Franci, J.; Bardaxoglou, E.; Ramee, M.P.; Paul, J.L.; Malledant, Y.; Campion, J.P. Total pancreatectomy for ductal adenocarcinoma of the pancreas with special reference to resection of the portal vein and multicentric cancer. *World J. Surg.* **1993**, *17*, 122–126, discussion 126–127. [CrossRef] [PubMed]
76. Schmidt, C.M.; Glant, J.; Winter, J.M.; Kennard, J.; Dixon, J.; Zhao, Q.; Howard, T.J.; Madura, J.A.; Nakeeb, A.; Pitt, H.A.; et al. Total pancreatectomy (r0 resection) improves survival over subtotal pancreatectomy in isolated neck margin positive pancreatic adenocarcinoma. *Surgery* **2007**, *142*, 572–578; discussion 578–580. [CrossRef] [PubMed]
77. Nathan, H.; Wolfgang, C.L.; Edil, B.H.; Choti, M.A.; Herman, J.M.; Schulick, R.D.; Cameron, J.L.; Pawlik, T.M. Peri-operative mortality and long-term survival after total pancreatectomy for pancreatic adenocarcinoma: A population-based perspective. *J. Surg. Oncol.* **2009**, *99*, 87–92. [CrossRef] [PubMed]
78. Satoi, S.; Murakami, Y.; Motoi, F.; Sho, M.; Matsumoto, I.; Uemura, K.; Kawai, M.; Kurata, M.; Yanagimoto, H.; Yamamoto, T.; et al. Reappraisal of total pancreatectomy in 45 patients with pancreatic ductal adenocarcinoma in the modern era using matched-pairs analysis: Multicenter study group of pancreatobiliary surgery in japan. *Pancreas* **2016**, *45*, 1003–1009. [CrossRef]
79. Johnston, W.C.; Hoen, H.M.; Cassera, M.A.; Newell, P.H.; Hammill, C.W.; Hansen, P.D.; Wolf, R.F. Total pancreatectomy for pancreatic ductal adenocarcinoma: Review of the national cancer data base. *HPB* **2016**, *18*, 21–28. [CrossRef]
80. Xiong, J.; Wei, A.; Ke, N.; He, D.; Chian, S.K.; Wei, Y.; Hu, W.; Liu, X. A case-matched comparison study of total pancreatectomy versus pancreaticoduodenectomy for patients with pancreatic ductal adenocarcinoma. *Int. J. Surg.* **2017**, *48*, 134–141. [CrossRef] [PubMed]
81. Passeri, M.J.; Baker, E.H.; Siddiqui, I.A.; Templin, M.A.; Martinie, J.B.; Vrochides, D.; Iannitti, D.A. Total compared with partial pancreatectomy for pancreatic adenocarcinoma: Assessment of resection margin, readmission rate, and survival from the U.S. National cancer database. *Curr. Oncol.* **2019**, *26*, e346–e356. [CrossRef]

82. Hashimoto, D.; Mizuma, M.; Kumamaru, H.; Miyata, H.; Chikamoto, A.; Igarashi, H.; Itoi, T.; Egawa, S.; Kodama, Y.; Satoi, S.; et al. Risk model for severe postoperative complications after total pancreatectomy based on a nationwide clinical database. *Br. J. Surg.* **2020**, *107*, 734–742. [CrossRef]
83. Stoop, T.F.; Ateeb, Z.; Ghorbani, P.; Scholten, L.; Arnelo, U.; Besselink, M.G.; Del Chiaro, M. Surgical outcomes after total pancreatectomy: A high-volume center experience. *Ann. Surg. Oncol.* **2020**, *28*, 1543–1551. [CrossRef]
84. Stoop, T.F.; Ateeb, Z.; Ghorbani, P.; Scholten, L.; Arnelo, U.; Besselink, M.G.; Del Chiaro, M. Impact of endocrine and exocrine insufficiency on quality of life after total pancreatectomy. *Ann. Surg. Oncol.* **2020**, *27*, 587–596. [CrossRef] [PubMed]
85. Wu, W.; Dodson, R.; Makary, M.A.; Weiss, M.J.; Hirose, K.; Cameron, J.L.; Ahuja, N.; Pawlik, T.M.; Wolfgang, C.L.; He, J. A contemporary evaluation of the cause of death and long-term quality of life after total pancreatectomy. *World J. Surg.* **2016**, *40*, 2513–2518. [CrossRef] [PubMed]
86. Pulvirenti, A.; Pea, A.; Rezaee, N.; Gasparini, C.; Malleo, G.; Weiss, M.J.; Cameron, J.L.; Wolfgang, C.L.; He, J.; Salvia, R. Perioperative outcomes and long-term quality of life after total pancreatectomy. *Br. J. Surg.* **2019**, *106*, 1819–1828. [CrossRef] [PubMed]
87. Truty, M.J.; Kendrick, M.L.; Nagorney, D.M.; Smoot, R.L.; Cleary, S.P.; Graham, R.P.; Goenka, A.H.; Hallemeier, C.L.; Haddock, M.G.; Harmsen, W.S.; et al. Factors predicting response, perioperative outcomes, and survival following total neoadjuvant therapy for borderline/locally advanced pancreatic cancer. *Ann. Surg.* **2021**, *273*, 341–349. [CrossRef]
88. Diener, M.K.; Mihaljevic, A.L.; Strobel, O.; Loos, M.; Schmidt, T.; Schneider, M.; Berchtold, C.; Mehrabi, A.; Muller-Stich, B.P.; Jiang, K.; et al. Periarterial divestment in pancreatic cancer surgery. *Surgery* **2020**. Oct 5. [CrossRef] [PubMed]
89. Cai, B.; Lu, Z.; Neoptolemos, J.P.; Diener, M.K.; Li, M.; Yin, L.; Gao, Y.; Wei, J.; Chen, J.; Guo, F.; et al. Sub-adventitial divestment technique for resecting artery-involved pancreatic cancer: A retrospective cohort study. *Langenbeck's Arch. Surg.* **2021**. [CrossRef]
90. Sabater, L.; Cugat, E.; Serrablo, A.; Suarez-Artacho, G.; Diez-Valladares, L.; Santoyo-Santoyo, J.; Martín-Pérez, E.; Ausania, F.; Lopez-Ben, S.; Jover-Navalon, J.M.; et al. Does the artery-first approach improve the rate of r0 resection in pancreatoduodenectomy?: A multicenter, randomized, controlled trial. *Annals of surgery* **2019**, *270*, 738–746. [CrossRef]
91. Habib, J.R.; Kinny-Köster, B.; van Oosten, F.; Javed, A.A.; Cameron, J.L.; Lafaro, K.J.; Burkhart, R.A.; Burns, W.R.; He, J.; Thompson, E.D.; et al. Periadventitial dissection of the superior mesenteric artery for locally advanced pancreatic cancer: Surgical planning with the "halo sign" and "string sign". *Surgery* **2020**. [CrossRef] [PubMed]
92. Del Chiaro, M.; Schulick, R.D. Commentary on: Divestment or skeletonization of the SMA or the hepatic artery for locally advanced pancreatic ductal cancer after neoadjuvant therapy. *Surgery* **2020**. [CrossRef] [PubMed]
93. Kim, P.T.; Wei, A.C.; Atenafu, E.G.; Cavallucci, D.; Cleary, S.P.; Moulton, C.A.; Greig, P.D.; Gallinger, S.; Serra, S.; McGilvray, I.D. Planned versus unplanned portal vein resections during pancreaticoduodenectomy for adenocarcinoma. *Br. J. Surg.* **2013**, *100*, 1349–1356. [CrossRef] [PubMed]
94. Oba, A.; Ito, H.; Ono, Y.; Sato, T.; Mise, Y.; Inoue, Y.; Takahashi, Y.; Saiura, A. Regional pancreatoduodenectomy versus standard pancreatoduodenectomy with portal vein resection for pancreatic ductal adenocarcinoma with portal vein invasion. *BJS Open* **2020**, *4*, 438–448. [CrossRef]
95. Del Chiaro, M.; Schulick, R.D. Use of total pancreatectomy and preoperative radiotherapy in patients undergoing pancreatectomy with artery resection. *J. Am. Coll. Surg.* **2019**, *228*, 131. [CrossRef] [PubMed]
96. Del Chiaro, M.; Rangelova, E.; Segersvärd, R.; Arnelo, U. Are there still indications for total pancreatectomy? *Updates Surg.* **2016**, *68*, 257–263. [CrossRef] [PubMed]
97. Ando, N.; Kato, H.; Igaki, H.; Shinoda, M.; Ozawa, S.; Shimizu, H.; Nakamura, T.; Yabusaki, H.; Aoyama, N.; Kurita, A.; et al. A randomized trial comparing postoperative adjuvant chemotherapy with cisplatin and 5-fluorouracil versus preoperative chemotherapy for localized advanced squamous cell carcinoma of the thoracic esophagus (jcog9907). *Ann. Surg. Oncol.* **2012**, *19*, 68–74. [CrossRef]
98. Fokas, E.; Allgäuer, M.; Polat, B.; Klautke, G.; Grabenbauer, G.G.; Fietkau, R.; Kuhnt, T.; Staib, L.; Brunner, T.; Grosu, A.L.; et al. Randomized phase ii trial of chemoradiotherapy plus induction or consolidation chemotherapy as total neoadjuvant therapy for locally advanced rectal cancer: Cao/aro/aio-12. *J. Clin. Oncol.* **2019**, *37*, 3212–3222. [CrossRef]
99. Kasi, A.; Abbasi, S.; Handa, S.; Al-Rajabi, R.; Saeed, A.; Baranda, J.; Sun, W. Total neoadjuvant therapy vs standard therapy in locally advanced rectal cancer: A systematic review and meta-analysis. *JAMA Netw. Open* **2020**, *3*, e2030097. [CrossRef]
100. Murphy, J.E.; Wo, J.Y.; Ryan, D.P.; Clark, J.W.; Jiang, W.; Yeap, B.Y.; Drapek, L.C.; Ly, L.; Baglini, C.V.; Blaszkowsky, L.S.; et al. Total neoadjuvant therapy with folfirinox in combination with losartan followed by chemoradiotherapy for locally advanced pancreatic cancer: A phase 2 clinical trial. *JAMA Oncol.* **2019**, *5*, 1020–1027. [CrossRef]
101. Jang, J.Y.; Han, Y.; Lee, H.; Kim, S.W.; Kwon, W.; Lee, K.H.; Oh, D.Y.; Chie, E.K.; Lee, J.M.; Heo, J.S.; et al. Oncological benefits of neoadjuvant chemoradiation with gemcitabine versus upfront surgery in patients with borderline resectable pancreatic cancer: A prospective, randomized, open-label, multicenter phase 2/3 trial. *Ann. Surg.* **2018**, *268*, 215–222. [CrossRef]
102. Unno, M.; Motoi, F.; Matsuyama, Y.; Satoi, S.; Matsumoto, I.; Aosasa, S.; Shirakawa, H.; Wada, K.; Fujii, T.; Yoshitomi, H.; et al. Randomized phase ii/iii trial of neoadjuvant chemotherapy with gemcitabine and s-1 versus upfront surgery for resectable pancreatic cancer (prep-02/jsap-05). *J. Clin. Oncol.* **2019**, *37*, 189. [CrossRef]
103. Uesaka, K.; Boku, N.; Fukutomi, A.; Okamura, Y.; Konishi, M.; Matsumoto, I.; Kaneoka, Y.; Shimizu, Y.; Nakamori, S.; Sakamoto, H.; et al. Adjuvant chemotherapy of s-1 versus gemcitabine for resected pancreatic cancer: A phase 3, open-label, randomised, non-inferiority trial (jaspac 01). *Lancet* **2016**, *388*, 248–257. [CrossRef]

104. Conroy, T.; Hammel, P.; Hebbar, M.; Ben Abdelghani, M.; Wei, A.C.; Raoul, J.L.; Choné, L.; Francois, E.; Artru, P.; Biagi, J.J.; et al. Folfirinox or gemcitabine as adjuvant therapy for pancreatic cancer. *N. Engl. J. Med.* **2018**, *379*, 2395–2406. [CrossRef] [PubMed]
105. Oettle, H.; Post, S.; Neuhaus, P.; Gellert, K.; Langrehr, J.; Ridwelski, K.; Schramm, H.; Fahlke, J.; Zuelke, C.; Burkart, C.; et al. Adjuvant chemotherapy with gemcitabine vs observation in patients undergoing curative-intent resection of pancreatic cancer: A randomized controlled trial. *JAMA* **2007**, *297*, 267–277. [CrossRef] [PubMed]
106. Neoptolemos, J.P.; Stocken, D.D.; Bassi, C.; Ghaneh, P.; Cunningham, D.; Goldstein, D.; Padbury, R.; Moore, M.J.; Gallinger, S.; Mariette, C.; et al. Adjuvant chemotherapy with fluorouracil plus folinic acid vs gemcitabine following pancreatic cancer resection: A randomized controlled trial. *JAMA* **2010**, *304*, 1073–1081. [CrossRef]

Article

Clinical Benefits of Conversion Surgery for Unresectable Pancreatic Ductal Adenocarcinoma: A Single-Institution, Retrospective Analysis

Yuko Mataki [1,*], Hiroshi Kurahara [1], Tetsuya Idichi [1], Kiyonori Tanoue [1], Yuto Hozaka [1], Yota Kawasaki [1], Satoshi Iino [1], Kosei Maemura [2], Hiroyuki Shinchi [3] and Takao Ohtsuka [1]

1. Department of Digestive Surgery, Breast and Thyroid Surgery, Graduate School of Medical and Dental Sciences, Kagoshima University, 8-35-1, Kagoshima 890-8520, Japan; h-krhr@m3.kufm.kagoshima-u.ac.jp (H.K.); k3352693@kadai.jp (T.I.); wilson@m.kufm.kagoshima-u.ac.jp (K.T.); yhozaka@kufm.kagoshima-u.ac.jp (Y.H.); k5968102@kadai.jp (Y.K.); iino@m2.kufm.kagoshima-u.ac.jp (S.I.); takao-o@kufm.kagoshima-u.ac.jp (T.O.)
2. Department of Digestive Surgery, Kagoshima Principal Hospital, Kagoshima 890-0055, Japan; maemura-k01@kch.kagoshima.jp
3. Department of health sciences, School of Medicine, Kagoshima University, Kagoshima 890-8520, Japan; shinchi@m.kufm.kagoshima-u.ac.jp
* Correspondence: mataki@m.kufm.kagoshima-u.ac.jp; Tel.: +81-99-275-5361; Fax: +81-99-265-7426

Simple Summary: Pancreatic ductal adenocarcinoma (PDAC) is a dismal disorder, but conversion surgery (CS) has provided possibilities of better prognosis for unresectable (UR-)PDAC. We retrospectively investigated the clinical benefits of CS in patients with UR-PDAC. We performed CS in 20 of the 398 UR-PDAC cases between 2006 and 2019(5.1%). Compared the overall survival (OS) period among patients undergoing CS, resectable (R), borderline resectable (BR), unresectable locally advanced cancer (UR-LA), and unresectable cancer with distant metastasis (UR-M) groups, the CS group had significantly better survival than R, BR, UR-LA, and UR-M groups (73.7, 32.7, 22.7, 15.7, and 8.8 months, respectively). Moreover, multivariate analysis revealed the presence of chemoraiotherapy and partial response/complete response in the Response Evaluation Criteria in Solid Tumors (RECIST) were statistically significant prognostic factors for OS among patients undergoing CS ($p = 0.004$ and 0.03, respectively). This study highlights importance of multidisciplinary treatment including CS for patients with UR-PDAC.

Abstract: Background: Unresectable pancreatic ductal adenocarcinoma (UR-PDAC) has a poor prognosis. Conversion surgery is considered a promising strategy for improving the prognosis of UR-PDAC. This study aimed to investigate the clinical benefits of conversion surgery in patients with UR-PDAC. Methods: We retrospectively evaluated patients with PDAC who were referred to our department for possible surgical resection between January 2006 and December 2019. Conversion surgery was performed only in patients with UR-PDAC who could expect R0 resection. We analyzed the prognostic factors for overall survival among patients who underwent conversion surgery. Results: Overall, 638 patients with advanced pancreatic cancer were enrolled in this study. According to resectability, resectable cancer (R) was present in 180 patients, borderline resectable cancer (BR) was present in 60 patients, unresectable locally advanced cancer (UR-LA) was present in 252 patients, and unresectable cancer with distant metastasis (UR-M) was present in 146 patients. Conversion surgery was performed in 20 of the 398 UR cases (5.1%). The median period between the initial therapy and conversion surgery was 15.5 months. According to the Response Evaluation Criteria in Solid Tumors (RECIST) evaluation, the treatment response was CR in one patient, PR in 13, SD in five, and PD in one. Downstaging was pathologically determined in all cases. According to the Evans grading system, grade I was observed in four patients (20%), grade IIb was observed in seven (35%), III was observed in seven (35%), and IV was observed in two (10%). We compared the overall survival period from initial treatment among patients undergoing conversion surgery; the median overall survival durations in the conversion surgery, R, BR, UR-LA, and UR-M groups were 73.7, 32.7, 22.7, 15.7, and 8.8 months, respectively. Multivariate analysis revealed that the presence or absence of chemoradiotherapy (CRT) and the RECIST partial response (PR)/complete response (CR) for the main tumor were statistically significant prognostic factors for overall survival among patients undergoing conversion surgery (p = 0.004 and 0.03, respectively). Conclusion: In UR-PDAC, it is important to perform multidisciplinary treatment, including CRT with conversion surgery.

Keywords: unresectable pancreatic ductal adenocarcinoma; conversion surgery; chemoradiotherapy

1. Introduction

Pancreatic ductal adenocarcinoma (PDAC) is a very dismal disease with a poor prognosis among malignant tumors in Japan [1]. Even in the United States, PDAC is the fourth leading cause of cancer-related deaths [2]. This disease has a 5-year survival rate of approximately 10%. Surgical resection is the only potentially curative therapy, but only 10–20% of patients with resectable PDAC are classified at the time of the initial diagnosis [3]. When we select the methodology of treatment for a patient with PDAC, the appropriate treatment is likely to decided based on the resectable classification rather than the stage classification. The National Comprehensive Cancer Network (NCCN) has proposed a resectable classification for PDAC and recommended optimal therapy based on each resectability [4]. Among them, pancreatic cancer patients with unresectable locally advanced cancer (UR-LA) and unresectable cancer with metastasis (UR-M) are recommended to receive chemotherapy if their performance status is good. Combination chemotherapy with fluorouracil, leucovorin, irinotecan, and oxaliplatin (FOLFIRINOX) or modified (mFOLFIRINOX), chemoradiation, gemcitabine plus nab-paclitaxel (PTX), and/or chemoradiation are listed as candidate regimens for chemotherapy. The Japanese Pancreas Society designed new and definite resectability criteria in 2019 based on the NCCN guideline [5]. Regarding resectable advanced pancreatic cancer, a prospective randomized trial in Japan compared surgical resection and chemoradiotherapy (CRT) after laparotomy was used to identify the localized pancreatic cancer invading the surrounding vasculature; this study showed that patients who underwent surgical resection had significantly longer survival than those treated with CRT alone [6].

In recent reports, multidisciplinary treatments, including surgical resection and chemotherapy or chemoradiation therapy, have improved the survival of patients with PDAC [7–9]. As for patients with resectable (R) PDAC, adjuvant chemotherapy has become standard even after curative resection [10,11]. Moreover, many studies have reported the effectiveness of neoadjuvant chemotherapy. In recent years, patients with UR-PDAC have been able to achieve treatment effects to be converted to surgical resection. This surgical strategy is called "conversion surgery". Therefore, several reports about conversion surgery have been published in selected patients with initially UR-PDAC, and the prognostic effect of conversion surgery has been reported [12–22]. However, it is unclear whether conversion surgery with a high treatment effect is truly advantageous in patients with UR-PDAC.

In this study, we aimed to clarify the clinical benefits and important factors of conversion surgery for patients with UR-PDAC who underwent CRT.

2. Methods

2.1. Ethics Statements

All research performed in studies involving human participants were according to discipline of the institutional research committee and with the 1964 Declaration of Helsinki. Written informed consent was obtained from all study participants.

2.2. Study Design and Patient Population

This retrospective study was performed using data from a prospective database. All patients with PDAC treated at the Department of Digestive Surgery, Breast and Thyroid Surgery, Kagoshima University between January 2006 and December 2019 were enrolled in our study. PDAC was diagnosed by cytology or pathology through endoscopic retrograde cholangiopancreatography or endoscopic ultrasound-guided fine-needle aspiration. PDAC progression was diagnosed using multidetector-row computed tomography, ethoxybenzyl-magnetic resonance imaging, and fluorine-18-2-deoxy-D-glucose positron emission tomography. All patients were divided into resectable cancer (R), borderline resectable cancer (BR), UR-LA, and UR-M, which was defined according to the NCCN Clinical Practice Guidelines version 2 from 2020 [4].

2.3. Therapy Method

The gemcitabine and S-1 (GS) regimen is as follows, that the daily dosage of S-1 chemotherapy was 60 mg/m^2 combined with 1000 mg/m^2 gemcitabine. Patients received gemcitabine intravenously on days 8 and 15 of a 21-day cycle and oral S-1, twice daily on days 1–14. The GEM plus nab-PTX regimen consisted of gemcitabine 1000 mg/m^2 and nab-PTX 125 mg/m^2 administered on days 1, 8, and 15, every 28 days. The modified FOLFIRINOX (m-FOLFIRINOX) regimen used in our study was the same as that of a Japanese phase II study and consisted of oxaliplatin at a dose of 85 mg/m^2, administered as a 2-h intravenous infusion, immediately followed by leucovorin at a dose of 200 mg/m^2, administered as a 2-h intravenous infusion, with the addition, after 30 min of irinotecan at a dose of 180 mg/m^2, administered as a 90-min intravenous infusion through a bypass line. This treatment was immediately followed by fluorouracil at a dose of 400 mg/m^2 administered via intravenous bolus, followed by a continuous intravenous infusion of 2400 mg/m^2 over a 46-h period, every 2 weeks. CRT regimens included hyper-fractionated accelerated radiotherapy administered with S-1 at 80 mg/m^2 for the first 21 days. A total of 50–58 Gy was administered in 40 fractions over 4 weeks. At 1 month after CRT completion, S-1 was administered for 2 weeks, followed by a 2 weeks period.

The GEM plus nab-PTX and FOLFIRINOX regimens were approved in Japan for the treatment of UR-PC in December 2014, and these regimens have been utilized since then.

2.4. Conversion Surgery

We discussed and decided the indication for conversion surgery for individual UR-PDAC patients at a multidisciplinary conference of pancreatic surgeons, medical oncologists, radiologists, and clinical pathologists. Among UR-PDAC patients who responded to various therapies, conversion surgery was permitted for only those who met the following conditions: patients showing adequate reduction of the main tumor, enabling complete removal inclusive of the major vessels and metastatic site, those with at least several months of local control, those with no metastasis, or those with controllable metastasis by surgical resection.

2.5. Adjuvant Chemotherapy

We basically consider adjuvant therapy after conversion surgery if the patient is in good condition. Furthermore, if new lesions are operable after conversion surgery, we consider additional resection for the lesions.

2.6. Assessment

The clinical treatment effect was assessed using RECIST version 1.1 [23], and the histologic assessment of the extent of response was evaluated using the Evans grading system [24]. R0 was defined as pathologically margin free in the resected specimen.

The Clavien–Dindo classification was used to evaluate postoperative complications [25]. Mortality was defined as death within 90 days after surgery.

2.7. Statistical Analysis

Associations between different categorical variables were properly assessed using the chi-square or Fisher exact test. Survival curves were estimated using the Kaplan–Meier method and analyzed using the log-rank test. Overall survival was calculated as the interval between initial treatment and death due to any cause (including death from other diseases), whereas progression-free survival was calculated as the interval between initial treatment and disease progression. The univariate Cox proportional hazard models were used to estimate the independent significant factors for the overall survival of patients with UR-PDAC. Relative risks were expressed as adjusted hazard ratios and corresponding 95% confidence intervals. Valuables with a p-value of < 0.05 on univariate analysis were calculated into the multivariate model. A p-value of < 0.05 was considered to be statistically significant. All statistical analyses were performed using SigmaPlot, version 12.5 for Windows (HULINKS, Inc., Tokyo, Japan).

3. Results

3.1. Patient Characteristics

During the above observation period, 638 patients were included. R was present in 180 patients, BR was present in 60, UR-LA was present in 252, and UR-M was present in 146. Overall, 398 consecutive patients with unresected pancreatic cancer were studied in terms of their unresectable status. Conversion surgery was performed in 20 patients (20/398, 5.0%; UR-LA, n = 9; UR-M, n = 11). The clinical characteristics of patients with and without conversion surgery are compared in Table 1.

Table 1. A comparison of the clinical characteristics between CS and non-CS patients.

Variables	Conversion Surgery		p-Value
	(+) (n = 20)	(−) (n = 378)	
age (years), median (range)	65 (44–83)	69 (33–87)	0.25
gender (M/F), n	(10/10)	(207/171)	0.656
tumor location (Ph/Pb,Pt), n	(14/6)	(218/160)	0.282
unresectability status (UR-LA vs UR-M), n	(9/11)	(243/135)	0.622
CEA, median (range) (U/mL)	3.4 (1.1–9.4)	4.0 (0.3–845)	0.51
CA19-9, median (range) (U/mL)	2577 (0.6–1985)	211 (0.6–50,000)	0.17
tumor size, median (range) (mm)	30 (18–50)	35 (8–116)	0.323
T(4/3), n	(16/4)	(332/46)	0.385
N(1/0), n	(7/13)	(136/252)	0.917
M(1/0), n	(11/9)	(197/181)	0.829

M, male; F, female; CS, conversion surgery; Ph, pancreatic head; Pb, pancreatic body; Pt, pancreatic tail; UR-LA, unresectable locally advanced cancer; UR-M, unresectable cancer with metastasis. T, N, and M were classified according to the Tumor-Node-Metastasis (TNM) classification.

There were no statistically significant differences in age, sex, the tumor location (pancreatic head versus (vs.) pancreatic body and tail), unresectability status (UR-LA vs. UR-M), serum carcinoembryonic antigen (CEA) level, cancer antigen 19-9 (CA19-9) level, tumor size, and T-, N-, and M-categories according to the Tumor-Node-Metastasis (TNM) classification before treatment between patients with and without conversion surgery.

The clinical characteristics of the 20 patients who underwent conversion surgery are shown in Figures 1 and 2 and Tables 2 and 3.

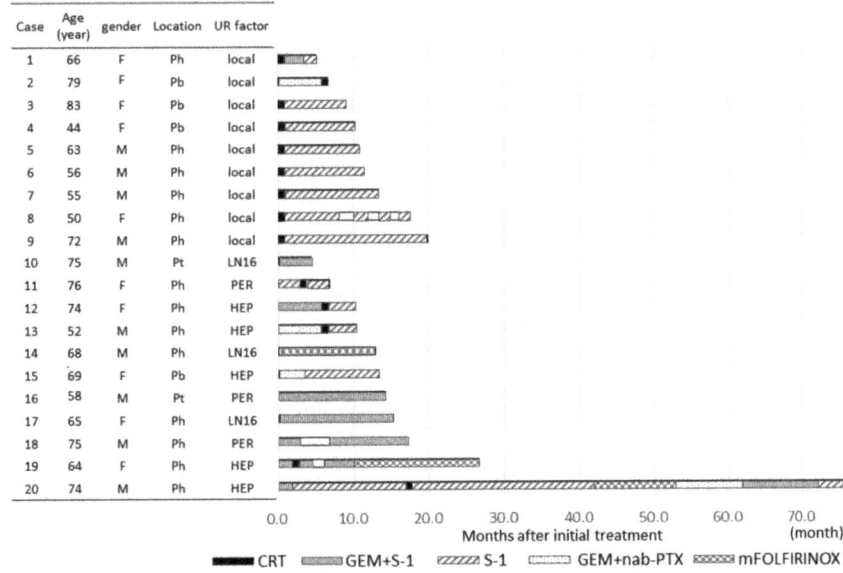

Figure 1. Clinical characteristics of the 20 patients who underwent conversion surgery including therapy before operation. Abbreviations: UR-LA, unresectable locally advanced cancer; UR-M, unresectable cancer with metastasis; M, male; F, female; Ph, pancreatic head; Pb, pancreatic body; Pt, pancreatic tail; LN16, para-aortic lymph node metastasis; PER, peritoneal disseminations; HEP, hepatic metastases; CRT, chemoradiotherapy; GEM, gemcitabine; S-1, oral administration of S-1; nabPXL, nab-paclitaxel; mFOLFIRINOX, modified FOLFIRINOX (combination chemotherapy with fluorouracil, leucovorin, irinotecan, and oxaliplatin).

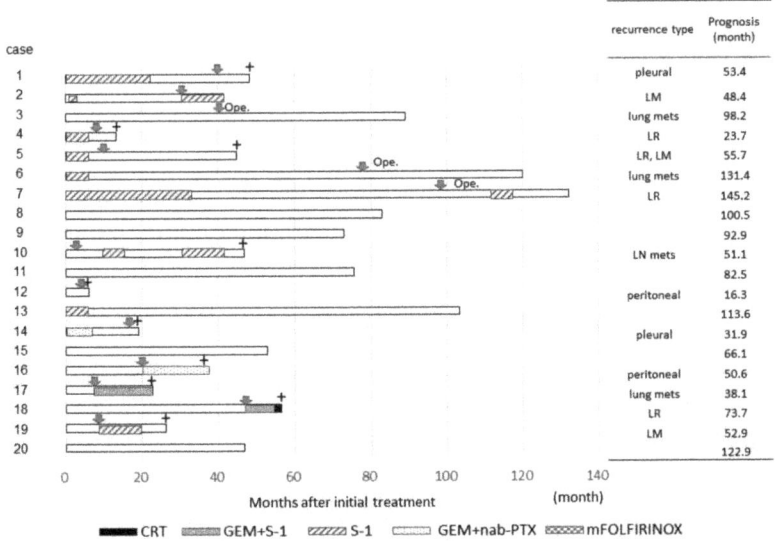

Figure 2. Clinical characteristics of the 20 patients who underwent conversion surgery including therapy after operation. Abbreviations: pleural, pleural disseminations; LM, liver metastasis; lung mets, lung metastasis; LR, local recurrence; peritoneal, peritoneal disseminations; directing arrow, recurrent or metastatic period; Ope, additional operation; +, period of death.

Table 2. Clinical characteristics of 20 patients who underwent conversion surgery.

Case	CEA (U/mL, Before)	CEA (U/mL, After)	CA19-9 (U/mL, Before)	CA19-9 (U/mL, After)	Tumor Size (mm, Before)	Tumor Size (mm, After)	Treatment Effect (RECIST)	Operative Method	Operative Time (min)	Bleeding Volume (mL)	Hospital Stay (Day)
1	2.4	2	25.9	9.9	27	13	PR	SSPPD	678	295	32
2	2.6	3.3	55.9	39	33	13	PR	DP	403	160	22
3	8	10.3	2789	24.9	32	23	PR	DP	373	260	50
4	1.1	5.1	81.4	34	50	50	SD	DP	438	1150	9
5	2.9	3.1	5103	19.9	23	12	PR	SSPPD + PVR	509	1250	11
6	9.4	4.4	92	10.9	29	13	PR	SSPPD	575	1220	23
7	6.4	2.4	253.5	49.6	24	9	PR	SSPPD + PVR	738	3010	16
8	2	2.7	9.2	11.4	42	10	PR	SSPPD	464	1030	10
9	1.5	1.6	1559	11.2	41	9	PR	SSPPD + PVR	574	1665	13
10	2.3	2.2	67.4	9	21	10	PR	DP	408	1075	11
11	3.4	3	20.6	7.4	30	16	PR	SSPPD + PVR	643	1390	9
12	2.5	3.2	1985	48.2	24	12	SD	SSPPD + HPR	841	2340	11
13	3.8	4.2	270	38.1	29	8	PR	SSPPD	729	2470	16
14	4.6	8	1515	16.4	41	34	PR	SSPPD + PVR	919	3600	47
15	5.1	3	1846	13.3	35	0	CR	DP	391	240	23
16	3.4	3.4	5.2	10.4	21	19	SD	DP	352	90	8
17	8	8.4	0.6	0.6	18	13	SD	SSPPD	623	1040	13
18	3	4.6	1047	10.7	32	11	PR	SSPPD	550	1020	8
19	1.8	2.1	516	17.8	30	9	PD	TP + PVR + HPR	613	460	14
20	2.9	9.5	330	99	24	25	SD	SSPPD + PVR	641	1695	13

UR-LA, unresectable locally advanced cancer; UR-M, unresectable cancer with metastasis; before, before initial therapy; after, after various therapy; PR, partial response; SD, stable disease; PR, partial response; SSPPD, substomach preserving pancreatoduodenectomy; DP, distal pancreatectomy; PVR, portal vein resection; HPR, hepatic partial resection; TP, total pancreatectomy.

Table 3. Clinical characteristics of 20 patients who underwent conversion surgery. Each stage was classified according to the TNM classification.

Case	Stage (Before)	Stage (After)	p-Stage	Pathological	Evans
1	3	3	2a	tub2	IIb
2	3	2a	2a	tub1	I
3	3	3	2b	tub2	III
4	3	2b	2a	muc	IIb
5	3	2a	2a	tub1	IIb
6	3	1a	1	por	III
7	3	3	2b	tub1	III
8	3	3	2a	similar to NEN	IIb
9	3	3	1	tub2	IIb
10	4	3	0	no neoplasm	IV
11	4	2a	2a	tub1	III
12	4	2a	2a	tub2	I
13	4	2b	1	a few	III
14	4	4	2a	tub2	IIb
15	4	0	0	no neoplasm	IV
16	4	2a	2b	tub1	I
17	4	2a	1	tub1	III
18	4	3	2b	tub2	III
19	4	4	4	tub2	IIb
20	4	3	2a	tub2	I

UR-LA, unresectable locally advanced cancer; UR-M, unresectable cancer with metastasis; before, before initial therapy; after, after various therapy; p-stage, pathological stage; tub1, tubular adenocarcinoma with high differentiation; tub2, tubular adenocarcinoma with moderate differentiation; por, poorly differentiated adenocarcinoma; muc, mucinous adenocarcinoma; NEN, neuroendocrine neoplasm; a few, a few neoplasms; Evans, Evans classification.

Among the 11 patients with UR-M, the type of metastasis at the time of initial diagnosis was hepatic metastasis in five patients, peritoneal dissemination in three, and para-aortic lymph node metastasis in three. Histological confirmation of the metastatic lesions was made in all patients with peritoneal disseminations and para-aortic lymph node metastasis, but this was not the case in three of five patients with liver metastasis.

The periods between initial treatment and conversion surgery were a median of 10.8 (range, 5.1–19.9) months in patients with UR-LA and median of 13.3 (range, 4.4–75.9) months in those with UR-M. There were no significant differences in the period between the groups.

The methods of therapy until conversion surgery varied, but CRT was performed in all patients with UR-LA. Among them, CRT was selected as the initial therapy in all patients except one (case 2, Figure 1), and CRT was performed after gemcitabine plus nab-PTX therapy as induction chemotherapy in the remaining case (case 2, Figure 1).

Chemotherapy of various types was performed in patients with UR-M, and additional CRT was carried out to perform local control in five of these cases. According to the RECIST evaluation, the treatment response after various therapies was complete response (CR) in one patient, partial response (PR) in 13, stable disease (SD) in five, and progressive disease (PD) in one.

The CA19-9 level at the time of conversion surgery was significantly lower than that at the time of initial diagnosis (median, 16.4 U/mL (range, 0.6–99) vs. median, 156 U/mL (range 0.6–1985), $p = 0.0065$), but the CEA level was not significantly different at the time between the initial diagnosis and conversion surgery ($p = 0.418$). The size of the main tumor at the time of conversion surgery was significantly smaller than that at the time of diagnosis (median, 13 mm (range, 0–50) vs. 30 mm (range, 18–50), $p < 0.001$). In cases 6, 17, and 19, the CEA level, CA19-9 level, and size of the main tumor after each therapy were reduced compared with those in the period before initial therapy, respectively (Table 2).

As for the operative method, substomach-preserving pancreaticoduodenectomy was performed in 13 patients, including concomitant portal vein resection (PVR) in six patients and hepatic resection (HPR) in one patient. Distal pancreatectomy and total pancreatectomy with PVR and HPR were performed in six patients and one patient, respectively (Table 2). The median operative time and volume of blood loss were 575 (range, 352–919) min and 1150 (range, 90–3600) mL, respectively. The median postoperative stay was 13 (range, 8–50) days. Major complications in the postoperative period (Clavien–Dindo classification class IIIa) occurred in three patients with chylous ascites, interstitial pneumonia, and intraabdominal abscess (cases 1, 3, and 14, respectively; Table 2); those complications caused patients' postoperative hospital stay to exceed 1 month. No perioperative mortality was observed. R0 resection of the main tumor was performed in all patients. Compared with before and after various therapies, clinical stage was downstaged in 13 cases, and the pathological stage was downstaged in 19 cases. Pathologically, tubular adenocarcinoma with high differentiation and tubular adenocarcinoma with moderate differentiation were the pathological forms of the residual tumor in six and eight cases, respectively. According to the Evans grading system, grade I was observed in four patients (20%), grade IIb in seven (35%), III in seven (35%), and IV in two (10%). A pathological CR was observed in two patients (cases 10 and 16, Table 2). The pathological assessment was difficult to perform in one case because of a few residual cancer cells (case 20, Table 2). In two patients who underwent hepatic resection combined with pancreatectomy, one patient had residual cancer cells in the resected liver.

3.2. Adjuvant Chemotherapy

Only eight patients (40%) received postoperative adjuvant chemotherapy, and S-1 was administered to all those patients. The reasons why 12 patients did not receive adjuvant chemotherapy were poorer performance status, severe perioperative complications, elderly age, and patient unwillingness. Recurrence occurred in 14 patients (70%) who underwent conversion surgery and received various therapies. The recurrence type varied: dissemination occurred in four patients, local recurrence, including metachronous double cancer, in three, liver metastasis in three, lung metastasis in three, and lymph node metastasis in one. Two patients with lung metastasis and one with metachronous double cancer of the remnant pancreas underwent additional resection of the metastatic lesion at 41, 78, and 97 months after conversion surgery, respectively (cases 3, 6 and 7; Figure 2).

We compared overall survival from the period of initial treatment between patients who underwent conversion surgery with UR-LA and those with UR-M and found no significant difference between these patient groups (median not reached vs. 52 months, $p = 0.20$) (Figure 3).

Moreover, we compared overall survival from the period from initial treatment between the conversion surgery, R, BR, UR-LA, and UR-M groups according to the NCCN guidelines. The median overall survival durations in the conversion surgery, R, BR, UR-LA, and UR-M groups were 73.7, 32.7, 22.7, 15.7, and 8.8 months, respectively (Figure 4). There were significant differences in the survival period between each group (p-value not shown).

By the univariate and multivariate logistic regression analyses, we researched the prognostic factors for overall survival among patients who underwent conversion surgery. Table 4 shows that the presence of CRT and RECIST PR/CR for the main tumor decreased the risk of death relative to the absence of CRT and RECIST SD/PD for the main tumor

(p = 0.002 and 0.015, respectively). Multivariate analysis revealed that the presence of CRT and RECIST PR/CR for the main tumor was a statistically significant prognostic factor for overall survival among patients undergoing conversion surgery (p = 0.004 and 0.03, respectively).

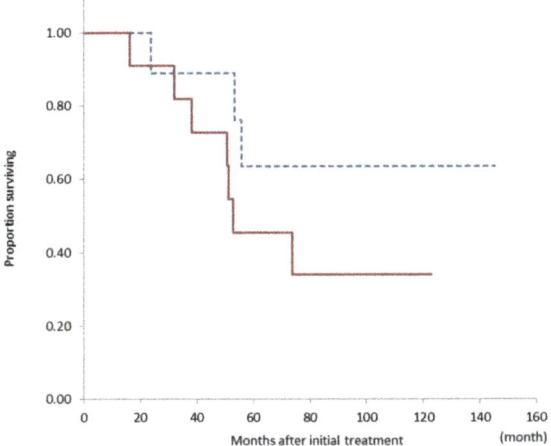

Figure 3. Comparison of the overall survival curves between patients with unresectable locally advanced cancer (dashed line, n = 9) and unresectable cancer with metastasis (solid line, n = 11) who underwent conversion surgery. There is no significant difference in overall survival between the groups (p = 0.20).

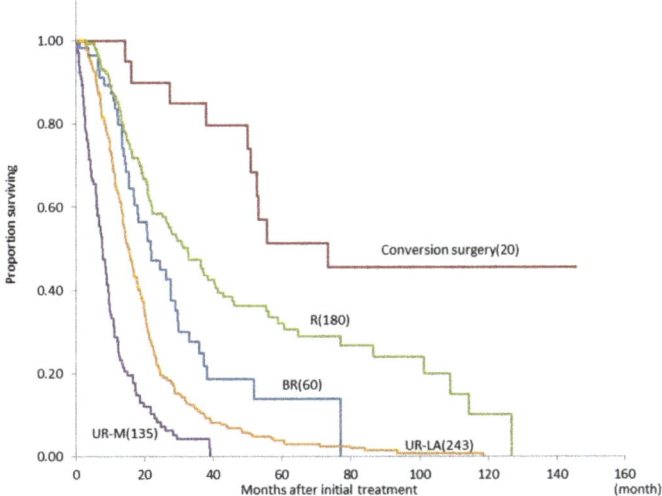

Figure 4. Comparison of the overall survival curves between patients with pancreatic ductal adenocarcinoma judged as R (n = 180), BR (n = 60), UR-LA (n = 243), or UR-M, (n = 135) according to the NCCN guideline, who underwent conversion surgery (n = 20). Abbreviations: R, resectable cancer; BR, borderline resectable cancer; UR-LA, unresectable locally advanced cancer; UR-M, unresectable cancer with metastasis; NCCN, National Comprehensive Cancer Network.

Table 4. Predictive factors for the overall survival of patients with unresectable pancreatic cancer (univariate and multivariate logistic regression analyses).

Variables	Univariate Analysis			Multivariate Analysis		
	HR	95%CI	p-Value	HR	95%CI	p-Value
Age (per year)	0.67	-	0.54	-	-	-
Sex (male vs. female)	0.75	0.19–2.39	0.65	-	-	-
Location (Ph vs. Pb,Pt)	1.47	0.22–2.61	0.59	-	-	-
Tumor size (> 30 mm vs. <30 mm)	0.64	0.37–5.80	0.49	-	-	-
CEA (> 3 U/mL vs. <3 U/mL)	0.32	0.18–2.27	0.32	-	-	-
CA19-9 (> 100 U/mL vs. <100 U/mL)	0.62	0.15–1.88	0.45	-	-	-
UR-M vs. UR-LA	2.38	0.18–2.16	0.21	-	-	-
CRT ((+) vs.(−))	8.06	0.61–9.24	0.002	8.54	2.03–35.97	0.004
Tumor size (> 30 mm vs. <30 mm)	0.77	2.15–30.18	0.68	-	-	-
CEA > 3 U/mL vs. <3 U/mL	1.23	0.22–2.69	0.76	-	-	-
CA19-9 (> 100 U/mL vs. <100 U/mL)	0.35	0.32–4.80	0.32	-	-	-
Change of tumor size (> 0.5 v.s. <0.5)	0.72	0.04–2.74	0.61	-	-	-
Change of CEA	1.5	0.20–2.55	0.56	-	-	-
Change of CA19-9	1	0.39–5.83	1	-	-	-
RECIST (PD,SD vs. PR,CR)	4.93	0.12–7.91	0.015	5.05	1.20–21.25	0.03
Period until operation (> 12 m vs. <12 m)	0.89	1.37–17.72	0.86	-	-	-
Operation time (> 600 min vs. <600 min)	1.36	0.26–3.09 0.39–4.70	0.63	-	-	-
Bleeding volume (> 1000 mL vs. <1000 mL)	0.89	0.23–3.52	0.87	-	-	-
Evans (I-IIa vs. IIb-V)	0.57	0.12–2.76	0.49	-	-	-
pT (1,2 vs.3,4)	2.14	0.55–8.31	0.27	-	-	-
LN mets ((+) vs.(−))	0.77	0.16–3.67	0.75	-	-	-
Adjuvant chemo. ((−) vs(+))	2.07	0.53–8.10	0.29	-	-	-

HR, hazard ratio; CI, confidential interval; Ph, pancreatic head; Pb, pancreatic body; Pt, pancreatic tail; UR-LA, unresectable locally advanced cancer; UR-M, unresectable cancer with metastasis; CRT, chemoradiotherapy; PD, progressive disease; SD, stable disease; PR, partial response; CR, complete response; LN mets, lymph node metastasis.

4. Discussion

The reports on conversion surgery for locally advanced pancreatic cancer have been increasing since the 2010s [12–22]. According to the recent NCCN guidelines (version 1.2021) [4], surgical resection of locally advanced cancer is a subsequent therapy option for patients with good performance status and no disease progression after first-line therapy. The present retrospective study found that conversion surgery for UR-PDAC after various therapy is relatively safe and feasible, because of no mortality and lower severe morbidity (C-D classification $\geq$ IIIa was 15% rate), and it may help improve long-term prognosis.

In the current study, the resection rate was only 5.0% (UR-LA, 3.6%; UR-M, 7.5%). However, this value was very low compared with that in previous reports; the reason for the resection rate might depend on policy whether we actively accepted conversion surgery when multidisciplinary treatment was performed for patients with UR-PDAC [16]. Many studies have focused on the effectiveness of conversion surgery, and although patients with UR-PDAC were not candidates for surgery, conversion surgery was performed for only an extremely limited number of patients who were super-responders to palliative therapy. Hackert et al. reported that among 575 patients with locally advanced PDAC receiving neoadjuvant therapy, 292 (50.8%) underwent pancreatic resection, which was a higher resection rate than that in our study [7]. However, the median survival time (MST) after adjuvant surgery was only 15.3 months. In the current study, the median overall survival was 73.7 months, which is better than that in previous reports [13,16,18]. The MST of patients with UR-LA treated with no resection was reported to be 15–17 months, which was similar to that in the present study. The median overall survival durations in PDAC patients with UR-LA and UR-M were 15.7 and 8.8 months, respectively. On the other hand, Lee et al. reported an excellent outcome, showing that 15 of 64 (23.4%) PDAC patients with UR-LA who underwent conversion surgery had an overall survival exceeding 40 months, although they did not clearly describe the indications for surgery [26]. Strict criteria similar to those in our study may lead to lower resectability but longer overall survival as a result of patient selection, so we may need to expand our surgical indication.

Conversion surgery has provided a surprising outcome for patients with UR-PDAC. In particular, the prognosis of patients with UR-PDAC who underwent conversion surgery was significantly better than that of patients with resectable PDAC. Several authors have previously reported the usefulness of conversion surgery in such patients, as well as favorable results on prognosis [19,27–30]. In the present study, the prognosis of PDAC patients with UR-LA and UR-M who underwent conversion surgery was not significantly different. Among the patients with UR-PDAC who underwent conversion surgery, we identified that RECIST CR/PR after the various treatments was an important prognostic factor by multivariate analysis. It may be important to perform multidisciplinary treatment aimed at tumor shrinkage and possible conversion surgery in order to obtain a better prognosis. However, recurrence and metastasis after conversion surgery were observed in 70% of patients, especially early recurrence within one year after surgery in 30% of patients. Uesaka et al. demonstrated the non-inferiority of S-1 to gemcitabine as adjuvant chemotherapy for pancreatic cancer in terms of overall survival in a randomized trial [10]. Chad et al. reported that adjuvant therapy was not required for all patients with localized pancreatic cancer who had received neoadjuvant therapy; the benefit of adjuvant therapy was limited to those with node-positive disease [31]. In the current study, adjuvant chemotherapy after conversion surgery was performed in only eight (40%) of 20 patients. In other reports, early recurrence after conversion surgery occurred in approximately 30% of cases [32,33]. The conversion surgery tended to have a long operative time and high bleeding volume in the present study, so it was considered a major invasive surgery. Therefore, it may be important to reduce morbidity in surgery as much as possible and to create an environment in which adjuvant chemotherapy can be easily performed. The early recurrence rate should be decreased as much as possible in patients undergoing conversion surgery [34]. Moreover, in the present study, during the follow-up after conversion surgery, additional surgical resection was performed in one patient with double cancer in the remnant pancreas and two patients with single lung metastasis. The surgical resection for multicentric cancer in the remnant pancreas and solitary lung metastasis may have possibilities to provide long-term survival. [35,36].

Satoi et al. previously performed multicenter joint research that focused on conversion surgery of initially unresectable PDAC [13]. This study included 58 PDAC patients (41 with UR-LA and 17 with UR-M). The MST in the conversion surgery group was significantly better than that in the control group (39.7 months vs. 20.8 months, $p < 0.0001$). The optimal timing of adjuvant surgery was 240 days after the initial treatment. Moreover, a multivariate analysis showed that for the adjuvant surgery group, significant favorable factors for overall survival included the dosage above a certain level of gemcitabine, a decrease in tumor markers until conversion surgery, and PR/CR evaluation by RECIST. Michelakos et al. reported that in resected patients with BR/locally advanced PDAC treated with FOLFIRINOX, a preoperative CA19-9 level >100 U/mL and >8 months between diagnosis and surgery predicted a shorter postoperative DFS [33]. Therefore, the optimal period between the initial diagnosis and conversion surgery is controversial.

As for the pathological examination, the Evans grade, which reflects the extent of tumor degeneration or necrosis after chemo(radio)therapy, has been extensively identified as a prognostic factor [19,37–39]. Chatterjee et al. reported that among the 223 patients with resectable PDAC who received neoadjuvant chemoradiation and had pancreaticoduodenectomy, pCR (grade IV, 2.7%) or minimal residual tumor (grade III, 16.1%) in posttreatment specimens of pancreaticoduodenectomy correlated with better survival [40]. Histologically, grades IIb, III, and IV, i.e., destroyed areas over 50%, were observed in the main tumor in 16 of the 20 patients who underwent conversion surgery in the present study. Moreover, the residual tumor tended to contain a wide range of highly differentiated cells, so this result suggests that cells with poorly differentiation may be highly effective for chemo(radio-)therapy.

In the present study of patients with UR-PDAC who underwent conversion surgery, we identified important prognostic factors from initial treatment in multivariate analysis: the use of chemoradiotherapy and RECIST CR/PR after various treatments. Of the treatment for UR-PDAC, radiation therapy combined with systemic chemotherapy is one of the recommended therapies in the NCCN [4] and Japanese guidelines [5]. In our institution, we reported the usefulness of the combination therapy with S-1 and radiation in patients with UR-PDAC; it is a well-tolerated regimen that can be recommended as an effective treatment in prospective phase II trials, and it showed favorable survival with a median survival time of 14.3 months [41]. Jang et al. reported on the benefit of neoadjuvant treatment in patients with BR-PDAC, and gemcitabine-based neoadjuvant chemoradiation provided oncological benefits compared to upfront surgery by the prospective randomized controlled trial [42]. A recent LAP-07 trial comparing chemotherapy and CRT for locally advanced PDAC failed to show any survival benefit of CRT [43]. However, CRT was associated with a decreased local progression rate and no increase in grade 3 or 4 toxicities. This result may indicate that CRT has potential as a more useful method in conversion surgery.

In the present study, we identified no significant difference in overall survival between patients who underwent conversion surgery with UR-LA and UR-M. Yanagimoto et al. reported no significant differences between the two groups, which is similar to our study finding [18]. There are few reports of surgical resection of pancreatic resection with synchronous metastases. Wright et al. reported 23 cases of surgical resection of stage IV pancreatic cancer after a favorable response to systematic chemotherapy [27]. The sites of metastasis included the liver ($n = 16$), lung ($n = 6$), and peritoneum ($n = 2$). The treated patients with stage IV disease were 1147 cases in all, so the resection rate was only 2.0%. The MST from the initial diagnosis was 34.1 months. Frigerio et al. reported that 24 (4.5%) of 535 patients diagnosed as pancreatic cancer with liver metastasis underwent surgical resection of the primary site and hepatic resection [44]. The MST after diagnosis in the study was 56 months. The limited number of patients with distant metastasis (super-responders) accounted for less than 5% of PDAC patients with UR-M. The effectiveness of conversion surgery for metastatic PDAC remains controversial; therefore, it is indispensable to identify powerful surrogate markers for predicting long survival after conversion surgery.

This research has some limitations. First, this was a single-institute, retrospective analysis with a limited number of cases. Second, the necessity of conversion surgery is debatable, even though CRT is successful. Patients receiving chemotherapy generally develop a tolerance to it, and surgical resection may be the most useful means of local control; however, there is no evidence to support this. In Japan, PREP-04 (UMIN000017793), which is a multi-institutional prospective observational study to investigate the effects of conversion surgery on patients with initial UR-PDAC, is ongoing. Given that only selected patients who responded favorably to non-surgical treatment were targeted among all patients with UR-PDAC, a selection bias existed. Conversion rates vary among reports on conversion surgery for patients with UR-PDAC. Nitshe et al. reported a conversion rate of 28.6% for FOLFIRINOX [29], while Hackert et al. reported that it was 50.8% [7]. Currently, FOLFIRINOX or gemcitabine plus nab-PTX is recommended for patients with UR-PDAC. It is still unclear which anticancer drug is optimal for conversion surgery. Moreover, the usefulness of adjuvant chemotherapy for resectable PDAC has been demonstrated in the JASPAC01 study, but the usefulness of adjuvant chemotherapy in conversion surgery has not yet been proven [10]. As for radiotherapy, it is controversial whether radiotherapy should be administered. Compared to resectable PDAC, the extent of surgical invasion for UR-PDAC is larger, and it is necessary to consider patients' physical status, the drug used as adjuvant chemotherapy, and the administration period. Furthermore, the most relevant limitation of this study is represented by the lack of biological predictive markers that could support the selection of PDAC patients suitable for conversion surgery.

5. Conclusions

In conclusion, it is important to perform multidisciplinary treatment, including CRT with conversion surgery in patients with UR-PADC. However, many questions remain unsolved regarding the necessity of the conversion surgery including CRT, the optimal regimen, the duration of preoperative therapy, and criteria for surgical therapy. It is essential to perform prospective studies to resolve the various problems.

Author Contributions: Conceptualization, Y.M. and H.K.; methodology, K.T.; software, Y.H.; validation, T.I., K.T. and Y.H.; formal analysis, Y.K. and K.M.; investigation, H.K.; data curation, S.I.; writing—original draft preparation, Y.M; supervision, T.O.; project administration, H.S. All authors have read and agreed to the published version of the manuscript.

Funding: This research received no external funding.

Institutional Review Board Statement: Not applicable

Informed Consent Statement: Informed consent was obtained from all subjects involved in the study. Written informed consent has been obtained from the patient(s) to publish this paper.

Data Availability Statement: Not applicable

Conflicts of Interest: The authors declare no conflict of interest.

References

1. In Cancer Statistics in Japan-2019, Foundation for Promotion of Cancer Research (FPCR). Available online: https://www.fpcr.or.jp/data_files/view/41/mode:inline (accessed on 1 December 2020).
2. Jonathan, D.M.; Rishi, S.; Juan, W.V.; Rachna, T.S. Pancreatic cancer. *Lancet* **2020**, *395*, 2008–2020.
3. Vincent, A.; Herman, J.; Schulick, R.; Hruban, R.H.; Goggins, M. Pancreatic cancer. *Lancet* **2011**, *378*, 607–620. [CrossRef]
4. NCCN. Clinical Practice Guidelines in Oncology (NCCN Guidelines): NCCN, Pancreatic Adenocarcinoma, Version 1. 2020. Available online: https://www.nccn.org/professionals/physician_gls/pdf/pancreatic.pdf (accessed on 17 January 2021).
5. Japan Pancreas Society. *General Rules for the Study of Pancreatic Cancer*, 7th ed.; Kanehara Shuppan: Tokyo, Japan, 2016.
6. Imamura, M.; Doi, R.; Imaizumi, T.; Funakoshi, A.; Wakasugi, H.; Sunamura, M.; Ogata, Y.; Hishinuma, S.; Asano, T.; Aikou, T.; et al. A randomized multicenter trial comparing resection and radiochemotherapy for resectable locally invasive pancreatic cancer. *Surgery* **2004**, *136*, 1003–1011. [CrossRef] [PubMed]

7. Hackert, T.; Sachsenmaier, M.; Hinz, U.; Schneider, L.; Michalski, C.W.; Springfeld, C.; Strobel, O.; Jäger, D.; Ulrich, A.; Büchler, M.W. Locally advanced pancreatic cancer: Neoadjuvant therapy with FOLFIRINOX results in resectability in 60% of the patients. *Ann. Surg.* **2016**, *264*, 457–463. [CrossRef] [PubMed]
8. Sui, K.; Okabayashi, T.; Shima, Y.; Morita, S.; Iwata, J.; Sumiyoshi, T.; Saisaka, Y.; Yasuhiro, H.; Yoshihiro, N.; Matsumoto, M.; et al. Clinical effects of chemoradiotherapy in pursuit of optimal treatment of locally advanced unresectable pancreatic cancer. *Br. J. Radiol.* **2017**, *90*, 20170165. [CrossRef]
9. Saito, T.; Ishido, K.; Kudo, D.; Kimura, N.; Wakiya, T.; Nakayama, Y.; Hakamada, K. Combination therapy with gemcitabine and nab-paclitaxel for locally advanced unresectable pancreatic cancer. *Mol. Clin. Oncol.* **2017**, *6*, 963–967. [CrossRef]
10. Uesaka, K.; Boku, N.; Fukutomi, A.; Okamura, Y.; Konishi, M.; Matsumoto, I.; Kaneoka, Y.; Shimizu, Y.; Nakamori, S.; Sakamoto, H.; et al. Adjuvant chemotherapy of S-1 versus gemcitabine for resected pancreatic cancer: A phase 3, open-label, randomised, non-inferiority trial (JASPAC 01). *Lancet* **2016**, *16*, 248–257. [CrossRef]
11. Ferrone, C.R.; Marchegiani, G.; Hong, T.S.; Ryan, D.P.; Deshpande, V.; McDonnell, E.I.; Sabbatino, F.; Santos, D.D.; Allen, J.N.; Blaszkowsky, L.S.; et al. Radiological and surgical implications of neoadjuvant treatment with FOLFIRINOX for locally advanced and borderline resectable pancreatic cancer. *Ann. Surg.* **2015**, *261*, 12–17. [CrossRef]
12. Klaiber, U.; Hackert, T. Conversion surgery for pancreatic cancer—The impact of neoadjuvant treatment. *Front Oncol.* **2020**, *14*, 1501. [CrossRef]
13. Satoi, S.; Yamaue, H.; Kato, K.; Takahashi, S.; Hirono, S.; Takeda, S.; Eguchi, H.; Sho, M.; Wada, K.; Shinchi, H.; et al. Role of adjuvant surgery for patients with initially unresectable pancreatic cancer with a long-term favorable response to non-surgical anti-cancer treatments: Results of a project study for pancreatic surgery by the Japanese society of hepato-biliary-pan. *J. HepatoBiliary-Pancreat. Sci.* **2013**, *20*, 590–600. [CrossRef]
14. Gillen, S.; Schuster, T.; Büschenfelde, C.M.Z.; Friess, H.; Kleeff, J. Preoperative/neoadjuvant therapy in pancreatic cancer: A systematic review and meta-analysis of response and resection percentages. *PLoS Med.* **2010**, *7*, e1000267. [CrossRef]
15. Yoshitomi, H.; Takano, S.; Furukawa, K.; Takayashiki, T.; Kuboki, S.; Ohtsuka, M. Conversion surgery for initially unresectable pancreatic cancer: Current status and unsolved issues. *Surg. Today* **2019**, *49*, 894–906. [CrossRef] [PubMed]
16. Natsume, S.; Shimizu, Y.; Senda, Y.; Hijioka, S.; Matsuo, K.; Ito, S.; Komori, K.; Abe, T.; Hara, K. Conversion surgery only for highly selected patients with unresectable pancreatic cancer: A satisfactory outcome in exchange for a lower resection rate. *Surg. Today* **2019**, *49*, 670–677. [CrossRef] [PubMed]
17. Furuse, J.; Shibahara, J.; Sugiyama, M. Development of chemotherapy and significance of conversion surgery after chemotherapy in unresectable pancreatic cancer. *J. Hepato Biliary Pancreat. Sci.* **2018**, *25*, 261–268. [CrossRef]
18. Yanagimoto, H.; Satoi, S.; Yamamoto, T.; Yamaki, S.; Hirooka, S.; Kotsuka, M.; Ryota, H.; Ishida, M.; Matsui, Y.; Sekimoto, M. Benefits of conversion surgery after multimodal treatment for unresectable pancreatic ductal adenocarcinoma. *Cancers (Basel)* **2020**, *12*, 1428. [CrossRef]
19. Asano, T.; Hirano, S.; Nakamura, T.; Okamura, K.; Tsuchikawa, T.; Noji, T.; Nakanishi, Y.; Tanaka, K.; Shichinohe, T. Survival benefit of conversion surgery for patients with initially unresectable pancreatic cancer who responded favorably to nonsurgical treatment. *J. Hepato-Biliary-Pancreat. Sci.* **2018**, *25*, 342–350. [CrossRef]
20. Kimura, Y.; Nakamura, T.; Hayashi, T.; Kuwatani, M.; Motoya, M.; Yoshida, M.; Imamura, M.; Nagayama, M.; Yamaguchi, H.; Yamakita, K.; et al. Clinical usefulness of conversion surgery for unresectable pancreatic cancer diagnosed on multidetector computed tomography imaging: Results from a multicenter observational cohort study by the Hokkaido Pancreatic Cancer Study Group (HOPS UR-01). *Ann. Gastroenterol. Surg.* **2019**, *3*, 523–533. [CrossRef] [PubMed]
21. Tsuchiya, N.; Matsuyama, R.; Murakami, T.; Yabushita, Y.; Sawada, Y.; Kumamoto, T.; Endo, I. Role of conversion surgery for unresectable pancreatic cancer after long-term chemotherapy. *World J. Surg.* **2020**, *44*, 2752–2760. [CrossRef] [PubMed]
22. Klaiber, U.; Schnaidt, E.S.; Hinz, U.; Gaida, M.M.; Heger, U.; Hank, U.; Strobel, O.; Neoptolemos, J.P.; Mihaljevic, A.L.; Büchler, M.W.; et al. Prognostic factors of survival after neoadjuvant treatment and resection for initially unresectable pancreatic cancer. *Ann. Surg.* **2021**, *273*, 154–162. [CrossRef]
23. Eisenhauer, E.A.; Therasse, P.; Bogaerts, J.; Schwartz, L.H.; Sargent, D.; Ford, R.; Dancey, J.; Arbuck, S.; Gwyther, S.; Mooney, M.; et al. New response evaluation criteria in solid tumours: Revised RECIST guideline (version 1.1). *Eur. J. Cancer* **2009**, *45*, 228–247. [CrossRef] [PubMed]
24. Evans, D.B.; Rich, T.A.; Byrd, D.R.; Cleary, K.R.; Connelly, J.H.; Levin, B.; Charnsangavej, C.; Fenoglio, C.J.; Ames, F.C. Preoperative chemoradiation and pancreaticoduodenectomy for adenocarcinoma of the pancreas. *Arch. Surg.* **1992**, *127*, 1335–1339. [CrossRef]
25. Dindo, D.; Demartines, N.; Clavien, P.-A. Classification of surgical complications: A new proposal with evaluation in a cohort of 6336 patients and results of a survey. *Ann. Surg.* **2004**, *240*, 205–213. [CrossRef]
26. Lee, J.; Lee, J.-C.; Gromski, M.A.; Kim, H.W.; Kim, J.; Kim, J.; Hwang, J.-H. Clinical outcomes of FOLFIRINOX in locally advanced pancreatic cancer: A single center experience. *Medicine (Baltimore)* **2018**, *97*, e13592. [CrossRef] [PubMed]
27. Kato, K.; Kondo, S.; Hirano, S.; Tanaka, E.; Shichinohe, T.; Tsuchikawa, T.; Matsumoto, J. Adjuvant surgical therapy for patients with initially-unresectable pancreatic cancer with long-term favorable responses to chemotherapy. *J. Hepato-Biliary-Pancreat. Sci.* **2011**, *18*, 712–716. [CrossRef] [PubMed]
28. Wright, G.P.; Poruk, K.E.; Zenati, M.; Steve, J.; Bahary, N.; Hogg, M.E.; Zuriekat, A.H.; Wolfgang, C.L.; Zeh, H.J.; Weiss, M. Primary tumor resection following favorable response to systemic chemotherapy in stage IV pancreatic adenocarcinoma with synchronous metastases: A Bi-institutional analysis. *J. Gastrointest. Surg.* **2016**, *20*, 1830–1835. [CrossRef]

29. Nitsche, U.; Wenzel, P.; Siveke, J.T.; Braren, R.; Holzapfel, K.; Schlitter, A.M.; Stöß, C.; Kong, B.; Esposito, I.; Erkan, M.; et al. Resectability after first-line FOLFIRINOX in initially unresectable locally advanced pancreatic cancer: A single-center experience. *Ann. Surg. Oncol.* **2015**, *22*, 1212–1220. [CrossRef] [PubMed]
30. Opendro, S.S.; Satoi, S.; Yanagimoto, H.; Yamamoto, T.; Toyokawa, H.; Hirooka, S.; Yamaki, S.; Inoue, K.; Matsui, Y.; Kwon, A.-H. Role of adjuvant surgery in initially unresectable pancreatic cancer after long-term chemotherapy or chemoradiation therapy: Survival benefit? *J. Hepato-Biliary-Pancreat. Sci.* **2014**, *21*, 695–702. [CrossRef]
31. Chad, A.B.; Ashley, N.K.; Mohammed, A.; Callisia, N.C.; Kathleen, K.C.; Abdul, H.K.; Bryan, C.H.; Paul, S.R.; Ben, G.; William, A.H.; et al. Is adjuvant therapy necessary for all patients with localized pancreatic cancer who have received neoadjuvant therapy? *J. Gastrointest. Surg.* **2017**, *21*, 1793–1803.
32. Yoo, C.; Shin, S.H.; Kim, K.P.; Jeong, J.H.; Chang, H.M.; Kang, J.H.; Lee, S.S.; Park, D.H.; Song, T.J.; Seo, D.W.; et al. Clinical outcomes of conversion surgery after neoadjuvant chemotherapy in patients with borderline resectable and locally advanced unresectable pancreatic cancer: A single-center, retrospective analysis. *Cancers* **2019**, *11*, 278. [CrossRef] [PubMed]
33. Michelakos, T.; Pergolini, I.; Castillo, C.F.-D.; Honselmann, K.C.; Cai, L.; Deshpande, V.; Wo, J.Y.; Ryan, D.P.; Allen, J.N.; Blaszkowsky, L.S.; et al. Predictors of resectability and survival in patients with borderline and locally advanced pancreatic cancer who underwent neoadjuvant treatment with FOLFIRINOX. *Ann. Surg.* **2019**, *269*, 733–740. [CrossRef] [PubMed]
34. Satoi, S.; Yamamoto, T.; Yamaki, S.; Sakaguchi, T.; Sekimoto, M. Surgical indication for and desirable outcomes of conversion surgery in patients with initially unresectable pancreatic ductal adenocarcinoma. *Ann. Gastroenterol. Surg.* **2019**, *4*, 6–13. [CrossRef]
35. Yamada, S.; Kobayashi, A.; Nakamori, S.; Baba, H.; Yamamoto, M.; Yamaue, H.; Fujii, T. Resection for recurrent pancreatic cancer in the remnant pancreas after pancreatectomy is clinically promising: Results of a project study for pancreatic surgery by the Japanese society of hepato-biliary-pancreatic surgery. *Surgery* **2018**, *164*, 1049–1056. [CrossRef]
36. Kurahara, H.; Maemura, K.; Mataki, Y.; Tanoue, K.; Iino, S.; Kawasaki, Y.; Idichi, T.; Arigami, T.; Mori, S.; Shinden, Y.; et al. Lung recurrence and its therapeutic strategy in patients with pancreatic cancer. *Pancreatology* **2020**, *20*, 89–94. [CrossRef] [PubMed]
37. White, R.R.; Xie, H.B.; Gottfried, M.R.; Czito, B.G.; Hurwitz, H.I.; Morse, M.A.; Blobe, G.C.; Paulson, E.K.; Baillie, J.; Branch, M.S.; et al. Significance of histological response to preoperative chemoradiotherapy for pancreatic cancer. *Ann. Surg. Oncol.* **2005**, *12*, 214–221. [CrossRef] [PubMed]
38. Tanaka, M.; Heckler, M.; Mihaljevic, A.; Sun, H.; Klaiber, U.; Heger, U.; Büchler, M.W.; Hackert, T. CT response of primary tumor and CA19-9 predict resectability of metastasized pancreatic cancer after FOLFIRINOX. *Eur. J. Surg. Oncol.* **2019**, *45*, 1453–1459. [CrossRef]
39. Moutardier, V.; Magnin, V.; Turrini, O.; Viret, F.; Hennekinne-Mucci, S.; Gonçalves, A.; Pésenti, C.; Guiramand, J.; Lelong, B.; Giovannini, M.; et al. Assessment of pathologic response after preoperative chemoradiotherapy and surgery in pancreatic adenocarcinoma. *Int. J. Radiat. Oncol.* **2004**, *60*, 437–443. [CrossRef] [PubMed]
40. Chatterjee, D.; Katz, M.H.; Rashid, A.; Varadhachary, G.R.; Wolff, R.A.; Wang, H.; Lee, J.E.; Pisters, P.W.T.; Vauthey, J.-N.; Crane, C.; et al. Histologic grading of the extent of residual carcinoma following neoadjuvant chemoradiation in pancreatic ductal adenocarcinoma: A predictor for patient outcome. *Cancer* **2012**, *118*, 3182–3190. [CrossRef] [PubMed]
41. Shinchi, H.; Maemura, K.; Mataki, Y.; Kurahara, H.; Sakoda, M.; Ueno, S.; Hiraki, Y.; Nakajo, M.; Natsugoe, S.; Takao, S. A phase II study of oral S-1 with concurrent radiotherapy followed by chemotherapy with S-1 alone for locally advanced pancreatic cancer. *J. Hepato Biliary Pancreat. Sci.* **2012**, *19*, 152–158. [CrossRef]
42. Jang, J.Y.; Han, Y.; Lee, H.; Kim, S.W.; Kwon, W.; Lee, K.H.; Oh, D.Y.; Chie, E.K.; Lee, J.M.; Heo, J.S.; et al. Oncological benefits of neoadjuvant chemoradiation with gemcitabine versus upfront surgery in patients with borderline resectable pancreatic cancer: A prospective, randomized, open-label, multicenter phase 2/3 trial. *Ann. Surg.* **2018**, *268*, 215–222. [CrossRef] [PubMed]
43. Hammel, P.; Huguet, F.; van Laethem, J.L.; Goldstein, D.; Glimelius, B.; Artru, P.; Borbath, I.; Bouché, O.; Shannon, J.; André, T.; et al. Effect of chemoradiotherapy vs. chemotherapy on survival in patients with locally advanced pancreatic cancer controlled after 4 months of gemcitabine with or without erlotinib: The LAP07 randomized clinical trial. *JAMA* **2016**, *315*, 1844–1853. [CrossRef]
44. Frigerio, I.; Regi, P.; Giardino, A.; Scopelliti, F.; Girelli, R.; Bassi, C.; Gobbo, S.; Martini, P.T.; Capelli, P.; D'Onofrio, M.; et al. Downstaging in stage IV pancreatic cancer: A new population eligible for surgery? *Ann. Surg. Oncol.* **2017**, *24*, 2397–2403. [CrossRef] [PubMed]

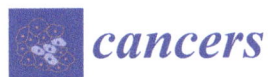

Article

Benefits of Conversion Surgery after Multimodal Treatment for Unresectable Pancreatic Ductal Adenocarcinoma

Hiroaki Yanagimoto [1], Sohei Satoi [1,*], Tomohisa Yamamoto [1], So Yamaki [1], Satoshi Hirooka [1], Masaya Kotsuka [1], Hironori Ryota [1], Mitsuaki Ishida [2], Yoichi Matsui [1] and Mitsugu Sekimoto [1]

1. Department of Surgery, Kansai Medical University, Hirakata 573-1010, Japan; yanagimh@med.kobe-u.ac.jp (H.Y.); tomot1226@yahoo.co.jp (T.Y.); yamakis@hirakata.kmu.ac.jp (S.Y.); ss_largehill@yahoo.co.jp (S.H.); kotsukam@hirakata.kmu.ac.jp (M.K.); ryoutahr@hirakata.kmu.ac.jp (H.R.); matsui@hirakata.kmu.ac.jp (Y.M.); sekimotm@hirakata.kmu.ac.jp (M.S.)
2. Department of Pathology and Laboratory Medicine, Kansai Medical University, Hirakata 573-1010, Japan; mitsuaki.ishida@gmail.com
* Correspondence: satoi@hirakata.kmu.ac.jp; Tel.: +81-72-804-0101; Fax: +81-72-804-2578

Received: 26 April 2020; Accepted: 28 May 2020; Published: 31 May 2020

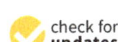

Abstract: Background: Traditionally, the treatment options for unresectable locally advanced (UR-LA) and metastatic (UR-M) pancreatic ductal adenocarcinoma (PDAC) are palliative chemotherapy or chemoradiotherapy. The benefits of surgery for such patients remains unknown. The present study investigated clinical outcomes of patients undergoing conversion surgery (CS) after chemo(radiation)therapy for initially UR-PDAC. Methods: We recruited patients with UR-PDAC who underwent chemo(radiation)therapy for initially UR-PDAC between April 2006 and September 2017. We analyzed resectability of CS, predictive parameters for overall survival, and early recurrence (within six months). Results: A total of 468 patients (108 with UR-LA and 360 with UR-M PDAC) were enrolled in this study, of whom, 17 (15.7%) with UR-LA and 15 (4.2%) with UR-M underwent CS. The median survival time (MST) and five-year survival of patients who underwent CS was 37.2 months and 34%, respectively; significantly better than non-resected patients (nine months and 1%, respectively, $p < 0.0001$). MST did not differ according to UR-LA or UR-M (50.5 vs. 29.0 months, respectively, $p = 0.53$). Early recurrence after CS occurred in eight patients (18.8%). Lymph node metastasis, positive washing cytology, large tumor size (>35 mm), and lack of postoperative adjuvant chemotherapy were statistically significant predictive factors for early recurrence. Moreover, the site of pancreatic lesion and administration of postoperative adjuvant chemotherapy were statistically significant prognostic factors for overall survival in the patients undergoing CS. Conclusion: Conversion surgery offers benefits in terms of increase survival for initially UR-PDAC for patients who responded favorably to chemo(radiation)therapy when combined with postoperative adjuvant chemotherapy.

Keywords: unresectable pancreatic ductal adenocarcinoma; conversion surgery; early recurrence

1. Introduction

In the present-day situation, successful treatment of pancreatic ductal adenocarcinoma (PDAC) remains a therapeutic challenge, and the prognosis is generally poor [1]. Approximately 70% of patients with PDAC are not eligible for surgery, due to locally advanced or metastatic disease at the time of diagnosis [2]. Current guidelines of the National Comprehensive Cancer Network (NCCN) recommend nab-paclitaxel combined with gemcitabine (GnP) or FOLFIRINOX regimens as standard treatments for unresectable (UR) PDAC [3,4]. However, the median survival time (MST) for UR-PDAC remains low (9.2–13.5 months) [5–7]. The result of remarkable therapeutic response may occasionally become an indication for conversion surgery (CS) [8,9], which is defined as additional surgery for patients with UR-PDAC who responded favorably to multimodal treatment. However, the incidence and clinical effects are unknown at present. In the present study, we evaluated the clinical outcomes of CS after chemo(radiation)therapy for UR-PDAC, predictive parameters for early recurrence (within six months after CS) and prognostic parameters for overall survival (OS).

2. Patients and Methods

2.1. Study Population

This retrospective study was conducted by using data from a prospective database. We recruited all consecutive patients undergoing chemotherapy or chemoradiotherapy for UR-PDAC who were to the Department of Surgery, Kansai Medical University, for any treatment between April 2006 and September 2017. All patients were diagnosed with PDAC by cytology or pathology through endoscopic retrograde cholangiopancreatography or endoscopic ultrasound-guided fine-needle aspiration. We have previously reported the details of multidetector-raw computed tomography (MDCT) imaging for the diagnosis of PDAC and to rule out distant metastasis, as well as staging laparoscopy techniques [10,11]. Moreover, multimodal image findings such as contrast-enhanced ultrasonography (CE-US), gadoxetic acid–enhanced magnetic resonance imaging (EOB-MRI), and positron emission tomography (PET) were considered, and we certainly confirmed that all patients had UR-PC initially, according to the National Comprehensive Cancer Network (NCCN) guideline version 2.2017 [3,4].

Ethical approval: All procedures performed in studies involving human participants were in accordance with the ethical standards of the institutional research committee and with the 1964 Declaration of Helsinki and its later amendments or comparable ethical standards. Informed consent: Written informed consent was obtained from all study participants.

2.2. Data Collection

The following data were collected: clinicopathological characteristics, type of chemotherapy or chemoradiotherapy, frequency of CS, rates of peri-operative morbidity and mortality, predictive parameters for early recurrence (defined as within 6 months after CS), and prognostic parameters for OS.

2.3. Statistical Analysis

Data are presented as median (range). Continuous or categorical variables were compared by using the Mann–Whitney U, chi-square, or Fisher's exact tests as appropriate. The OS and recurrence-free survival curves were estimated by using the Kaplan–Meier method and compared by using the log-rank test. Predictive factors identified by the univariate analysis were further examined by multivariate logistic regression analysis, to determine significant factors for OS and early recurrence among patients undergoing CS. The hazard ratio and 95% confidence intervals were calculated for all estimates. A two-tailed p-value of <0.05 was considered to be statistically significant. Calculations were performed by using JMP software, version 10 (SAS Inc., Cary, NC, USA).

3. Results

3.1. Patient Characteristics

Between April 2006 and September 2017, a total of 758 patients received treatment at our department; 290 of those patients underwent surgical resection. The remaining 468 patients with unresectable (UR) PDAC were finally enrolled in this study. Diagnoses were confirmed by using MDCT for 189 patients (40.4%) with unresectable locally advanced (UR-LA) PDAC and 279 (59.6%) with unresectable metastatic (UR-M) PDAC. We performed staging laparoscopy for 133 patients (28.4%) and palliative gastrojejunostomy for 20 patients (4.3%) with radiologically defined locally advanced disease.

Positive peritoneal lavage cytology was identified in 30 patients (6.4%), peritoneal dissemination in 25 (5.3%), liver metastasis in 20 (4.3%), and other metastases in six (1.3%). In total, we treated 108 patients (23%) with UR-LA and 360 patients (77%) with UR-M (Figure 1).

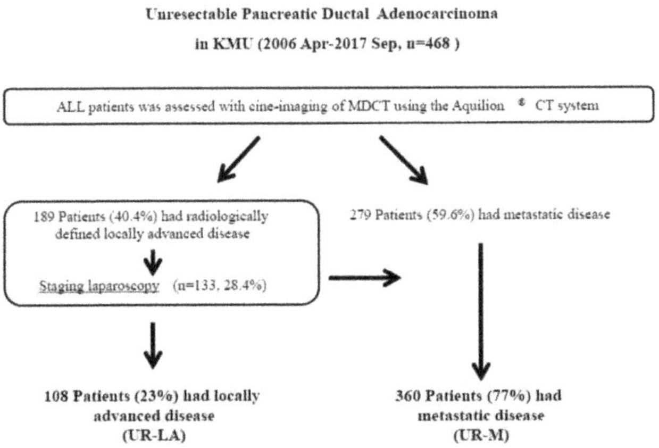

Unresectable Pancreatic Ductal Adenocarcinoma in KMU (2006 Apr-2017 Sep, n=468)

ALL patients was assessed with cine-imaging of MDCT using the Aquilion ® CT system

189 Patients (40.4%) had radiologically defined locally advanced disease

Staging laparoscopy (n=133, 28.4%)

279 Patients (59.6%) had metastatic disease

108 Patients (23%) had locally advanced disease (UR-LA)

360 Patients (77%) had metastatic disease (UR-M)

Figure 1. Study flow diagram. Diagnoses were made, using multidetector-raw computed tomography. In total, 189 patients were diagnosed with unresectable locally advanced pancreatic ductal adenocarcinoma (UR-LA PDAC), and 279 patients were diagnosed with unresectable metastatic (UR-M) PDAC. We performed staging laparoscopy for 133 patients with radiologically defined locally advanced disease. We finally enrolled 108 patients with UR-LA PDAC and 360 patients with UR-M PDAC in the present study. Abbreviations: KMU, Kansai Medical University; MDCT, multidetector-raw computed tomography; UR-LA, unresectable locally advanced; UR-M, unresectable metastatic.

Baseline characteristics of the study population and regimens that were selected as first-line treatment are listed in Table 1. The most frequently used regimen was gemcitabine (GEM), followed by GEM combined with S-1 and GEM combined with nab-paclitaxel.

Table 1. Baseline patient characteristics.

Variables	UR-LA (n = 108)	UR-M (n = 360)	p-Value
Age (years), median (range)	69(38–84)	67(33–86)	0.15
Male/female, n (%)	54(50)/54(50)	210(58.3)/150(41.7)	0.12
ECOG PS, n (%): 0/1/2	86(79.6)/18(16.6)/4(3.8)	218(60.5)/127(35.2)/15(4.2)	0.0004
Tumor location, n (%)			
Head/Body-tail	73(67.6)/35(32.4)	148(41.1)/212(58.9)	<0.0001
Tumor size (mm)	38(20-76)	40(15-83)	0.062
CA19-9 (U/L)	237(1.1-8949)	580(1-12219)	<0.0001
Extent of disease, n (%)			
Localized			
Metastatic site	108(100)		
Liver		193(53.6)	
Peritoneum		123(34.2)	
Lung/LN/Other		15(4.2)/23(6.4)/6(1.6)	
Treatment, n (%)			
GEM	17(15.7)	125(34.7)	
GEM + Erlotinib	2(1.9)	14(3.9)	
S-1	5(4.6)	38(10.6)	

Table 1. Cont.

Variables	UR-LA (n = 108)	UR-M (n = 360)	p-Value
GS	31(28.7)	42(11.6)	
GnP	13(12.0)	63(17.5)	
FOLFIRINOX	12(11.1)	21(5.8)	
S-1or GnP or GS plus PTX (i.p. + i.v.)	0(0)	43(11.9)	
Chemoradiotherapy	27(25)	10(2.8)	
Other	1(0.9)	4(1.1)	

UR-LA: unresectable locally advanced pancreatic cancer, UR-M: metastatic pancreatic cancer, PS: performance status, GEM: gemcitabine, GS: S-1 combined with gemcitabine, GnP: nab-paclitaxel combined with gemcitabine, PTX: paclitaxel.

The standard treatment for advanced pancreatic cancer has changed to gemcitabine since 2001, FOLFIRINOX since 2010, and GnP since 2013 in Japan. Moreover, gemcitabine combined with S-1 was often used as a treatment option. There was liver metastasis in 193 patients, peritoneal metastasis in 123 patients, and LA in 108 patients, respectively. Standardized regimen of chemotherapy in each time has been used in patients with UR-M PDAC. Patients with peritoneal metastasis were treated with S-1 + intravenous and intraperitoneal paclitaxel [12]. Moreover, we have implemented additional radiation therapy in UR-LA patients who still had the low-density area around celiac artery or superior mesenteric artery just before the planned conversion surgery for expecting the margin-negative resection. Positive peritoneal washing cytology was not defined as M1 at that time. Therefore, chemoradiation therapy was implemented for UR-LA with positive cytology.

3.2. Best Response After First-Line Treatment

Radiographic partial responses (PR) according to Response Evaluation Criteria in Solid Tumors (RECIST) criteria were observed in 45 patients (42%) with UR-LA and 86 (24%) with UR-M. Stable disease (SD) was observed in 38 patients (35%) with UR-LA and 119 (34%) with UR-M, and disease progression observed in 25 patients (23%) and 155 (42%), respectively. Disease control was achieved in 83 patients (77%) with UR-LA and 205 (58%) with UR-M. Furthermore, patients who could maintain PR or SD for more than eight months were shown in 44 patients (40.7%) with UR-LA and in 85 patients (23.6%) with UR-M, respectively.

3.3. Conversion Surgery

The major eligibility criteria for surgical exploration were as follows: clinical response (PR/CR) on CT imaging, reduction of tumor markers, fine performance status with patient's willingness for surgery, and an interval of at least eight months since initial treatment [13]. In patients with peritoneal metastasis, disappearance of occult distant organ metastasis was confirmed by second-look staging laparoscopy in the context of the above criteria. In patients with liver metastasis, a maximum of three occult metastases on the liver surface were resected. In cases where tumor extension to the major vessels with attachment was observed, these patients were indicated for resection. Clinical staging and surgical exploration were re-evaluated at multidisciplinary team meetings.

During the study period, 36 patients were planned to undergo CS, and four underwent exploratory laparotomy for occult distant organ metastasis. Finally, CS was performed on 17 patients (15.7%) with UR-LA and 15 (4.2%) with UR-M. Some reasons were raised in 99 patients who had PR but did not undergo conversion surgery due to still UR-LA status on CT imaging and poor performance status. We performed subtotal stomach-preserving pancreaticoduodenectomy for 13 patients (40.6%), distal pancreatectomy for 11 (34.4%), total pancreatectomy for four (12.5%), and distal pancreatectomy with en-bloc celiac axis resection (DP-CAR) on four patients (12.5%) (Table 2). Concomitant CHA resection was done in four patients (12.5%), and concomitant portal vein resection was in 15 patients (46.9%). R0 resection was achieved in 29 patients (90.6%). The median operative time for the total study population was 441 (range 223–866) min, and the median intraoperative blood loss was 1250 (range 207–6301) mL. Although the complication of Clavien–Dindo classification ≥IIIa [14] was reported for eight patients (25.0%), there was no mortality. The median postoperative hospital stay was 14 (range 7–116) days. Histopathologically, Evans grade ≥III was noted in nine patients (28.1%), one of whom exhibited pathological complete response (pCR). The 23 patients (71.9%) received postoperative adjuvant chemotherapy; S-1 was administered to 13 patients (40.6%), GEM to three (9.4%), GEM plus S-1 to one (3.1%), and intraperitoneal infusion and intravenous administration of paclitaxel combined with S-1 to six (18.8%). Twenty-two patients (68.8%) completed adjuvant chemotherapy. The nine patients (28.1%) did not receive postoperative adjuvant chemotherapy, because of our policy of non-adjuvant chemotherapy in the first four patients, patient's willingness ($n = 3$), or insufficient nutritional condition ($n = 2$).

Table 2. Patient characteristics of conversion surgery.

Variables	$n = 32$	UR-LA ($n = 17$)	UR-M ($n = 15$)	p-Value
Age(years), median (range)	66 (36–84)	65 (38–75)	69 (50–83)	0.135
Male: Female, n (%)	14 (44): 18 (56)	7(41):10(59)	7(47):8(53)	0.754
Ph: Pbt, n (%)	14 (44): 18 (56)	9 (53): 8 (47)	5 (33): 10 (67)	0.264
Tumor Size(mm), median (range)	36 (25–74)	35 (25–55)	40 (27–74)	0.747
Mets site: None:L:P, n (%)	17 (53): 4 (13):11 (34)	17 (100): 0 (0):0 (0)	0(0): 4 (27):11 (73)	<0.0001
CA19-9; U/mL, median (range)	278 (1.2–3400)	126 (8.4–2200)	984 (6.6–1953)	0.209
Preoperative CA19-9	29.1(1.0–181.9)	39.7(1.0–181.9)	19(1.0–73.9)	0.42
Primary Treatment				
GEM or GS	7	4	3	
GEM + nab-PTX (GnP)	7	4	3	
S1 or GEM based + ip PTX	8	0	8	
FOLFIRINOX	3	3	0	
GEM or S-1 or GS + RT (50.4 Gy)	7	6	1	
Radiation, n (%)	13(41)	11(65)	2(13)	0.002
Pretreatment period to op; (median, range)	9.5(4–28)	10 (4–28)	9 (6–16)	0.6207
RECIST (CR: PR), n (%)	1 (3.1%): 31(96.9%)	0(0):17(100)	1(7):14(63)	0.153
Operative time(min)	454(223–866)	441(223–655)	467(227–866)	0.36
Intraoperative blood loss(mL)	1229(207–6301)	1087(237–2931)	1255(207–6301)	0.58
Blood transfusion (U)	0(0–12)	0(0–7)	0(0–12)	0.42
PD: DP: DP-CAR: TP, n (%)	13 (40): 11(34): 4(13): 4(13)	9(52):4(24):2(12):2(12)	5(33):7(47):2(13):1(7)	0.257
-CHA/CA/PV resection-	-3(9)/4(13)/15(47)-	-3(18)/2(12)/9(52)-	-0(0)/2(13)/6(40)-	
Residual tumor (R0: R1), n (%)	29(91): 3(9)	16(94):1(6)	13(87):2(13)	0.471
Postop comp/Mortality (%)	8(25)/0(0)	2(12)/0(0)	6(40)/0(0)	0.066/0
Hospital stay (median, range)	14 (7–114)	11 (7–41)	14 (7–114)	0.271
Evans (I/IIa/IIb/III/IV, (%))	1(3)/12(38)/10(31)/8(25)/1 (3)	1(6)/7(41)/5(29)/4(24)/0 (0)	0(0)/5(33)/5(33)/4 (27)/1(7)	0.695

Ph: pancreas head, Pbt: pancreas body and tail, Mets: metastasis, L: liver, P: peritoneum, GEM: gemcitabine, GS: S-1 combined with gemcitabine, GnP: nab-paclitaxel combined with gemcitabine, PTX: paclitaxel, RT: radiation, PD: pancreaticoduodenectomy, DP: distal pancreatectomy, DP-CAR: distal pancreatectomy with en-bloc celiac axis resection, CHA: common hepatic artery, CA: celiac artery, PV: portal vein.

3.4. Survival Analysis

The MST of the entire study population was 10 months, and the one- and two-year survival rates were 39% and 12%, respectively (Figure 2). Patients who achieved PR ($n = 99$) and did not undergo CS exhibited significantly increased survival in comparison with other patients (15 vs. 7.5 months, $p < 0.0001$; Figure 2). The MST following initial treatment of patients who underwent CS ($n = 32$) was 37.2 months, and the one-, three-, and five-year survival rates were 100%, 51%, and 34%, respectively. These patients also exhibited significantly increased survival than those who achieved PR (37.2 vs. 18 months, $p < 0.0001$; Figure 2).

When long PR/SD was defined as PR/SD persisting for eight months or more, survival was significantly better among patients who underwent CS compared with those with long PR/SD who did not undergo CS ($n = 97$) (37.2 vs. 19.5 months, $p < 0.0001$).

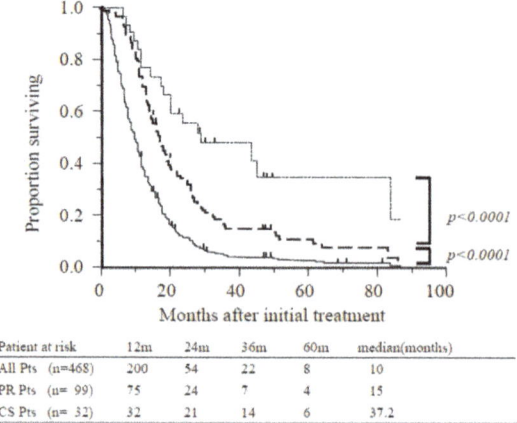

Figure 2. Overall survival of all patients, patients with radiographic partial response, and patients who underwent conversion surgery. The median overall survival (OS) for the study population (solid line, $n = 468$) was 10 months. Survival was significantly better among patients with partial response (dashed line, $n = 99$) compared with other cases ($p < 0.0001$). Survival of patients who underwent conversion surgery (dotted line, $n = 32$) was significantly better than those with partial response ($p < 0.0001$). Abbreviations: CS, conversion surgery; Pts, patients; PR, partial response.

3.5. Comparison between Patients with Unresectable Locally Advanced and Metastatic Disease

Age, gender, tumor location, tumor diameter, tumor markers, pretreatment period to operation, postoperative complications, mortality, and length of hospital stay were not significantly different patients with UR-LA who underwent CS and those with UR-M who underwent CS (Table 2). Significant differences were identified in metastatic site and requirement of additional radiation therapy. There was no significant difference in survival from the time of initial treatment or from the time of CS between patients who underwent CS with UR-LA and those with UR-M (50.5 vs. 29.0 months, $p = 0.53$; 25.0 vs. 21.0 months, $p = 0.61$, respectively; Figure 3).

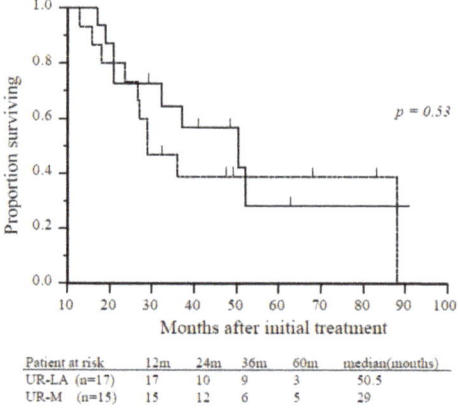

Figure 3. Overall survival of patients with unresectable locally advanced or metastatic disease who underwent conversion surgery. There was no significant difference in overall survival between patients with unresectable locally advanced (solid line, $n = 17$) and unresectable-metastatic disease (dashed line, $n = 15$) ($p = 0.53$). Abbreviations: UR-LA, unresectable locally advanced; UR-M, unresectable metastatic.

3.6. Recurrence-Free Survival

The MST from CS was 23 months, and the median recurrence-free survival time was 13 months (Figure 4).

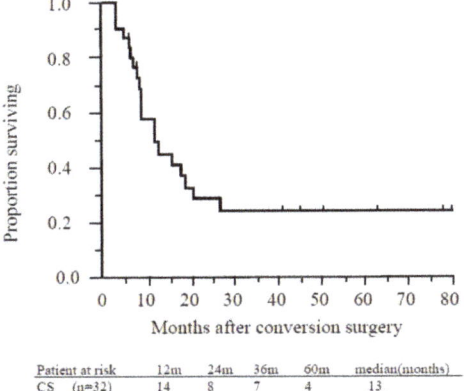

Figure 4. Recurrence-free survival of patients who underwent conversion surgery. The median recurrence-free survival time of patients who underwent conversion surgery was 13 months. Abbreviations: CS, conversion surgery.

Recurrence was confirmed in 20 (62.5%) of 32 patients who underwent CS, presenting as peritoneal dissemination in seven patients, locoregional recurrence in six, liver metastasis in five, and lung metastasis in two. Recurrence within six months after CS was observed in six patients (18.8%), presenting as liver metastasis in three patients, peritoneal dissemination in two, and local recurrence in one. One of those patients received GEM, and four patients received S-1 as adjuvant chemotherapy after CS. After relapse was confirmed, two of the six patients received the same regimen as was administered for initial treatment; these patients survived 23 and 32 months after CS. Patients who suffered recurrence within six months after CS had relatively poorer prognoses than non-recurrent patients (25.5 vs. 50.5 months, $p = 0.22$). Multivariate logistic regression analyses revealed that lymph node metastasis, washing cytology positive, large tumor (>35 mm), and lack of postoperative adjuvant chemotherapy were predictive factors for early recurrence (Table 3).

Table 3. Predictive factor for the recurrence within six months after CS (Univariate and multivariate logistic regression analyses).

Variables	Univariate Analysis		p-Value	Multivariate Analysis		p-Value
	HR	95% CI		HR	95% CI	
UR-M vs. UR-LA	1.16	0.19–7.37	0.87			0.07
Pbt vs. Ph	4.99	0.68–102	0.12			0.07
Tumor Size (>35 mm vs. <35 mm)	5.83	0–0.40	0.007	2.16	0–2.31	0.003
Pretreatment period (<8 m vs. >8 m)	2.22	0.29–46.22	0.47			0.38
Reduction of CA19-9 or DUPAN-2 (<70% vs. >70%)	5.99	0.80–50.84	0.08			0.38
LN mets (+) vs. (−)	4.29	0.58–88.2	0.16	4.5	0.40–11.10	0.01
R0 vs. R1	3.11	0–4.00	0.25			0.99
CY (+) vs. (−)	2.74	0.31–20.3	0.34	1.11	0.56–1.70	<0.0001
Evans I-IIa vs. IIb-IV	1.47	0.24–11.9	0.68			0.46
Adjuvant Tx (−) vs. (+)	1.36	0.16–8.74	0.76	2.96	0.32–3.06	0.0029

CS: conversion surgery, HR: hazard ratio, CI: confidential interval, LN: lymph node, R: residual tumor, CY: washing cytology, Tx: chemotherapy.

3.7. Prognostic Factors for Overall Survival Among Patients Who Underwent Conversion Surgery

The multivariate analysis revealed the site of pancreatic lesion and postoperative adjuvant chemotherapy to be statistically significant prognostic factors for OS among patients undergoing CS ($p = 0.0092$ and $p < 0.0001$, respectively). Other parameters, including reduction of tumor markers and Evans grading, were not significantly risk factors (Table 4).

Table 4. Univariate and multivariate analysis of prognostic factor of overall survival in CS group.

Variables	Univariate Analysis		p-Value	Multivariate Analysis		p-Value
	HR	95% CI		HR	95% CI	
UR-M vs. UR-LA	1.34	0.53–3.54	0.53			0.44
Pbt vs. Ph	1.24	0.49–3.40	0.65	14.14	1.86–182	0.0092
Tumor Size (>35 mm vs. <35 mm)	2.47	0.89–7.53	0.08			0.61
Pretreatment period (<8 m vs. >8 m)	0.79	0.22–2.25	0.68			0.27
Reduction of CA19-9 or DUPAN-2 (<70% vs. >70%)	1.08	0.38–3.89	0.89			0.086
LN mets (+) vs. (−)	1.07	0.38–2.86	0.89			0.5
R1 vs. R0	1.76	0.27–6.41	0.49			0.19
CY (+) vs. (−)	2.91	0.98–7.71	0.05			0.08
Evans I-IIa vs. IIb-IV	1.77	0.65–4.71	0.26			0.05
Adjuvant Tx (−) vs. (+)	4.63	1.76–12.13	0.0024	367.22	20.16–15093	<0.0001

CS: conversion surgery, HR: hazard ratio, CI: confidential interval, LN: lymph node, R: residual tumor, CY: washing cytology, Tx: chemotherapy.

4. Discussion

Despite recent advances in diagnostic medicine, detection of pancreatic cancer while it is within the resectable stage remains a clinical challenge. According to systematic reviews, the condition is not detected until it has reached the locally advanced or metastatic stage in 30–40% and 40–50% of patients, respectively [15–17]. Thus, despite the development of chemotherapy, the prognosis of patients with UR-PDAC remains poor, with a median survival of 9.2–13.5 months and low rates of long-term survival. [5–7]

Favorable outcomes may be achieved for a certain period of time, through the use of chemo(radiation)therapy for patients with unresectable malignancies, and this treatment can be converted to surgical resection, as required. Conversion surgery represents a new therapeutic strategy which may improve short- and long-term outcomes of patients with UR-PDAC. Several articles have reported the utility of CS in such patients, as well as the positive effects on prognosis [17–26]. In the present study, the rate of CS among patients with UR-LA and UR-M was similar to that reported previously [25]. We found the long-term prognosis; one-, three-, and five-year OS rates from initial treatment; and MST were significantly better among patients with long PR/SD who did not undergo CS, although there were no significant differences in survival with relation to UR-LA or UR-M. Therefore, CS should be considered even for patients initially diagnosed with UR-M if they exhibit surgical indicators. Considering the favorable long-term survival of patients who underwent CS in the present study, our suggestion of tumor extension to the major vessels with attachment as an indication for surgery appears reasonable. However, early recurrence was observed in almost 20% of patients, in line with the findings of Wright et al., who reported that seven out of 23 patients (30.4%) with metastatic PDAC who underwent CS experienced early recurrence. Other studies have also reported early recurrence rates after conversion surgery of approximately 30% [27–29]. This would suggest that patients cannot be expected to survive longer than patients who receive non-surgical treatment, and conversion surgery may be harmful to patients because of the high risk of mortality and morbidity associated with extensive pancreatectomy. The early recurrence rate should be decreased as much as possible for patients undergoing CS [30]. Thus, although CS can prolong OS, early recurrence remains a considerable risk. Appropriate preoperative selection of patients for CS is absolutely necessary in order to improve prognosis. The relatively strict surgical indication employed in the present study resulted in prolonged survival and a reduced incidence of early recurrence. In contrast, a review article reported that some authors recommend patients with UR-PDAC who did not experience progression after chemo(radiation) therapy should be offered surgical exploration [30]. The resectability and MST of patients in these studies who underwent CS ranged from 20% to 69% (median, 52%) and from 19.5 to 33 months (median, 21.9 months), respectively. Strict criteria may lead to lower resectability but longer OS, as a result of patient selection. Broad criteria may be associated with higher resectability but shorter OS, due to the risk of early recurrence after conversion surgery. Surgical indications for CS should be carefully decided through discussion in a multidisciplinary meeting.

To the best of our knowledge, there have been no previous studies on predictive factors of early recurrence after CS. The present study demonstrates that lymph node metastasis, positive washing cytology, large tumor size (>35 mm), and lack of postoperative adjuvant chemotherapy are significant predictive factors for early recurrence after CS. Thus, tumor size and washing cytology may be important preoperative factors which should be considered during patient selection for CS. Staging laparoscopy should be routinely performed before proceeding with CS in order to exclude patients with positive washing cytology. Metastatic site, decreased CA19-9 level, and performance status are not significant predictive factors for early recurrence. Several articles have reported that decreased CA19-9 levels after multimodal therapy represent a reliable predictive factor for resectability, OS, and DFS [21,29–35]. In most patients of the present study, CA19-9 decreased to within normal limits after multimodal treatment. Although the optimal selection criteria for surgical exploration or resection remain controversial for patients with initially UR-PDAC, it may be appropriate to base decision-making for CS on clinical response (defined by RECIST criteria) and decreased CA19-9 level after multimodal therapy [30].

Regarding pathological examination, the utility of Evans classification reflecting the extent of tumor degeneration or necrosis has been extensively studied as a prognostic factor after preoperative treatment [24,35–38]. There have been reports of the association between histopathological responses to chemo(radiation)therapy and the prognosis of patients with PDAC [24,35–38]. Chaterjee et al [36]. reported that 42 (18.8%) of 223 patients with resectable PDAC who received neoadjuvant chemotherapy were classified as Evans grade ≥III and had better survival rates than patients classified as Evans grade <III. Moreover, White et al. [37] suggested histologic response to be a useful surrogate marker for treatment efficacy, but Evans grade was not found to be a prognostic factor of CS in the present study.

The present study has some limitations which should be acknowledged. Firstly, it is a single-institute and retrospective study involving a small number of patients. All studies on this subject, to date, are retrospective studies, and so we believe that a prospective study is necessary to define the efficacy of CS. In Japan, the results of the PREP-04 trial (UMIN000017793)—a multi-institutional prospective cohort study investigating clinical outcomes of CS on patients with initially UR-PDAC— will be published in the near future. Given that only patients who responded favorably to chemo(radiation)therapy were analyzed among all patients with UR-PDAC, a selection bias exists. The development of an effective therapeutic strategy involving combined multimodal treatment with surgical resection is critical.

5. Conclusions

In conclusion, CS can provide clinical benefits, including increased survival for patients with initially UR-PDAC who have responded favorably to chemo(radiation)therapy. In addition to CS, postoperative adjuvant chemotherapy is necessary to prolong survival. It is essential that efforts are made to reduce early recurrence and to investigate surrogate markers in order to determine appropriate indications for surgery.

Author Contributions: Data curation, S.Y., S.H., M.K., and H.R.; methodology, M.I.; supervision, Y.M. and M.S.; writing—original draft, H.Y.; writing—review and editing, S.S., T.Y., and M.S. All authors have read and agreed to the published version of the manuscript.

Funding: No funding was received for this work.

Conflicts of Interest: All authors declare that they have no conflict of interest. Human and animal rights: This article does not contain any studies with animals performed by any of the authors.

References

1. Hackert, T.; Büchler, M.W. Pancreatic Cancer: Advances in Treatment, Results and Limitations. *Dig. Dis.* **2013**, *31*, 51–56. [CrossRef]
2. Egawa, S.; Toma, H.; Ohigashi, H.; Okusaka, T.; Nakao, A.; Hatori, T.; Maguchi, H.; Yanagisawa, A.; Tanaka, M. Japan Pancreatic Cancer Registry; 30th year anniversary: Japan Pancreas Society. *Pancreas* **2012**, *41*, 985–992. [CrossRef] [PubMed]
3. Network NCC. National Comprehensive Cancer Network NCCN Clinical Practice Guidelines in Oncology (NCCN Guidelines). 2017. Available online: https://www.nccn.org/professionals/physician_gls/default.aspx (accessed on 11 September 2017).
4. Tempero, M.A.; Malafa, M.P.; Al-Hawary, M.; Asbun, H.; Bain, A.; Behrman, S.W.; Benson, A.B., 3rd; Binder, E.; Cardin, D.B.; Cha, C.; et al. Pancreatic adenocarcinoma, Version 2.2017, NCCN clinical practice guidelines in oncology. *J. Natl. Compr. Cancer Netw.* **2017**, *15*, 1028–1061. [CrossRef] [PubMed]
5. Mukherjee, S.; Hurt, C.; Bridgewater, J.; Falk, S.; Cummins, S.; Wasan, H.; Crosby, T.; Jephcott, C.; Roy, R.; Radhakrishna, G.; et al. Gemcitabine-based or capecitabine-based chemoradiotherapy for locally advanced pancreatic cancer (SCALOP): A multicentre, randomised, phase 2 trial. *Lancet Oncol.* **2013**, *14*, 317–326. [CrossRef]
6. Von Hoff, D.D.; Ervin, T.; Arena, F.P.; Chiorean, E.G.; Infante, J.; Moore, M.; Seay, T.; Tjulandin, S.A.; Ma, W.W.; Saleh, M.N.; et al. Increased survival in pancreatic cancer with nab-paclitaxel plus gemcitabine. *N. Engl. J. Med.* **2013**, *369*, 1691–1703. [CrossRef]
7. Conroy, T.; Desseigne, F.; Ychou, M.; Bouche, O.; Guimbaud, R.; Bécouarn, Y.; Adenis, A.; Raoul, J.-L.; Gourgou-Bourgade, S.; De La Fouchardiere, C.; et al. FOLFIRINOX versus Gemcitabine for Metastatic Pancreatic Cancer. *N. Engl. J. Med.* **2011**, *364*, 1817–1825. [CrossRef]
8. Fukuchi, M.; Ishiguro, T.; Ogata, K.; Suzuki, O.; Kumagai, Y.; Ishibashi, K.; Ishida, H.; Kuwano, H.; Mochiki, E. Prognostic Role of Conversion Surgery for Unresectable Gastric Cancer. *Ann. Surg. Oncol.* **2015**, *22*, 3618–3624. [CrossRef]
9. Yokota, T.; Kato, K.; Hamamoto, Y.; Tsubosa, Y.; Ogawa, H.; Ito, Y.; Hara, H.; Ura, T.; Kojima, T.; Chin, K.; et al. Phase II study of chemoselection with docetaxel plus cisplatin and 5-fluorouracil induction chemotherapy and subsequent conversion surgery for locally advanced unresectable oesophageal cancer. *Br. J. Cancer* **2016**, *115*, 1328–1334. [CrossRef]
10. Satoi, S.; Yanagimoto, H.; Toyokawa, H.; Inoue, K.; Wada, K.; Yamamoto, T.; Hirooka, S.; Yamaki, S.; Yui, R.; Mergental, H.; et al. Selective Use of Staging Laparoscopy Based on Carbohydrate Antigen 19-9 Level and Tumor Size in Patients With Radiographically Defined Potentially or Borderline Resectable Pancreatic Cancer. *Pancreas* **2011**, *40*, 426–432. [CrossRef]
11. Satoi, S.; Yanagimoto, H.; Yamamoto, T.; Toyokawa, H.; Hirooka, S.; Yamaki, S.; Opendro, S.S.; Inoue, K.; Michiura, T.; Ryota, H.; et al. A clinical role of staging laparoscopy in patients with radiographically defined locally advanced pancreatic ductal adenocarcinoma. *World J. Surg. Oncol.* **2016**, *14*, 14. [CrossRef]
12. Satoi, S.; Fujii, T.; Yanagimoto, H.; Motoi, F.; Kurata, M.; Takahara, N.; Yamada, S.; Yamamoto, T.; Mizuma, M.; Honda, G.; et al. Multicenter Phase II Study of Intravenous and Intraperitoneal Paclitaxel With S-1 for Pancreatic Ductal Adenocarcinoma Patients With Peritoneal Metastasis. *Ann. Surg.* **2017**, *265*, 397–401. [CrossRef] [PubMed]
13. Satoi, S.; Yamaue, H.; Kato, K.; Takahashi, S.; Hirono, S.; Takeda, S.; Eguchi, H.; Sho, M.; Wada, K.; Shinchi, H.; et al. Role of adjuvant surgery for patients with initially unresectable pancreatic cancer with a long-term favorable response to non-surgical anti-cancer treatments: Results of a project study for pancreatic surgery by the Japanese Society of Hepato-Biliary-Pan. *J. Hepato-Biliary-Pancreat. Sci.* **2013**, *20*, 590–600. [CrossRef] [PubMed]
14. Dindo, D.; Demartines, N.; Clavien, P.-A. Classification of surgical complications: A new proposal with evaluation in a cohort of 6336 patients and results of a survey. *Ann. Surg.* **2004**, *240*, 205–213. [CrossRef]
15. Ferrone, C.R.; Brennan, M.; Gonen, M.; Coit, D.G.; Fong, Y.; Chung, S.; Tang, L.; Klimstra, D.; Allen, P.J. Pancreatic Adenocarcinoma: The Actual 5-Year Survivors. *J. Gastrointest. Surg.* **2007**, *12*, 701–706. [CrossRef] [PubMed]
16. Gillen, S.; Schuster, T.; Büschenfelde, C.M.Z.; Friess, H.; Kleeff, J. Preoperative/Neoadjuvant Therapy in Pancreatic Cancer: A Systematic Review and Meta-analysis of Response and Resection Percentages. *PLoS Med.* **2010**, *7*, e1000267. [CrossRef] [PubMed]

17. He, J.; Ahuja, N.; Makary, M.A.; Cameron, J.L.; Eckhauser, F.E.; Choti, M.A.; Hruban, R.H.; Pawlik, T.M.; Wolfgang, C.L. 2564 resected periampullary adenocarcinomas at a single institution: Trends over three decades. *HPB* **2013**, *16*, 83–90. [CrossRef]
18. Kato, K.; Kondo, S.; Hirano, S.; Tanaka, E.; Shichinohe, T.; Tsuchikawa, T.; Matsumoto, J. Adjuvant surgical therapy for patients with initially-unresectable pancreatic cancer with long-term favorable responses to chemotherapy. *J. Hepato-Biliary-Pancreat. Sci.* **2011**, *18*, 712–716. [CrossRef]
19. Wright, G.P.; Poruk, K.E.; Zenati, M.; Steve, J.; Bahary, N.; Hogg, M.E.; Zuriekat, A.H.; Wolfgang, C.L.; Zeh, H.J.; Weiss, M. Primary Tumor Resection Following Favorable Response to Systemic Chemotherapy in Stage IV Pancreatic Adenocarcinoma with Synchronous Metastases: A Bi-institutional Analysis. *J. Gastrointest. Surg.* **2016**, *20*, 1830–1835. [CrossRef]
20. Nitsche, U.; Wenzel, P.; Siveke, J.T.; Braren, R.; Holzapfel, K.; Schlitter, A.M.; Stöß, C.; Kong, B.; Esposito, I.; Erkan, M.; et al. Resectability After First-Line FOLFIRINOX in Initially Unresectable Locally Advanced Pancreatic Cancer: A Single-Center Experience. *Ann. Surg. Oncol.* **2015**, *22*, 1212–1220. [CrossRef]
21. Hackert, T.; Sachsenmaier, M.; Hinz, U.; Schneider, L.; Michalski, C.W.; Springfeld, C.; Strobel, O.; Jäger, D.; Ulrich, A.; Büchler, M.W. Locally advanced pancreatic cancer: Neoadjuvant therapy with FOLFIRINOX results in resectability in 60% of the patients. *Ann. Surg.* **2016**, *264*, 457–463. [CrossRef]
22. Kenta, S.; Okabayashi, T.; Shima, Y.; Morita, S.; Iwata, J.; Sumiyoshi, T.; Saisaka, Y.; Yasuhiro, H.; Yoshihiro, N.; Matsumoto, M.; et al. Clinical effects of chemoradiotherapy in pursuit of optimal treatment of locally advanced unresectable pancreatic cancer. *Br. J. Radiol.* **2017**, *90*, 20170165.
23. Saito, T.; Ishido, K.; Kudo, D.; Kimura, N.; Wakiya, T.; Nakayama, Y.; Hakamada, K. Combination therapy with gemcitabine and nab-paclitaxel for locally advanced unresectable pancreatic cancer. *Mol. Clin. Oncol.* **2017**, *6*, 963–967. [CrossRef] [PubMed]
24. Asano, T.; Hirano, S.; Nakamura, T.; Okamura, K.; Tsuchikawa, T.; Noji, T.; Nakanishi, Y.; Tanaka, K.; Shichinohe, T. Survival benefit of conversion surgery for patients with initially unresectable pancreatic cancer who responded favorably to nonsurgical treatment. *J. Hepato-Biliary-Pancreat. Sci.* **2018**, *25*, 342–350. [CrossRef] [PubMed]
25. Natsume, S.; Shimizu, Y.; Senda, Y.; Hijioka, S.; Matsuo, K.; Ito, S.; Komori, K.; Abe, T.; Hara, K. Conversion surgery only for highly selected patients with unresectable pancreatic cancer: A satisfactory outcome in exchange for a lower resection rate. *Surg. Today* **2019**, *49*, 670–677. [CrossRef]
26. Opendro, S.S.; Satoi, S.; Yanagimoto, H.; Yamamoto, T.; Toyokawa, H.; Hirooka, S.; Yamaki, S.; Inoue, K.; Matsui, Y.; Kwon, A.-H. Role of adjuvant surgery in initially unresectable pancreatic cancer after long-term chemotherapy or chemoradiation therapy: Survival benefit? *J. Hepato-Biliary-Pancreat. Sci.* **2014**, *21*, 695–702. [CrossRef]
27. Yoo, C.; Shin, S.H.; Kim, K.P.; Jeong, J.H.; Chang, H.M.; Kang, J.H.; Lee, S.S.; Park, D.H.; Song, T.J.; Seo, D.W.; et al. Clinical outcomes of conversion surgery after neoadjuvant chemotherapy in patients with borderline resectable and locally advanced unresectable pancreatic cancer: A single-center, retrospective analysis. *Cancers* **2019**, *11*, 278. [CrossRef]
28. Michelakos, T.; Pergolini, I.; Castillo, C.F.-D.; Honselmann, K.C.; Cai, L.; Deshpande, V.; Wo, J.Y.; Ryan, D.P.; Allen, J.N.; Blaszkowsky, L.S.; et al. Predictors of Resectability and Survival in Patients With Borderline and Locally Advanced Pancreatic Cancer who Underwent Neoadjuvant Treatment With FOLFIRINOX. *Ann. Surg.* **2019**, *269*, 733–740. [CrossRef]
29. Klaiber, U.; Schnaidt, E.S.; Hinz, U.; Gaida, M.M.; Heger, U.; Hank, T.; Strobel, O.; Neoptolemos, J.P.; Mihaljevic, A.L.; Büchler, M.W. Prognostic Factors of Survival After Neoadjuvant Treatment and Resection for Initially Unresectable Pancreatic Cancer. *Ann. Surg.* **2019**, in press. [CrossRef]
30. Satoi, S.; Yamamoto, T.; Yamaki, S.; Sakaguchi, T.; Sekimoto, M. Surgical indication for and desirable outcomes of conversion surgery in patients with initially unresectable pancreatic ductal adenocarcinoma. *Ann. Gastroenterol. Surg.* **2019**, *4*, 6–13. [CrossRef]
31. Van Veldhuisen, E.; Vogel, J.A.; Klompmaker, S.; Busch, O.R.; Van Laarhoven, H.W.M.; Van Lienden, K.P.; Wilmink, J.W.; Marsman, H.A.; Besselink, M.G. Added value of CA19-9 response in predicting resectability of locally advanced pancreatic cancer following induction chemotherapy. *HPB* **2018**, *20*, 605–611. [CrossRef]
32. Murphy, J.E.; Wo, J.Y.; Ryan, D.P.; Clark, J.W.; Jiang, W.; Yeap, B.Y.; Drapek, L.C.; Ly, L.; Baglini, C.V.; Blaszkowsky, L.S.; et al. Total Neoadjuvant Therapy With FOLFIRINOX in Combination With Losartan Followed by Chemoradiotherapy for Locally Advanced Pancreatic Cancer: A Phase 2 Clinical Trial. *JAMA Oncol.* **2019**, *5*, 1020–1027. [CrossRef] [PubMed]

33. Rangelova, E.; Wefer, A.; Persson, S.; Valente, R.; Tanaka, K.; Orsini, N.; Segersvärd, R.; Arnelo, U.; Del Chiaro, M. Surgery improves survival after neoadjuvant therapy for borderline and locally advanced pancreatic cancer: A single institution experience. *Ann. Surg.* **2019**, in press. [CrossRef] [PubMed]
34. Heger, U.; Sun, H.; Hinz, U.; Klaiber, U.; Tanaka, M.; Liu, B.; Sachsenmaier, M.; Springfeld, C.; Michalski, C.W.; Büchler, M.W.; et al. Induction chemotherapy in pancreatic cancer: CA 19-9 may predict resectability and survival. *HPB* **2020**, *22*, 224–232. [CrossRef] [PubMed]
35. Tanaka, M.; Heckler, M.; Mihaljevic, A.; Sun, H.; Klaiber, U.; Heger, U.; Büchler, M.W.; Hackert, T. CT response of primary tumor and CA19-9 predict resectability of metastasized pancreatic cancer after FOLFIRINOX. *Eur. J. Surg. Oncol.* **2019**, *45*, 1453–1459. [CrossRef] [PubMed]
36. Chatterjee, D.; Katz, M.H.; Rashid, A.; Varadhachary, G.R.; Wolff, R.A.; Wang, H.; Lee, J.E.; Pisters, P.W.; Vauthey, J.N.; Crane, C.; et al. Histologic grading the extent of residual carcinoma following neoadjuvant chemoradiation in pancreatic ductal adenocarcinoma: A predictor for patient outcome. *Cancer* **2012**, *118*, 3182–3190. [CrossRef]
37. White, R.R.; Xie, H.B.; Gottfried, M.R.; Czito, B.G.; Hurwitz, H.I.; Morse, M.A.; Blobe, G.C.; Paulson, E.K.; Baillie, J.; Branch, M.S.; et al. Significance of Histological Response to Preoperative Chemoradiotherapy for Pancreatic Cancer. *Ann. Surg. Oncol.* **2005**, *12*, 214–221. [CrossRef]
38. Moutardier, V.; Magnin, V.; Turrini, O.; Viret, F.; Hennekinne-Mucci, S.; Gonçalves, A.; Pésenti, C.; Guiramand, J.; Lelong, B.; Giovannini, M.; et al. Assessment of pathologic response after preoperative chemoradiotherapy and surgery in pancreatic adenocarcinoma. *Int. J. Radiat. Oncol.* **2004**, *60*, 437–443. [CrossRef]

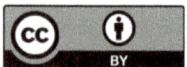

© 2020 by the authors. Licensee MDPI, Basel, Switzerland. This article is an open access article distributed under the terms and conditions of the Creative Commons Attribution (CC BY) license (http://creativecommons.org/licenses/by/4.0/).

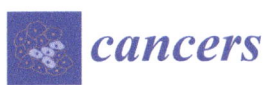

Systematic Review

Systematic Review and Meta-Analysis of Surgical Treatment for Isolated Local Recurrence of Pancreatic Cancer

Simone Serafini [1], Cosimo Sperti [1,*], Alberto Friziero [1], Alessandra Rosalba Brazzale [2], Alessia Buratin [3], Alberto Ponzoni [4] and Lucia Moletta [1]

1. Department of Surgery, Oncology and Gastroenterology, 3rd Surgical Clinic, University of Padua, Via Giustiniani 2, 35128 Padua, Italy; simone.serafini@ymail.com (S.S.); alberto.friziero@aopd.veneto.it (A.F.); lucia.moletta@unipd.it (L.M.)
2. Department of Statistical Sciences, University of Padua, Via Cesare Battisti 241, 35121 Padua, Italy; brazzale@stat.unipd.it
3. Department of Biology, University of Padua, Viale G. Colombo 3, 35131 Padua, Italy; buratin.alessia1@gmail.com
4. Department of Radiology, Padua General Hospital, Via Giustiniani 2, 35128 Padua, Italy; alberto.ponzoni@aopd.veneto.it
* Correspondence: csperti@libero.it; Tel.: +39-04-9821-8845; Fax: +39-04-9821-8821

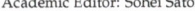

Citation: Serafini, S.; Sperti, C.; Friziero, A.; Brazzale, A.R.; Buratin, A.; Ponzoni, A.; Moletta, L. Systematic Review and Meta-Analysis of Surgical Treatment for Isolated Local Recurrence of Pancreatic Cancer. *Cancers* **2021**, *13*, 1277. https://doi.org/10.3390/cancers13061277

Academic Editor: Sohei Satoi

Received: 11 February 2021
Accepted: 10 March 2021
Published: 13 March 2021

Publisher's Note: MDPI stays neutral with regard to jurisdictional claims in published maps and institutional affiliations.

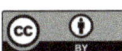

Copyright: © 2021 by the authors. Licensee MDPI, Basel, Switzerland. This article is an open access article distributed under the terms and conditions of the Creative Commons Attribution (CC BY) license (https://creativecommons.org/licenses/by/4.0/).

Simple Summary: Recurrences after primary resection of pancreatic cancer are generally treated with chemotherapy or best supportive care. Despite some reports of encouraging results after the re-resection of recurrences, the real role of surgery in this setting remains unclear. The aim of our systematic review and meta-analysis was to define the benefit of surgery in the case of isolated local recurrence. The data collected on 431 patients suggest an overall survival benefit of 29 months for patients re-operated compared to patients given medical therapies. In selected patients with recurrent pancreatic cancer, resection is safe and feasible, and may offer a survival advantage.

Abstract: Purpose: To perform a systematic review and meta-analysis on the outcome of surgical treatment for isolated local recurrence of pancreatic cancer. Methods: A systematic review and meta-analysis based on Preferred Reporting Items for Systematic Reviews and Meta-analyses (PRISMA) guidelines was conducted in PubMed, Scopus, and Web of Science. Results: Six studies concerning 431 patients with recurrent pancreatic cancer met the inclusion criteria and were included in the analysis: 176 underwent redo surgery, and 255 received non-surgical treatments. Overall survival and post-recurrence survival were significantly longer in the re-resected group (ratio of means (ROM) 1.99; 95% confidence interval (CI), 1.54–2.56, I^2 = 75.89%, p = 0.006, and ROM = 2.05; 95% CI, 1.48–2.83, I^2 = 76.39%, p = 0.002, respectively) with a median overall survival benefit of 28.7 months (mean difference (MD) 28.7; 95% CI, 10.3–47.0, I^2 = 89.27%, p < 0.001) and median survival benefit of 15.2 months after re-resection (MD 15.2; 95% CI, 8.6–21.8, I^2 = 58.22%, p = 0.048). Conclusion: Resection of isolated pancreatic cancer recurrences is safe and feasible and may offer a survival benefit. Selection of patients and assessment of time and site of recurrence are mandatory.

Keywords: isolated local recurrence; pancreatectomy; pancreatic cancer; pancreatic remnant; recurrence; redo surgery

1. Introduction

Pancreatic ductal adenocarcinoma (PDAC) was the fourth cause of cancer-related death in the United States and in Italy in 2018, with an estimated 55.440 and 13.300 new cases diagnosed, and 44.300 and 11.463 related deaths, respectively [1,2]. Surgical resection continues to be the only chance of cure, but the 5-year survival rate remains low, ranging from 19% to 27% [3,4]. Such disappointing results are justified by the aggressive biology of pancreatic cancer and the high rate of recurrence (up to 80%) even after radical resections [5]. Recurrent pancreatic cancer poses a challenge for clinicians and is commonly treated with chemotherapy or best supportive care. Unlike other cancers, re-surgery for relapsing pancreatic cancer is not generally considered an option because evidence regarding its benefits is lacking, and isolated tumor recurrences amenable to resection are relatively uncommon. An isolated local recurrence (ILR) is usually defined as a tumoral recurrence localized to the posterior resection margin, the pancreatic remnant, or the locoregional lymph nodes. Some authors have recently reported encouraging results of surgical management of pancreatic cancer recurrence in selected patients [6–9].

The aim of the present study was to conduct a systematic review and meta-analysis of the outcome of redo-surgery for patients with isolated local recurrent PDAC after initial pancreatectomy.

2. Materials and Methods

2.1. Study Selection

A systematic literature search was conducted using PubMed, Scopus, and Web of Science to identify all studies published up to 30 November 2020 regarding the recurrence of pancreatic cancer after surgery. The search terms used were "pancreatic cancer/neoplasm/adenocarcinoma", "recurrence", "surgery/pancreatectomy/redo surgery/completion pancreatectomy". The articles found were used to broaden the search, and all emerging abstracts, studies, and citations were reviewed. The reference lists of all the studies considered were also screened for any other potentially relevant papers.

2.2. Inclusion and Exclusion Criteria

The following inclusion criteria were considered for the studies: (1) they reported on patients with histologically proven ILR PDAC treated surgically with curative intent, with or without (neo) adjuvant chemotherapy and/or radiotherapy; (2) they provided data on patients reoperated for recurrent PDAC after initial pancreatectomy, and their long-term outcomes; (3) they were written in English. The following exclusion criteria were considered: (1) reviews without original data or animal studies; (2) absence of individual patient data; (3) duplications; (4) lack of long-term data; and (5) in the event of successive publications by the same group, only the most detailed study was included.

Three independent reviewers (SS, ARB, AB) extracted the data using standardized data forms. All data from each eligible study were entered in a dedicated spreadsheet (Excel 2007, Microsoft Corporation®, Padua, Italy). Disagreements between the reviewers were solved by discussion and consensus. The following data were collected: title, first author, year of publication, characteristics of study population, study design, number of patients who underwent re-resection, disease-free interval (DFI), overall survival (OS), and post-recurrence survival (PRS). The articles included in this review were chosen in accordance with the Preferred Reporting Items for Systematic Reviews and Meta-Analyses (PRISMA) guidelines [10].

2.3. Terminology and Definitions

Disease-free interval (DFI) was defined as the interval between the date of primary tumor resection and the date of recurrence. Overall survival (OS) was defined as the time between the primary tumor resection and death or latest follow-up. Post-recurrence survival (PRS) was the time interval between recurrence detection or reoperation and death or latest follow-up.

2.4. Statistical Analysis

The statistical methods of this study were reviewed by two authors (BAR and BA). Two meta-analyses were conducted in line with the Cochrane Collaboration guidelines on the Meta-analysis of Observational Studies in Epidemiology [11,12]. The first analysis focused on OS in months; the second focused on survival in months after the recurrence of PDAC. The data used for the meta-analyses are summarized in Table 1. Survival was retrieved from the published studies as median values and ranges. Where not stated explicitly, these values were calculated from the data reported in the papers or extrapolated from the Kaplan-Meier (K-M) plots. Since all articles used in this analysis reported only the size of the study groups (without standard errors), all median survival times were converted into means and variances using a dedicated statistical algorithm [13].

The survival data were pooled for the analysis of either the mean difference (MD) or the logarithm of the ratio of means (ROM) [14]. Values of MD > 0 or ROM > 1 indicate a higher survival rate for patients who underwent re-resection. Cochran's Q statistic and the I^2 statistic were used to test between-study heterogeneity [15]. If the Q statistic was significant at the 0.1 level, the summary effect and corresponding 95% confidence interval (CI) were obtained with the Mantel-Haenszel random effects model [16]. For I^2 < 50%, between-study heterogeneity was judged to be low moderate; for $I^2 \geq 50\%$, it was considered substantial. The point estimate of MD and ROM was considered statistically significant when p was < 0.05. A cumulative meta-analysis was also run to test the stability of the pooled endpoint estimates. Publication bias was assessed visually using a funnel plot, and the number of missing studies was estimated using the trim-and-fill method [17,18]. All analyses were conducted using R version 3.5.2 [19].

Table 1. Studies included in the meta-analysis. OS and PFR are compared for each study (significant difference for p value < 0.05). Pts: number of patients; OS: overall survival; PRS: post recurrence survival; * extrapolated from K-M plot; ^ extrapolated from confidence interval; NR: not reported.

Author	Treatment	Pts	OS (Range)	p Value	PRS (Range)	p Value
Strobel et al. [20]	RESECTED *	41	NR	NR	26 (1–60)	<0.01
	UNRESECTED *	16	NR		10.8 (1–36)	
Miyazaki et al. [21]	RESECTED *	11	78.2 (17–107)	<0.001	25 (3–61)	<0.01
	UNRESECTED *	159	20.3 (5–103)		9.3 (3–75)	
Hashimoto et al. [22]	RESECTED	8	72 (36–129)	NR	17 (10–85)	NR
	UNRESECTED	2	30 (28–32)		10 (9–11)	
Nakayama et al. [23]	RESECTED ^	11	70 (19–70)	=0.02	44 (11–44)	=0.01
	UNRESECTED ^	35	25 (15–35)		11 (6–25)	
Yamada et al. [24]	RESECTED *	90	26 (4–60)	=0.012	NR	NR
	UNRESECTED *	24	14 (2–60)		NR	
Kim et al. [25]	RESECTED *	15	NR	NR	28 (5–57)	=0.01
	UNRESECTED *	19	NR		12 (4.5–35)	

3. Results

The study search and selection strategy are shown in the flow chart in Figure 1. The preliminary literature search identified 1326 studies matching the initial search criteria. After screening, six studies were ultimately included in the quantitative synthesis (meta-analysis) [20–25].

It was not possible to include DFI in this analysis because this information was lacking in most studies. Likewise, due to the lack and fragmentation of precise data about the time to recurrence, it was not possible to estimate and compare conditional survival of resected and non-resected patients. Four reports [21–24] were included for OS and five for PRS [20–23,25] analysis. All six studies were retrospective and concerned a total of 431 patients with recurrent pancreatic cancer after primary pancreatic resection: 176 treated with re-resection, and 255 given non-surgical removal of recurrence. The characteristics of the selected studies are summarized in Table 1.

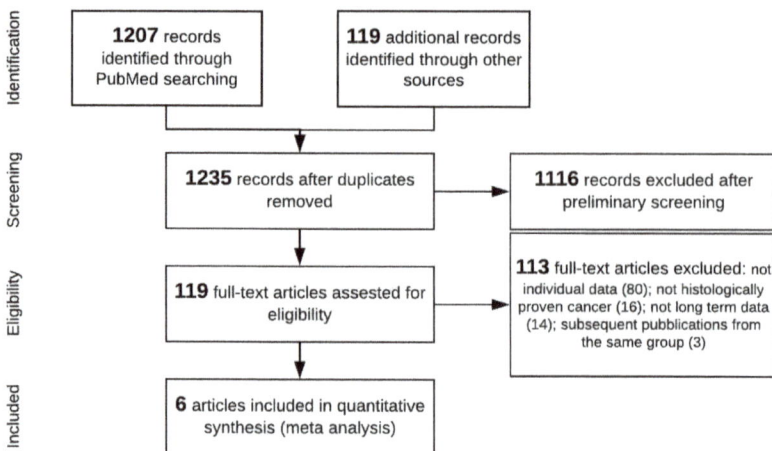

Figure 1. Preferred Reporting Items for Systematic Reviews and Meta-Analyses (PRISMA) flow diagram.

After surgery for recurrent PDAC, the mortality rate reported was 1.1% (2/176 patients) [20,25]; the morbidity rate ranged from 6% [25] to 33% [24].

A random-effects meta-analytical model was used for all variables. The random-effects method was always chosen because Cochran's Q statistic proved statistically significant at the $p < 0.05$ level for all meta-analyses, with a borderline situation for the analysis focusing on mean survival after recurrent PDAC, for which it was $p = 0.048$.

OS was almost twice as long in patients reoperated for ILR PDAC than in patients given non-surgical treatments (ROM 1.99; 95% CI, 1.54–2.56, $I^2 = 75.89\%$, $p = 0.006$). The median survival benefit for patients who underwent re-resection was 28.7 months (MD 28.7; 95% CI, 10.3–47.0, $I^2 = 89.27\%$, $p < 0.001$), as shown in Figure 2.

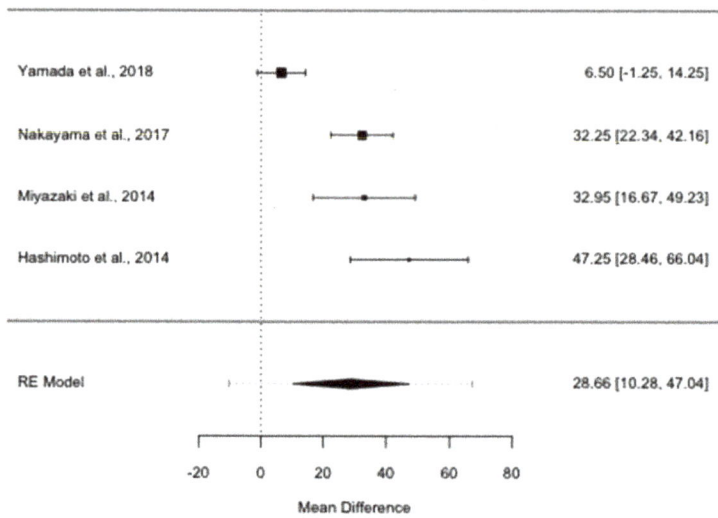

Figure 2. Forest plot for overall survival mean difference in months. RE: random-effects.

Median PRS was significantly longer for the group treated surgically than for the patients not re-resected (ROM = 2.05; 95% CI, 1.48–2.83, $I^2 = 76.39\%$, $p = 0.002$): it was

15.2 months longer in the former than in the latter group (MD 15.2; 95% CI, 8.6–21.8, $I^2 = 58.22\%$, $p = 0.048$) (Figure 3).

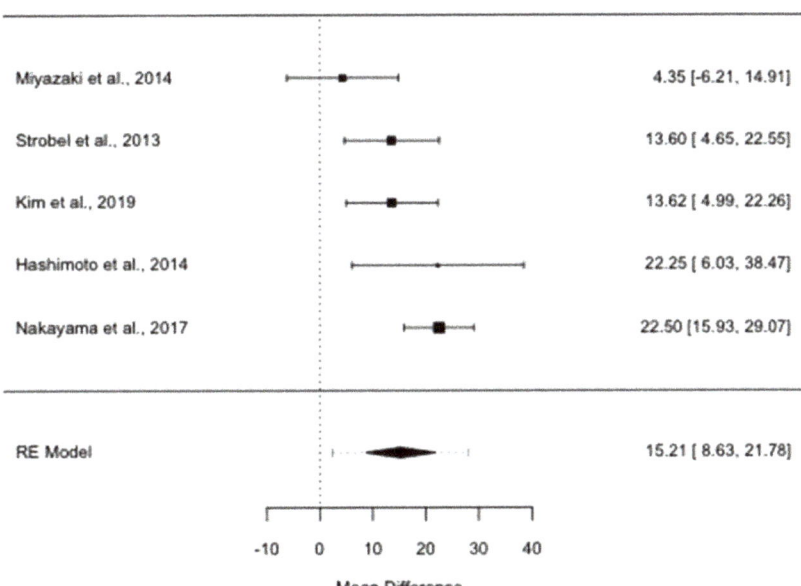

Figure 3. Forest plot for post recurrence survival mean difference in months. RE: random-effects.

The cumulative meta-analysis demonstrated that the benefit after pancreatic re-resection settles very quickly for both OS and PRS. Funnel plots provided some evidence of publication bias. One study was estimated to be missing on the left for OS, while no study seems to be missing for PRS (Figures 4 and 5).

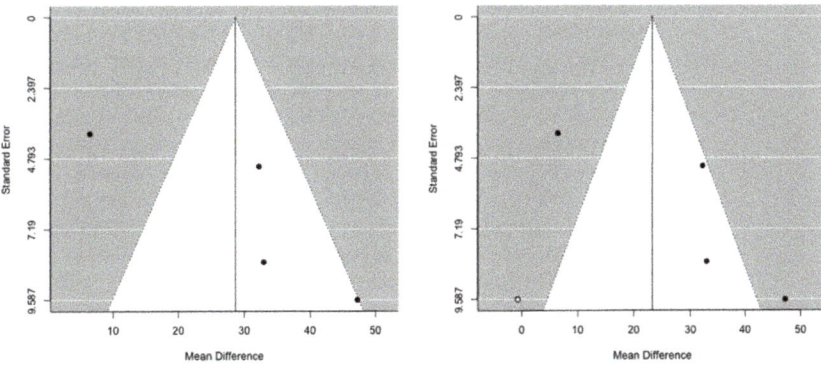

Figure 4. Funnel plots for mean difference in overall survival. Left: original data; Right: imputation of missing studies.

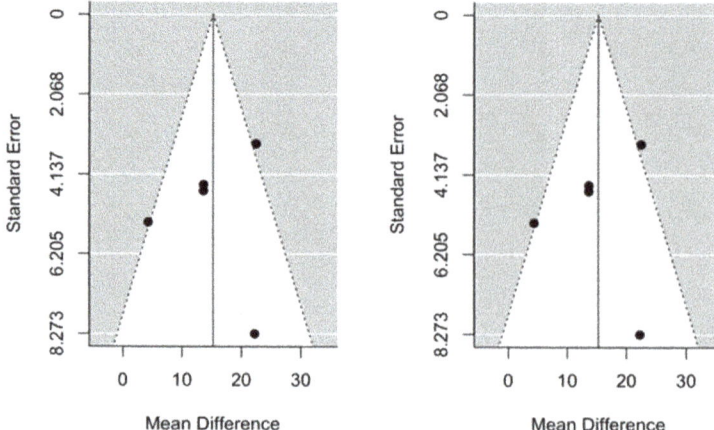

Figure 5. Funnel plots for mean difference in post recurrence survival. Left: original data; Right: imputation of missing studies.

4. Discussion

Pancreatic ductal adenocarcinoma is recognized as a major cause of cancer-related deaths for early metastasis, extensive invasion, and poor prognosis. At diagnosis, 50% of patients present with synchronous metastases, and further 30% present with locally advanced disease, who are not suitable for upfront surgery [1]. Moreover, despite radical resection, PDAC frequently relapses, and the clinical management of recurrences is troublesome. The well-accepted treatment for recurrent PDAC is still chemotherapy, whenever feasible. Recent studies on the surgical treatment of recurrent PDAC in selected patients reported encouraging results in terms of survival, with negligible surgical morbidity and mortality rates.

Strobel et al. [20] conducted a prospective cohort study with patients with pancreatic cancer recurrence and assessed perioperative outcome, survival, and prognostic parameters. In this series, 57 patients underwent surgery for histologically proven ILR after R0/R1 resection of PDAC. ILR was resected in 41 patients. Most resections were carried out for extrapancreatic recurrences. A pancreatic re-resection was performed in 24 patients (44%). In 19 cases, a total pancreatectomy was necessary; segmental resections were possible in only 5 patients. In 11 (20%) patients with ILR in paracaval or interaortocaval lymph nodes, a simple excision with lymphadenectomy was performed. A total of 36 (63%) patients with ILR had a recurrence in close touch with visceral arteries (SMA or the celiac trunk). In these cases resection was only attempted if the arteries were not directly involved. No data about the number of R1/R0 resection after the first operation were reported. The authors [20] also assessed the potential effect of intraoperative radiation therapy (IORT). A total of 22 patients underwent surgical resection and IORT. In 16 patients, the ILR was considered not resectable because of infiltration of the mesenteric vessels; 10 of these patients received IORT (10–15 Gray). In patients with resection of ILR, the subgroup with IORT demonstrated a shorter survival than patients without IORT (17.0 vs. 29.6 months of median survival). In contrast, patients with unresectable ILR had significantly better survival with IORT (15.1 vs. 4.3 months of median survival). They concluded that benefit of percutaneous and intraoperative radiotherapy warrants further evaluation.

Miyazaki et al. [21] reported on 284 consecutive patients with pancreatic cancer who underwent initial pancreatectomy with curative intent (R0 and R1 resection). A total of 170 patients were diagnosed with recurrent pancreatic cancer, but only 11 (16.4%) developed ILR. Two out of eleven were R1 at the time of the first operation.

Hashimoto et al. [22] retrospectively analysed the survival and pathological findings of 10 patients who developed remnant pancreatic cancer. The authors performed a pyrosequencing assay for KRAS (codon 12) mutations and immunohistochemistry for MUC1/MUC2, and compared the histological diagnosis of the initial tumor and the remnant pancreatic cancer in the resected group. The results indicated that four cases might have developed local recurrence of the primary lesions, and the other four cases might have developed new primary lesions. It is important to point out that only one case out of ten was R1 resection at the time of the first operation.

Nakayama et al. [23] compared the survival outcomes of patients who developed isolated local vs. distant recurrence. In this subset of patients, only 3 out of 46 patients were considered R1 after the first pancreatic resection. Median survival after the recurrence was longer in the patients with ILR than in those with distant metastasis (44 vs. 13 months, p-value < 0.05).

Yamada et al. [24] conducted a multicenter survey of patients diagnosed with ILR in the remnant pancreas. Data from 114 patients were collected in a retrospective manner. Although their multivariate analysis could not identify any independent prognostic factors, the univariate analysis showed that excision of ILR, age (<65 years), body mass index (>20 kg/m^2), tumor dimensions (<20 mm), and distance from the pancreatic resection margin (>10 mm) were statistically significant positive prognostic factors. In this study, there was no correlation between the R1 margin at the time of first operation and distance to the pancreatic stump of ILR, which implies that the onset of a tumor in the remnant pancreas should not always be considered as a consequence of intrapancreatic colonization of the primitive cancer, as supported by Hashimoto et al. [22].

Kim et al. [25] reported on a cohort of 1610 consecutive patients with pancreatic cancer who underwent initial pancreatectomy with curative intent between January 2000 and December 2014 at Asian Medical Centre, Seoul, Korea. A total of 1346 patients were diagnosed with recurrent pancreatic cancer, but only 197 (14.6%) and 34 (2.5%) of these patients had isolated recurrence and ILR, respectively. Moreover, the authors performed a survival analysis according to the recurrence pattern. Survival after recurrence was better in patients who underwent resection of isolated recurrence in the remnant pancreas (median 28 vs. 12 months) and lung (median 36.5 vs. 9.5 months) than in those who did not undergo resection.

In a previously published systematic review by Moletta et al. [26] about the role of surgical resection for recurrent PDAC, an overall survival benefit after resection compared to non-resected patients was reported.

This raises some questions. First, is surgery for recurrent PDAC definitely worthwhile? If so, can it be proposed for all sites of recurrence? Which is the optimal treatment for recurrent PDAC: chemotherapy or surgery?

In this study, we confirmed the potential benefit of surgery, applying a quantitative analysis and statistical significance to the data previously reviewed. We analyzed six studies and compared the results of surgery vs. medical treatment (chemotherapy or best supportive care) for patients with recurrent PDAC. The results of our analysis confirmed that redo surgery for recurrent tumor offers a survival advantage for selected patients with a very low risk of perioperative mortality and an acceptable morbidity rate. The survival benefit (patients re-operated for ILR compared to patients given medical therapies) was estimated as about 29 and 15 months in terms of OS and PRS, respectively.

The resection of recurrent disease seems to be feasible and safe, and should be considered for selected patients with isolated pancreatic cancer local recurrences. Among the various sites affected, surgery for recurrences in the pancreatic remnant seems to be associated with a better outcome. Zhou et al. [8] reviewed the English literature until June 2016, collecting 19 articles on 55 patients who had complete pancreatectomy for relapsing PDAC. The 1, 3, and 5-year OS rates after second pancreatectomy were 82.2%, 49.2%, and 40.6%, respectively.

To date, only some reports and case series that investigate the benefit of surgery in isolated distant recurrence or in oligo metastatic patients have been published. Despite advances in surgical techniques, pancreatic surgery often results in a positive resection margin status (R). In particular, R0 was defined as a distance from the tumor to the closest resection margin of >1 mm, whereas R1 as a distance of ≤1 mm to the resection margin or margin involved without macroscopic involvement. R1 resection and medial/posterior margin due to perineural invasion, regional lymph node metastases, and systemic spreading at the time of surgery resulted in early recurrences. Based on today's knowledge, it is not possible to define if ILR are de novo tumors or recurrence of the primary ones. Encouraging survival rates have been reported for isolated lung metastases: the median survival time after lung metastasectomy ranged from 18.6 [9] to 47 months [27]. On the other hand, poor outcomes have been reported after the resection of liver or peritoneal metastases [28,29]. New randomized clinical trials should be conducted to better define the role of surgery in this setting.

We cannot clearly answer the question regarding the optimal treatment for recurrent PDAC because of the lack of controlled studies comparing the outcomes of patients who undergo surgery with those given chemotherapy. In the era of multi-agent systemic therapy, survival for pancreatic cancer has globally increased. However, even if many different randomized clinical trials for borderline, locally advanced, and "de novo" metastatic PDAC are published confirming the survival benefit of new regimen, in the case of recurrent PDAC, such studies are missing, and there is currently no scientific evidence supporting a specific treatment. Some authors have shown improvement in survival after treatment of recurrent PDAC with intensified regimes including FOLFIRINOX (FFN) and nab-paclitaxel plus gemcitabine (GEMNAB) compared with single agent chemotherapy. Gbolahan et al. [30] reported that administration of FFN or GEMNAB compared with single agent chemotherapy was associated with a statistically significant survival benefit, with a median OS of 14 (95% CI 9–17) vs. 8 (95% CI 6–12) months. Javed et al. [31], in a recent retrospective multi-center European study, did not report any significant differences in terms of survival between FFN/GEMNAB and any other combination of gemcitabine- or 5-fluorouracil-based regimen: polichemotherapy was always superior when compared with gemcitabine monotherapy with a variable median OS of 7.9–9.9 vs. 4.9 (95% CI 4.4–5.6) months. Kawaida et al. [32] reported an objective response rate of 13.6% and a progression-free survival of 7.2 months after administration of GEMNAB with an important hematological toxicity rate of 72.7% (grade 3–4).

It is reasonable to believe that the combination of new chemotherapy regimens and surgery in fit patients could improve the outcome of recurrent PDAC. Given the heterogeneous chemotherapy regimens used, the small numbers of patients included in different studies, and the fact that most patients present with multiple sites of relapse and frequently in poor health, inevitably, the surgical option can only be offered to a few, very selected patients.

Our study has some limitations to consider. The relatively small number of studies analyzed and their heterogeneity and retrospective nature entail a significant risk of selection bias. The lack of data in some studies also prevented us from measuring disease-free interval and compare conditional survival to obtain a more accurate picture of patients' outcomes. We therefore were unable to investigate the potential role of a number of factors including patient's characteristics, baseline tumor burden and stage, neoadjuvant chemotherapy, morbidity from surgical resection and adjuvant therapy, comorbidity, and functional status on failure to receive therapy. All these aspects can lead to a selection bias that it is difficult to avoid, according to the rarity of ILR in PDAC. These important questions should be further addressed in new prospective and multicentric studies.

5. Conclusions

To our knowledge, this is the first meta-analysis comparing the outcome of patients with ILR PDAC following resection or sequential chemotherapies. In selected patients with recurrent pancreatic cancer, resection is safe and feasible, and may offer a survival advantage. Surgery should be considered as part of the multimodality management of relapsing pancreatic cancer. An accurate patient selection, considering the site and time of recurrence, and a multidisciplinary approach are essential to choose the best appropriate treatment.

Author Contributions: S.S. acquisition of data, analysis and interpretation of data, drafting the article, final approval; C.S. conception and design of the study, critical revision, final approval; A.F. interpretation of data, drafting the article, final approval; A.R.B. acquisition of data, analysis and interpretation of data, drafting the article, final approval; A.B. acquisition of data, analysis and interpretation of data, drafting the article, final approval; A.P., interpretation of data, drafting the article, final approval; L.M. conception and design of the study, critical revision, final approval. All authors have read and agreed to the published version of the manuscript.

Funding: This research received no external funding.

Conflicts of Interest: The authors declare no conflict of interest.

References

1. Siegel, R.L.; Miller, K.D.M.; Jemal, A. Cancer statistics, 2018. *CA Cancer J. Clin.* **2018**, *68*, 7–30. [CrossRef] [PubMed]
2. AIOM. *Cancer Numbers in Italy Italian Association of Medical Oncology*; AIOM: Milano, Italy, 2018; Available online: https://www.aiom.it/wp-content/uploads/2018/10/2018_NumeriCancro-operatori.pdf (accessed on 11 February 2021).
3. Ferrone, C.R.; Pieretti-Vanmarcke, R.; Bloom, J.P.; Zheng, H.; Szymonifka, J.; Wargo, J.A.; Thayer, S.P.; Lauwers, G.Y.; Deshpande, V.; Mino-Kenudson, M.; et al. Pancreatic ductal adenocarcinoma: Long-term survival does not equal cure. *Surgery* **2012**, *152*, S43–S49. [CrossRef] [PubMed]
4. Katz, M.H.G.; Hwang, R.F.; Fleming, J.B.; Sun, C.C.; Wolff, R.A.; Varadhachary, G.; Abbruzzese, J.L.; Crane, C.H.; Krishnan, S.; Vauthey, J.-N.; et al. Long-Term Survival After Multidisciplinary Management of Resected Pancreatic Adenocarcinoma. *Ann. Surg. Oncol.* **2009**, *16*, 836–847. [CrossRef] [PubMed]
5. Dunne, R.F.; Hezel, A.F. Genetics and Biology of Pancreatic Ductal Adenocarcinoma. *Hematol. Clin. N. Am.* **2015**, *29*, 595–608. [CrossRef]
6. Kleeff, J.; Reiser, C.; Hinz, U.; Bachmann, J.; Debus, J.; Jaeger, D.; Friess, H.; Büchler, M.W. Surgery for Recurrent Pancreatic Ductal Adenocarcinoma. *Ann. Surg.* **2007**, *245*, 566–572. [CrossRef]
7. Thomas, R.M.; Truty, M.J.; Nogueras-Gonzalez, G.M.; Fleming, J.B.; Vauthey, J.-N.; Pisters, P.W.T.; Lee, J.E.; Rice, D.C.; Hofstetter, W.L.; Wolff, R.A.; et al. Selective Reoperation for Locally Recurrent or Metastatic Pancreatic Ductal Adenocarcinoma Following Primary Pancreatic Resection. *J. Gastrointest. Surg.* **2012**, *16*, 1696–1704. [CrossRef]
8. Zhou, Y.; Song, A.; Wu, L.; Si, X.; Li, Y. Second pancreatectomy for recurrent pancreatic ductal adenocarcinoma in the remnant pancreas: A pooled analysis. *Pancreatology* **2016**, *16*, 1124–1128. [CrossRef]
9. Arnaoutakis, G.J.; Rangachari, D.; Laheru, D.A.; Iacobuzio-Donahue, C.A.; Hruban, R.H.; Herman, J.M.; Edil, B.H.; Pawlik, T.M.; Schulick, R.D.; Cameron, J.L.; et al. Pulmonary Resection for Isolated Pancreatic Adenocarcinoma Metastasis: An Analysis of Outcomes and Survival. *J. Gastrointest. Surg.* **2011**, *15*, 1611–1617. [CrossRef] [PubMed]
10. Moher, D.; Liberati, A.; Tetzlaff, J.; Altman, D.G.; PRISMA Group. Preferred reporting items for systematic reviews and meta-analyses: The PRISMA statement. *BMJ* **2009**, *339*, b2535. [CrossRef]
11. Clarke, M.; Horton, R. Bringing it all together: Lancet-Cochrane collaborate on systematic reviews. *Lancet* **2001**, *357*, 1728. [CrossRef]
12. Stroup, D.F.; Berlin, J.A.; Morton, S.C.; Olkin, I.; Williamson, G.D.; Rennie, D.; Moher, D.; Becker, B.J.; Sipe, T.A.; Thacker, S.B.; et al. Meta-analysis of Observational Studies in EpidemiologyA Proposal for Reporting. *JAMA* **2000**, *283*, 2008–2012. [CrossRef] [PubMed]
13. Hozo, S.P.; Djulbegovic, B.; Hozo, I. Estimating the mean and variance from the median, range, and the size of a sample. *BMC Med Res. Methodol.* **2005**, *5*, 13. [CrossRef]
14. Messori, A.; Maratea, D.; Fadda, V.; Trippoli, S. Using risk difference as opposed to odds-ratio in meta-analysis. *Int. J. Cardiol.* **2013**, *164*, 127. [CrossRef]
15. Higgins, J.P.T.; Thompson, S.G. Quantifying heterogeneity in a meta-analysis. *Stat. Med.* **2002**, *21*, 1539–1558. [CrossRef]
16. Mantel, N.; Haenszel, W. Statistical aspects of the analysis of data from retrospective studies of disease. *J. Natl. Cancer Inst.* **1959**, *22*, 719–748.
17. Egger, M.; Smith, G.D.; Schneider, M.; Minder, C. Bias in meta-analysis detected by a simple, graphical test. *BMJ* **1997**, *315*, 629–634. [CrossRef] [PubMed]
18. Duval, S.J. The trim and fill method. In *Publication Bias in Meta-Analysis: Prevention, Assessment, and Adjustments*; Rothstein, H.R., Sutton, A.J., Borenstein, M., Eds.; Wiley: Chichester, UK, 2005; pp. 127–144.
19. R Core Team. *R: A Language and Environment for Statistical Computing*; R Foundation for Statistical Computing: Vienna, Austria, 2017.
20. Strobel, O.; Hartwig, W.; Hackert, T.; Hinz, U.; Berens, V.; Grenacher, L.; Bergmann, F.; Debus, J.; Jäger, D.; Büchler, M.; et al. Re-resection for Isolated Local Recurrence of Pancreatic Cancer is Feasible, Safe, and Associated with Encouraging Survival. *Ann. Surg. Oncol.* **2012**, *20*, 964–972. [CrossRef]

21. Miyazaki, M.; Yoshitomi, H.; Shimizu, H.; Ohtsuka, M.; Yoshidome, H.; Furukawa, K.; Takayasiki, T.; Kuboki, S.; Okamura, D.; Suzuki, D.; et al. Repeat pancreatectomy for pancreatic ductal cancer recurrence in the remnant pancreas after initial pancreatectomy: Is it worthwhile? *Surgery* **2014**, *155*, 58–66. [CrossRef] [PubMed]
22. Hashimoto, D.; Chikamoto, A.; Ohmuraya, M.; Sakata, K.; Miyake, K.; Kuroki, H.; Watanabe, M.; Beppu, T.; Hirota, M.; Baba, H. Pancreatic cancer in the remnant pancreas following primary pancreatic resection. *Surg. Today* **2013**, *44*, 1313–1320. [CrossRef]
23. Nakayama, Y.; Sugimoto, M.; Gotohda, N.; Konishi, M.; Takahashi, S. Efficacy of completion pancreatectomy for recurrence of adenocarcinoma in the remnant pancreas. *J. Surg. Res.* **2018**, *221*, 15–23. [CrossRef]
24. Yamada, S.; Kobayashi, A.; Nakamori, S.; Baba, H.; Yamamoto, M.; Yamaue, H.; Fujii, T. Resection for recurrent pancreatic cancer in the remnant pancreas after pancreatectomy is clinically promising: Results of a project study for pancreatic surgery by the Japanese Society of Hepato-Biliary-Pancreatic Surgery. *Surg.* **2018**, *164*, 1049–1056. [CrossRef] [PubMed]
25. Kim, Y.I.; Song, K.B.; Lee, Y.; Park, K.; Hwang, D.W.; Lee, J.H.; Shin, S.H.; Kwon, J.W.; Ro, J.; Kim, S.C. Management of isolated recurrence after surgery for pancreatic adenocarcinoma. *BJS* **2019**, *106*, 898–909. [CrossRef]
26. Moletta, L.; Serafini, S.; Valmasoni, M.; Pierobon, E.S.; Ponzoni, A.; Sperti, C. Surgery for Recurrent Pancreatic Cancer: Is It Effective? *Cancers* **2019**, *11*, 991. [CrossRef]
27. Kawai, N.; Yasukawa, M.; Kawaguchi, T.; Tojo, T.; Taniguchi, S. Surgical Treatment for Pulmonary Metastasis of Pancreatic Ductal Adenocarcinoma: Study of 12 Cases. *Anticancer Res.* **2017**, *37*, 5573–5576. [CrossRef]
28. Hackert, T.; Niesen, W.; Hinz, U.; Tjaden, C.; Strobel, O.; Ulrich, A.; Michalski, C.; Büchler, M. Radical surgery of oligometastatic pancreatic cancer. *Eur. J. Surg. Oncol. (EJSO)* **2017**, *43*, 358–363. [CrossRef] [PubMed]
29. Zanini, N.; Lombardi, R.; Masetti, M.; Giordano, M.; Landolfo, G.; Jovine, E. Surgery for isolated liver metastases from pancreatic cancer. *Updat. Surg.* **2015**, *67*, 19–25. [CrossRef]
30. Gbolahan, O.B.; Tong, Y.; Sehdev, A.; O'Neil, B.; Shahda, S. Overall survival of patients with recurrent pancreatic cancer treated with systemic therapy: A retrospective study. *BMC Cancer* **2019**, *19*, 1–9. [CrossRef] [PubMed]
31. Javed, M.A.; Beyer, G.; Le, N.; Vinci, A.; Wong, H.; Palmer, D.; Morgan, R.D.; Lamarca, A.; Hubner, R.A.; Valle, J.W.; et al. Impact of intensified chemotherapy in metastatic pancreatic ductal adenocarcinoma (PDAC) in clinical routine in Europe. *Pancreatology* **2019**, *19*, 97–104. [CrossRef]
32. Kawaida, H.; Kono, H.; Amemiya, H.; Saitou, R.; Yamamoto, A.; Hosomura, N.; Watanabe, M.; Kimura, A.; Furuya, S.; Shimizu, H.; et al. Feasibility of Combination Therapy with Nab-paclitaxel Plus Gemcitabine in Patients with Recurrent Pancreatic Cancer. *Anticancer Res.* **2018**, *38*, 6537–6542. [CrossRef] [PubMed]

Systematic Review

Meta-Analysis of Circulating Cell-Free DNA's Role in the Prognosis of Pancreatic Cancer

Jelena Milin-Lazovic [1,†], Petar Madzarevic [1,†], Nina Rajovic [1], Vladimir Djordjevic [2,3], Nikola Milic [3], Sonja Pavlovic [4], Nevena Veljkovic [5,6], Natasa M. Milic [1,7,‡] and Dejan Radenkovic [2,3,*,‡]

1. Institute for Medical Statistics and Informatics, Faculty of Medicine, University of Belgrade, 11000 Belgrade, Serbia; jelena.milin@med.bg.ac.rs (J.M.-L.); petar.madzarevic@gmail.com (P.M.); nina.rajovic@med.bg.ac.rs (N.R.); milic.natasa@mayo.edu (N.M.M.)
2. Department of Surgery, University Clinical Center of Serbia, 11000 Belgrade, Serbia; vladimir.djordjevic@kcs.ac.rs
3. Faculty of Medicine, University of Belgrade, 11000 Belgrade, Serbia; nmilic1996@gmail.com
4. Institute of Molecular Genetics and Genetic Engineering, University of Belgrade, 11000 Belgrade, Serbia; sonya@imgge.bg.ac.rs
5. Vinca Institute of Nuclear Sciences, National Institute of the Republic of Serbia, University of Belgrade, 11000 Belgrade, Serbia; nevena.veljkovic@heliant.rs
6. Heliant Ltd., 11000 Belgrade, Serbia
7. Department of Internal Medicine, Division of Nephrology and Hypertension, Mayo Clinic, Rochester, MN 55902, USA
* Correspondence: dejan.radenkovic@med.bg.ac.rs
† First co-authors.
‡ Senior co-authors.

Simple Summary: Pancreatic cancer is an aggressive disease with a poor prognosis. The analysis of cell-free DNA (cfDNA) for genetic abnormalities is a promising new approach for the diagnosis and prognosis of pancreatic cancer patients. In this study, we conducted a systematic review and meta-analysis of studies that reported cfDNA in pancreatic ductal adenocarcinoma (PDAC). In total, 48 studies were included in the qualitative synthesis, while 44 were assessed in the quantitative synthesis, including 3524 PDAC patients. An overall negative impact of cfDNA and *KRAS* mutations on the overall (OS) and progression free survival (PFS) (HR = 2.42, 95% CI: 1.95–2.99 and HR = 2.46, 95% CI: 2.01–3.00, respectively) were found. The performance of molecular studies to assess the presence of *KRAS* mutation by liquid biopsy may support global efforts to improve outcomes for PDAC patients.

Abstract: Introduction: The analysis of cell-free DNA (cfDNA) for genetic abnormalities is a promising new approach for the diagnosis and prognosis of pancreatic cancer patients. Insights into the molecular characteristics of pancreatic cancer may provide valuable information, leading to its earlier detection and the development of targeted therapies. Material and Methods: We conducted a systematic review and a meta-analysis of studies that reported cfDNA in pancreatic ductal adenocarcinoma (PDAC). The studies were considered eligible if they included patients with PDAC, if they had blood tests for cfDNA/ctDNA, and if they analyzed the prognostic value of cfDNA/ctDNA for patients' survival. The studies published before 22 October 2020 were identified through the PubMED, EMBASE, Web of Science and Cochrane Library databases. The assessed outcomes were the overall (OS) and progression-free survival (PFS), expressed as the log hazard ratio (HR) and standard error (SE). The summary of the HR effect size was estimated by pooling the individual trial results using the Review Manager, version 5.3, Cochrane Collaboration. The heterogeneity was assessed using the Cochran Q test and I^2 statistic. Results: In total, 48 studies were included in the qualitative review, while 44 were assessed in the quantitative synthesis, with the total number of patients included being 3524. Overall negative impacts of cfDNA and *KRAS* mutations on OS and PFS in PDAC (HR = 2.42, 95% CI: 1.95–2.99 and HR = 2.46, 95% CI: 2.01–3.00, respectively) were found. The subgroup analysis of the locally advanced and metastatic disease presented similar results (HR = 2.51, 95% CI: 1.90–3.31). In the studies assessing the pre-treatment presence of *KRAS*, there was a moderate to high degree of heterogeneity ($I^2 = 87\%$ and $I^2 = 48\%$, for OS and PFS, respectively), which was remarkably decreased in the analysis of the studies measuring post-treatment *KRAS* ($I^2 = 24\%$ and $I^2 = 0\%$, for OS and PFS, respectively). The patients who were *KRAS* positive before but *KRAS* negative after treatment had a better prognosis than the persistently *KRAS*-positive patients (HR = 5.30, 95% CI: 1.02–27.63). Conclusion: The assessment of *KRAS* mutation by liquid biopsy can be considered as an additional tool for the estimation of the disease course and outcome in PDAC patients.

Keywords: cell-free DNA; pancreatic ductal adenocarcinoma; survival; meta-analysis

1. Introduction

Pancreatic cancer is an aggressive disease with a poor prognosis. Despite the constantly evolving therapeutic and diagnostic techniques, the survival rate for pancreatic cancer still remains low compared to other malignant tumors [1]. According to the American Cancer Society (ACS) and the National Cancer Institute (NCI), the overall 5-year survival rate for pancreatic cancer is below 9% [2]. Even the small percentage of people diagnosed with the local disease (10%) experience an aberrant 5-year survival rate of 37%. The vast majority see a fate of being diagnosed at the distant stage of the disease (53%), where the survival rate is 3% [2]. Pancreatic cancer's low survival rates are attributed to late diagnosis, the lack of effective chemotherapy, and surgical limitations [3]. In 2017, there were 447,700 new cases diagnosed worldwide, and 441,082 deaths due to pancreatic cancer were recorded in the same year [4,5]. Pancreatic cancer accounts for 1.8% of all cancers, but causes 4.6% of all cancer deaths, thus resulting in it being the seventh highest cause of cancer death worldwide [2].

Cell-free DNA (cfDNA) has gained attention as a potential biomarker for a large variety of malignancies (lung, breast, liver, etc.) due to the increased levels of apoptosis, necrosis, pyroptosis, mitotic catastrophes, autophagy and phagocytosis present in cancer patients [6]. Thus, the detection of cfDNA changes in serum or plasma and the uncovering of genetic abnormalities being released from malignant tumors has been considered as promising candidate technique for cancer diagnosis through liquid biopsy [6,7]. The analysis of cell-free DNA (cfDNA) for genetic abnormalities is also a new promising approach for the diagnosis and prognosis of pancreatic cancer patients. Insights into the molecular characteristics of the pancreatic cancer may provide valuable information, leading to its earlier detection and the development of targeted therapies. The identification of a circulating biomarker for pancreatic cancer, in a non-invasive manner, is an exciting area of exploration, which may lead to personalized prognosis and therapeutic optimization from simple blood tests [8]. Previous studies have suggested that the vast majority of pancreatic ductal adenocarcinoma (PDAC) harbor mutations in the *KRAS* gene, with cfDNA mutant *KRAS* being an early marker of disease recurrence [9,10]. Tumor-derived cfDNA, known as circulating tumor DNA (ctDNA), has been the subject of extensive research. However, ctDNA's clinical usability still has not been established due to the non-standardized technique for its quantification. With the introduction of digital droplet polymerase chain reaction (ddPCR), new insights in this area have been acquired [11,12]. ddPCR's ability to aid in the determination of cfDNA and ctDNA's size and level has been shown to yield prognostic value in pancreatic cancer [13]. In this study, we performed (1) a systematic review incorporating prior studies that explored the association between cfDNA and the prognosis of patients with PDAC, and (2) a meta-analysis which quantifies the association between the presence of *KRAS* mutation and overall survival (OS) and progression-free survival (PFS) in these patients.

2. Material and Methods

A systematic review was performed in accordance with the Preferred Reporting Items for Systematic Reviews [14] and the Meta-analysis of Observational Studies in Epidemiology [15]. The standardized protocol was specifically developed for the purpose of this review, and was used by independent reviewers.

2.1. Study Selection

The publications were screened for inclusion in the systematic review in two phases, and all of the disagreements were resolved by discussion at each stage with the inclusion of a third reviewer or by consensus. Studies were included based on the following criteria: (1) studies including patients with pancreatic cancer, (2) studies with blood tests for cfDNA/ctDNA, and (3) studies analyzing the prognostic value of cfDNA/ctDNA for patients' survival results. Articles containing any of the following were excluded: (1) cfDNA/ctDNA extracted from tumor tissue; (2) studies without survival outcomes, such as OS and PFS; (3) studies lacking key data for the extraction of HR; or (4) diagnostic articles.

2.2. Search Strategy

A biostatistician with expertise in conducting systematic reviews and meta-analyses (N.M.M.) and a pancreatic cancer surgeon (D.R.) developed the search strategy. Searches of the PubMed, EMBASE, Web of Science and Cochrane Library databases until 22 October 2020 were performed for studies containing key words for cfDNA and pancreatic cancer: "cell-free DNA" or "ctDNA" or "cfDNA" or "circulating DNA" or "circulating tumor DNA" or "KRAS", and "pancreatic cancer" or "pancreatic carcinoma" or "pancreatic adenocarcinoma". There were no restrictions on the publication language or status. The authors of relevant studies were contacted in an attempt to obtain missing data, and to confirm the information on the study methodology and the results. The authors of relevant abstracts were contacted in order to identify eligible unpublished datasets. Reference lists of the articles that are included in the analysis were searched manually, as well as relevant reviews and editorials. Experts in the field were asked to provide information on potentially eligible studies.

2.3. Article Screening and Selection

Two reviewers (J.M.L., P.M.) independently evaluated the eligibility of all of the titles and abstracts, and performed full-text screening according to the inclusion and exclusion criteria. Disagreements were resolved by consensus (J.M.L., P.M.) or arbitration (N.M.M, D.R.).

2.4. Data Abstraction and Quality Assessment

Two reviewers (J.M.L., P.M.) independently extracted the following data: the first author's name, year of publication, country, number of patients, study design, inclusion and exclusion criteria, TNM stage, sample origin, time of the sample collected, methods of DNA detection, detection markers, and information needed to assess the articles' quality. The authors were contacted to clarify and confirm the accuracy of the abstracted data. The extraction of the survival outcome data included OS, PFS, disease-free survival (DFS), recurrence-free survival (RFS) and disease-specific survival (DSS). Hazard ratios (HR) with a corresponding 95% confidence interval (95% CI) were also obtained from the related articles.

2.5. Risk of Bias

The risk of bias in the individual studies was assessed according to the following criteria proposed by the GRADE (Grading of Recommendations, Assessment, Development and Evaluations) Working Group [16]: (1) failure to develop and apply appropriate eligibility criteria (the inclusion of a control population), (2) flawed measurements of both exposure and outcome, (3) failure to adequately control for confounding variables, and (4) incomplete follow-up. Two reviewers (J.M.L., P.M.) independently evaluated the risk of bias within and across the studies, and the overall quality of the gathered evidence. An adapted version of the Newcastle–Ottawa tool for observational studies was used [17].

2.6. Statistical Analysis

The assessed outcomes were OS and PFS expressed as the log HR and standard error (SE). For articles without explicit data for the HR and 95% CI, the logHR and SE were calculated by extracting the survival rates from Kaplan Meier curves using the WebPlotDigitizer v4.4 [18]. The HR was than estimated using a calculator formulated by Tierney et al. [19]. The number of patients at risk was extracted when available; if not, the numbers were calculated taking into account the total number of patients included in the survival analysis and selected time points accounting for the censored data [6,20–31]. In addition, if the HR data were not available, but were presented in the individual-level data, the HR with corresponding 95% CI were calculated by IBM SPSS, version 25 [32]. The summary HR effect size was estimated by pooling the individual trial results using the Review Manager, version 5.3, Cochrane Collaboration. The heterogeneity was assessed using the Cochran Q test and I^2 statistic. According to Higgins and Thompson [33], the heterogeneity was defined as $I^2 > 50\%$ or p value < 0.10. A random effect model was used due to presence of heterogeneity in all of the analysis [33]. The weight of each study was calculated by the inverse variance method and adjusted by effect models, which determined how much each study contributed to the pooled HR. Sensitivity analyses were performed in order to evaluate the effect of the sample origin and different survival outcome measures. A subgroup analysis was performed for locally advanced and metastatic disease. A separate forest plot was constructed for each analysis showing the HR (box), 95% CI (lines) and weight (size of box) for each trial. The diamond presented the overall effect size. The presence of publication bias was assessed by a linear regression test of the funnel plot asymmetry. $p < 0.05$ was considered to be statistically significant.

3. Results

3.1. Systematic Review

A total of 5768 potentially eligible articles were found. After duplicates were removed, 3997 titles and abstracts were screened. After reading the titles and abstracts, 3694 articles were excluded because they were not original studies, examined populations other than humans (animals, cell lines), examined other diseases, did not measure ctDNA/cfDNA, or were retracted studies, author corrections or abstracts. Of the 303 reviewed full text articles, 255 were excluded because they were not written in the English language, had no survival data, had no liquid biopsy data, were methodological studies, were ongoing clinical trials, or the full-text version of the article was not available. A total of 48 articles were selected for inclusion in the systematic review, and 44 studies were included in the meta-analysis. The flow chart presenting the steps of the study selection in detail is shown in Figure 1.

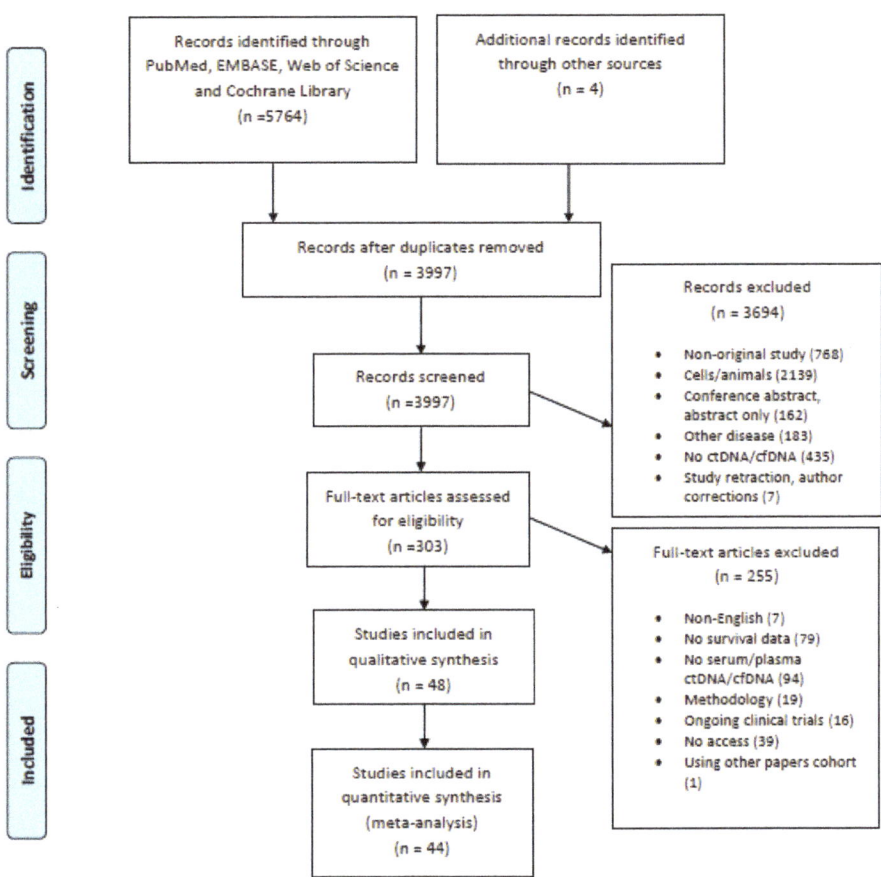

Figure 1. Flow chart of the study selection.

The characteristics of all of the 48 publications included in the systematic review are presented in detail in Table 1. Most of the studies were conducted in China or Japan (Figure 2). The studies were published between 1996 and 2020, with a minimum sample size of 10 [20] and a maximum of 210 patients [34]. The UICC/AJCC TNM classification was given by an exact number of patients in each stage in 18 of the studies [23,25,28,30,34–48], while the UICC/AJCC TNM classification was not reported for a subgroup of patients for which the ctDNA was measured, but was instead given for a total number of patients included in the study in four studies [20,49–51]. In total, 42 studies measured the cfDNA in plasma [9,13,21,24–31,34–36,38–46,48–66], three studies measured it from serum [37,47,67], two studies measured it from blood [20,22] and one study examined the cfDNA both in serum and plasma [23]. The time of the sampling was pre-treatment in 29 studies [9,13,23,24,26,29,34,36–40,43,44,46,49,52–55,57,58,60,62–67], pre/post-treatment in 10 studies [25,27,28,30,35,41,42,45,47,59], post-treatment only in two studies [48,50], pre/post and during treatment in one study [22], and six studies did not report the time of sampling [20,21,31,51,56,61]. KRAS was explicitly measured in 41 studies [9,20–31,34–39,41–50,52–55,57–64,67], the cfDNA/ctDNA total concentration was measured in four studies [13,52,56,65], cfDNATFx was measured in one study [66], hypermethylation was measured in one study [40], TP53 was measured in one study [62], ERBB exon 17 was measured in one study [58], and SPARC MI, UCHL1 MI, PENK M and NPTX2 MI were measured in one study [51].

Table 1. Overview of the current literature on circulating tumor DNA in pancreatic cancer, with survival endpoints and patient group data.

Reference (Year)	Country	n	TNM or Other Tumor Stage Classification Available	Median Follow up *	Sample Origin	Time of Sample Origin	Method	Marker	Endpoints
Nomoto [20] (1996)	Japan	10	II–IV, numbers not reported	not reported	blood	not reported	PCR	KRAS	OS
Mulcahy [51] (1998)	England	21	21 unresectable disease	5.5 (1.2–16.7)	plasma	pre-treatment	RFLP-PCR	KRAS	OS
Yamada [35] (1998)	Japan	30	I = 3, II = 6, III = 7, IV = 5	12.2 (1.3–43.5)	plasma	pre/post treatment	MASA-PCR	KRAS codon 12	OS
Castells [36] (1999)	Spain	44	I = 4, II = 11, III = 5, IV = 23, unknown = 1	9 (6–17)	plasma	pre-treatment	RFLP-PCR	KRAS	OS
Chen [50] (2010)	China	91	unresectable	7 (3–21)	plasma	pre-treatment	Nested PCR	KRAS	OS
Earl [52] (2015)	Spain	31	resectable = 10, locally advanced = 8, metastatic = 13	not reported	plasma	pre-treatment	ddPCR	KRAS	OS
Kinugasa [37] (2015)	Japan	75	II = 2, III = 5, IV = 68	not reported	serum	pre-treatment	ddPCR	KRAS, G12V	OS
Sausen [53] (2015)	USA and Denmark	51	I–III, numbers not reported	32	plasma	pre-treatment	ddPCR	KRAS	PFS
Semrad [21] (2015)	USA	28	locally advanced and metastatic, numbers not reported	not reported	plasma	not reported	ARMS PCR	KRAS	OS, PFS
Singh [54] (2015)	India	110	resectable and unresectable, numbers not reported	not reported	plasma	not reported	Nested PCR	ctDNA concentration	OS
Hadano [38] (2016)	Japan	105	I–II = 84, III–IV = 21	54 (14–96)	plasma	pre-treatment	ddPCR	KRAS	OS
Tjensvoll [22] (2016)	Norway	14	locally advanced = 2, metastatic = 12	3.7	blood	pre/post and during treatment	PNA directed PCR clamping	KRAS B1, B2	OS, PFS
Adamo [55] (2017)	United Kingdom	26	resectable = 6, non-resectable = 5, metastatic = 15	not reported	plasma	pre-treatment	tNGS and ddPCR	KRAS	DSS
Ako [23] (2017)	Japan	40	UICC1 = 22, UICC2 = 7, UICC3 = 9, not clear = 2	7.8 (0.3–30.2)	plasma/serum	pre-treatment	ddPCR	KRAS, G12D, G12V	OS

Table 1. *Cont.*

Reference (Year)	Country	n	TNM or Other Tumor Stage Classification Available	Median Follow up *	Sample Origin	Time of Sample Origin	Method	Marker	Endpoints
Allenson [24] (2017)	USA, Czech and Slovakia	85	Localized = 33, localized postsurgical = 20, locally advanced = 13, metastatic = 19	not reported	plasma	pre-treatment	ddPCR	KRAS	OS
Chen [39] (2017)	Denmark	189	III = 40, IV = 149	not reported	plasma	pre-treatment	NGS and PCR	KRAS	OS
Cheng [56] (2017)	China	188	Metastatic = 188	no reported	plasma	pre-treatment	NGS/ddPCR	KRAS G12V, ERBB2, exon 17	OS
Del Re [25] (2017)	Italy	27	III = 4, IV = 23	not reported	plasma	pre/post treatment	ddPCR	KRAS	PFS
Henriksen [40] (2017)	Denmark	95	I = 11, II = 29, III = 13, IV = 42	not reported	plasma	pre-treatment	PCR	Hypermethylation	OS
Pietrasz [57] (2017)	France	135	resectable, locally advanced and stage IV	34.2	plasma	pre/post treatment	ddPCR/NGS	KRAS	OS, PFS
Sefrioui [26] (2017)	France	58	resectable = 16, locally advanced = 18, metastatic = 24	7.5 (1–64)	plasma	pre-treatment	ddPCR	KRAS ctDNA	OS
Van Laethem [58] (2017)	Belgium	60	II-IV, numbers not reported	not reported	plasma	post treatment	BEAMing	KRAS	OS
Kim [59] (2018)	Korea	106	resectable = 41, locally advanced = 25, metastatic = 40	10.3 (0.07–19.96)	plasma	pre-treatment	ddPCR	KRAS concentration	OS, PFS
Kruger [27] (2018)	Germany	54	locally advanced = 7, metastatic = 47	not reported	plasma	pre/post treatment	BEAMing	KRAS	OS, PFS
Lapin [13] (2018)	Norway	61	locally advanced = 6, metastatic = 55	7.7 months (0.3–25.8)	plasma	pre-treatment and during	Agilent 2100 Bioanalyzer and Agilent High Sensitivity DNA kit	cfDNA concentration and size	PFS, OS
Levy [28] (2018)	USA	35	I = 3, II = 16, III = 7, IV = 9	11.2 (5.48–13.2)	plasma	pre/post treatment	ddPCR	KRAS	OS

Table 1. *Cont.*

Reference (Year)	Country	n	TNM or Other Tumor Stage Classification Available	Median Follow up *	Sample Origin	Time of Sample Origin	Method	Marker	Endpoints
Lin [46] (2018)	China	65	UICCI/II = 5, UICCIII/IV = 60	21	plasma	pre-treatment	ddPCR	KRAS codon 12	OS
Nakano [47] (2018)	Japan	45	I = 2, II = 43	not reported	serum	pre/post treatment	PNA directed PCR clamping	KRAS codon12/13	OS, DFS
Perets [29] (2018)	Israel	17	metastatic = 14	not reported	plasma	pre-treatment	PCR	KRAS	OS
Yang [41] (2018)	China	35	I = 3, II = 29, III = 3	12.4 (6.1–17.2)	plasma	pre/post treatment	ddPCR	KRAS	OS, PFS
Bernard [49] (2019)	USA	104	Metastatic = 104	187 days	plasma	pre-treatment	ddPCR	ctDNA, KRAS	PFS
Groot [30] (2019)	USA	59	I–II = 43, III–IV = 16	16 (13–19)	plasma	pre/post treatment	ddPCR	KRAS	OS, PFS, RFR
Lee [42] (2019)	Australia, New Zealand and Singapore	131	I = 1, II = 3, III = 33	38.4	plasma	pre/post treatment	PCR	KRAS	RFS, OS
Liu [43] (2019)	China	112	I/II = 58, III/IV = 22	not reported	plasma	pre-treatment	PCR	KRAS	OS
Mohan [9] (2019)	England	55	locally advanced disease = 24, metastatic = 31	no reported	plasma	pre-treatment	NGS/ddPCR	KRAS	OS
Patel [61] (2019)	USA	94	Advanced = 94	18.2 (95% CI, 13.7–22.7).	plasma	not reported	NGS	KRAS	OS
Shi [44] (2019)	China	113	I = 49, II = 57, III = 7	23.6	plasma	pre-treatment	NGS/ddPCR	KRAS	RFS, OS
Watanabe [45] (2019)	Japan	78	locally advanced = 13, metastasis = 20, recurrence = 4, peritoneal dissemination = 2. I = 3, II = 33, III = 1, IV = 1	16.2	plasma	pre/post treatment	ddPCR	KRAS (C12V, G12D, G12R, and Q61H)	OS
Bachet [62] (2020)	Multicenter	113	advanced = 113	not reported	plasma	pre-treatment	NGS	KRAS, TP53	OS, PFS
Cheng [34] (2020)	China	210	III = 71, IV = 139	not reported	plasma	pre-treatment	ddPCR	KRAS G12V, G12D	OS
Jiang [48] (2020)	China	27	I = 13, II = 9, IV = 5	18.6 months (12.4–28.9)	plasma	post treatment	PCR/NGS	KRAS	DFS

Table 1. Cont.

Reference (Year)	Country	n	TNM or Other Tumor Stage Classification Available	Median Follow up *	Sample Origin	Time of Sample Origin	Method	Marker	Endpoints
Okada [31] (2020)	Japan	96	resectable = 66 unresectable = 30	not reported	plasma	not reported	ddPCR	KRAS	DFS
Singh [60] (2020)	India	61	I–IV, numbers not reported	36	plasma	not reported	qMSP PCR	SPARC MI, UCHL1 MI, PENK M, NPTX2 MI	OS
Strijker [63] (2020)	The Netherlands and Italy	58	no metastases on baseline imaging or distant lymph only = 10, liver metastases = 37, metastases other than liver = 10	12.3 (2.3–27.7)	plasma	pre-treatment	NGS/ddPCR	KRAS codon 12/13	OS
Sugimori [67] (2020)	Japan	47	locally advanced = 17, peritoneal metastasis = 9, liver/lung metastasis = 21	not reported	serum	pre-treatment	ddPCR/NGS	KRAS G12/13	PFS
Toledano [64] (2020)	Spain	61	distant metastasis = 61	not reported	plasma	pre-treatment	BEAMing	KRAS	OS, PFS
Uesato [65] (2020)	Japan	104	advanced and liver metastasis = 104	not reported	plasma	pre-treatment	NGS	ctDNA	OS, PFS
Wei [66] (2020)	China	70	no liver metastasis = 12, liver metastasis = 51	not reported	plasma	pre-treatment	WGS/PCR	ctDNATFx	OS

BEAMing, beads, emulsions, amplification and magnetics; ddPCR, digital droplet polymerase chain reaction; NGS, next-generation sequencing; PCR, polymerase chain reaction; RFLP-PCR, restriction fragment length polymorphism polymerase chain reaction; MASA-PCR, mutant allele-specific polymerase chain reaction; PNA-clamping PCR, peptide nucleic acid-mediated clamping polymerase chain reaction; NGS, next-generation sequencing; WGS, whole-genome sequencing; ARMS PCR, amplification-refractory mutation system; TFx, tumor fraction; OS, overall survival; RFR, relapse free rate; PFS, progress-free survival; DSS, disease specific survival; DFS, disease free survival; qMSP PCR, quantitative methylation specific polymerase chain reaction. * median follow up in months.

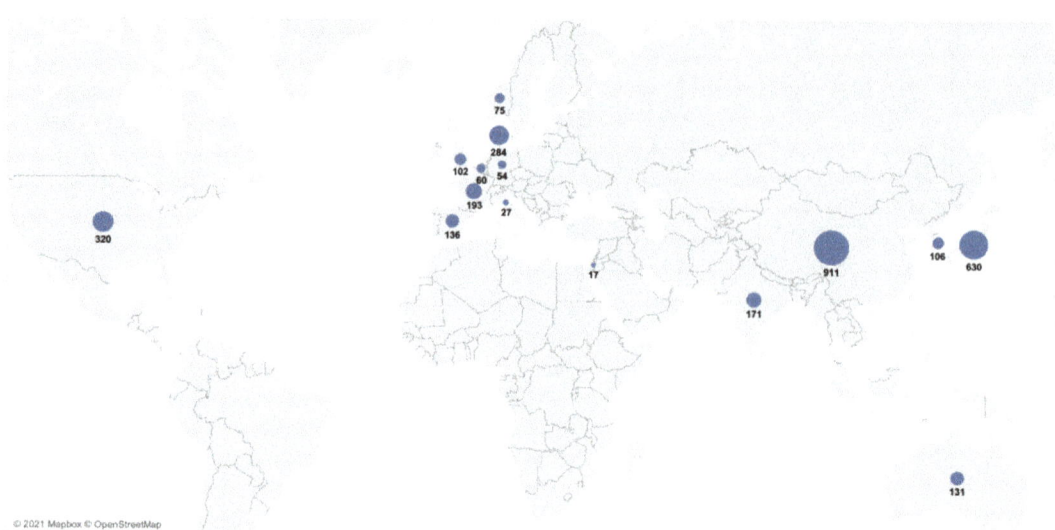

Figure 2. Geographical overview of the patient cases included in the meta-analyses. Data from multicenter and multicountry studies were excluded.

A total of 44 studies used polymerase chain reaction (PCR) (ddPCR in 24 [9,23–26,28,30,31,34,37,38,41,44–46,49,52,55,57–60,63,67]; two used restriction fragment length-PCR (RFLP-PCR) [36,54]; two used nested PCR [53,56]; two used peptide nucleic acid-mediated clamping (PNA clamping) [22,47]; three used beads, emulsions, amplification and magnetics (BEAMing) [27,50,64]; one used mutant allele-specific PCR (MASA PCR) [35]; one used amplification-refractory mutation system PCR (ARMS PCR) [21]; one used quantitative methylation specific polymerase chain reaction (qMSP PCR) [51]; and an explicit PCR method was not reported in eight studies [20,29,39,40,42,46,48,66]). Next-generation sequencing (NGS) was used in three studies [61,62,65], and a bioassay was used as a primary method in one study [13].

3.2. Pre-Treatment KRAS Mutation, and Overall and Progression-Free Survival

A meta-analysis was performed in order to assess the relationship between the presence of *KRAS* mutations in PDAC patients and OS before treatment. A total of 35 studies had OS as an outcome. Four studies were excluded from the overall HR effect size calculation due to measuring hypermethylation in ctDNA [40] or only post-treatment cfDNA, [48,50] or performing cfDNA TFx analysis [66]. Finally, 31 studies were included in the meta-analysis. The presence of pre-treatment *KRAS* mutations had significant prognostic value for OS in PDAC (HR = 2.42, 95% CI: 1.95–2.99) (Figure 3). There was a high degree of heterogeneity in the OS analysis (I^2 = 87%) and a significant presence of publication bias (p = 0.021) (Supplemental Figure S1). The sensitivity analysis, excluding two studies which examined ctDNA in serum, showed a similar HR (HR = 2.49, 95% CI: 2.00–3.10) (Supplemental Figure S2).

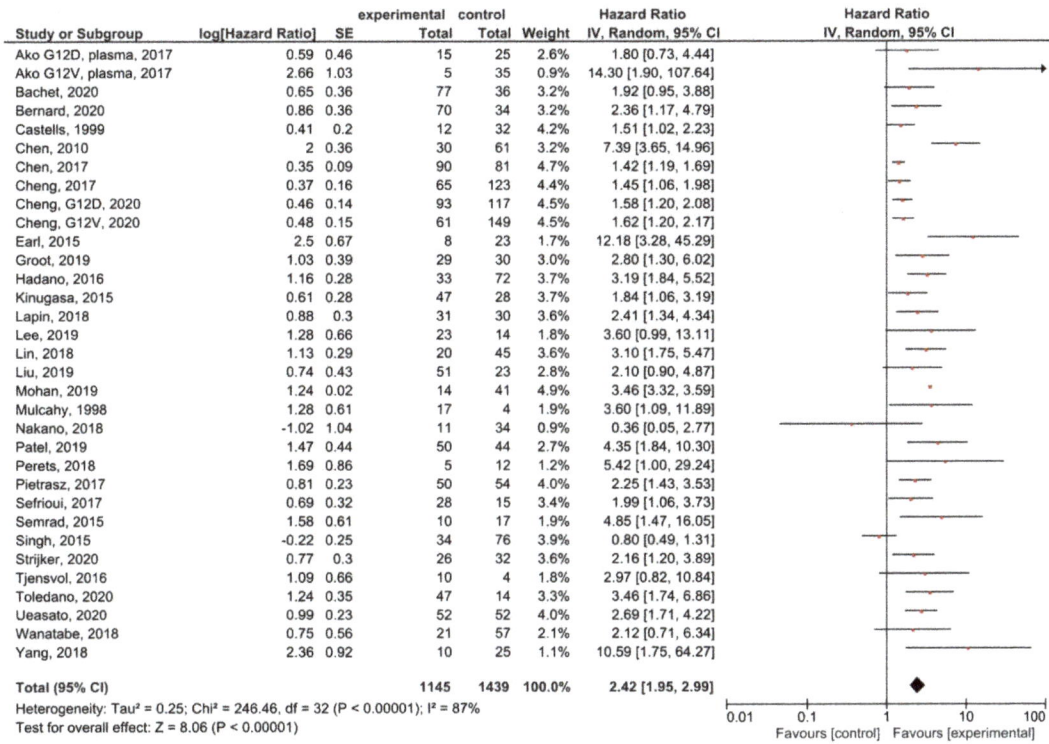

Figure 3. Forest plot presenting the relationship between the presence of *KRAS* mutations before treatment in PDAC patients and OS.

A meta-analysis was performed in order to assess the relationship between the presence of *KRAS* mutations in PDAC patients and PFS before treatment. A total of 19 studies had PFS, DFS, RFS or DSS as an outcome. The presence of pre-treatment *KRAS* mutations demonstrated a significant prognostic value for PFS in PDAC patients (HR = 2.46, 95% CI: 2.01–3.00, n = 19) (Figure 4). There was a high degree of heterogeneity in the PFS analysis (I^2 = 48%) %) and a significant presence of publication bias (p < 0.001) (Supplemental Figure S3). The sensitivity analysis including only PFS as an outcome resulted in a similar HR (HR = 2.27, 95% CI: 1.83–2.82, n = 14) (Supplemental Figure S4).

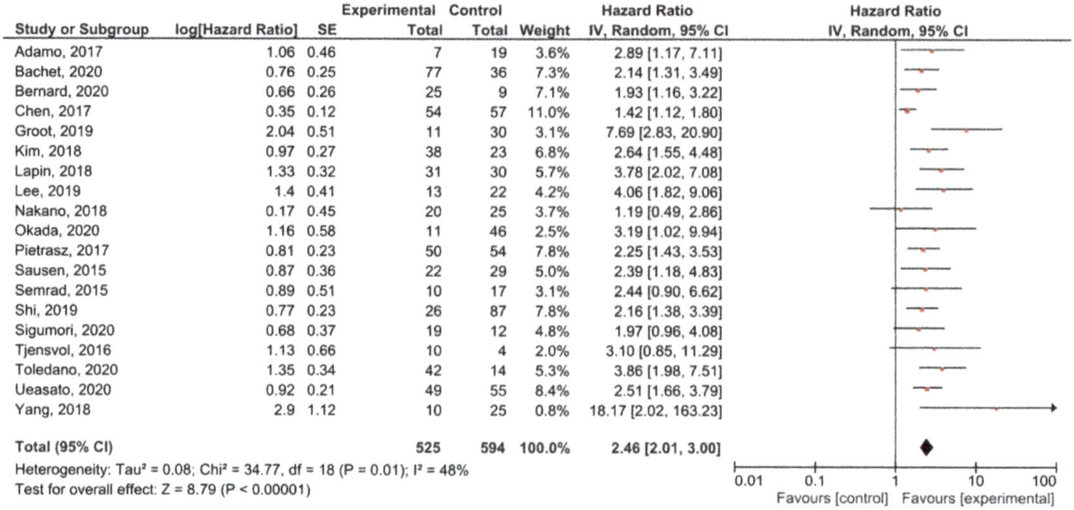

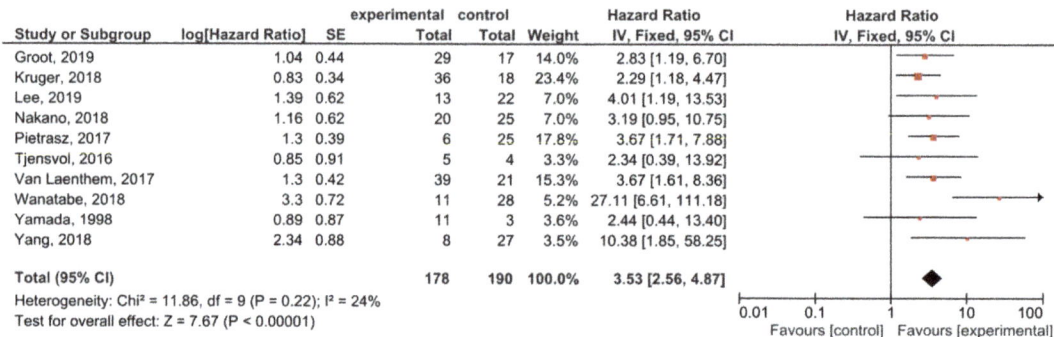

Figure 4. Forest plot presenting the relationship between the presence of *KRAS* mutations before treatment in PDAC patients and PFS.

3.3. Post-Treatment KRAS Mutation and Overall and Progression-Free Survival

A total of 10 studies examined ctDNA post-treatment; the presence of post-treatment *KRAS* mutations demonstrated significant prognostic value for OS in PDAC patients (HR = 3.53, 95% CI: 2.56–4.87, n = 10) (Figure 5). There was a low degree of heterogeneity in the OS analysis (I^2 = 24%) and no publication bias (p = 0.186) (Supplemental Figure S5). Patients in nine studies underwent different regimes of chemotherapy; in six studies, surgery was performed, and combined radiotherapy was performed in one study.

Figure 5. Forest plot presenting the relationship between the presence of *KRAS* mutations after treatment in PDAC patients and OS.

The presence of post-treatment *KRAS* mutations demonstrated significant prognostic value for PFS in PDAC patients (HR = 3.53, 95% CI: 2.49–4.99, n = 10) (Figure 6). There was no heterogeneity in the PFS analysis (I^2 = 0%) and no publication bias (p = 0.247) (Supplemental Figure S6). Patients in nine studies underwent different regimes of chemotherapy, and in six studies surgery was performed.

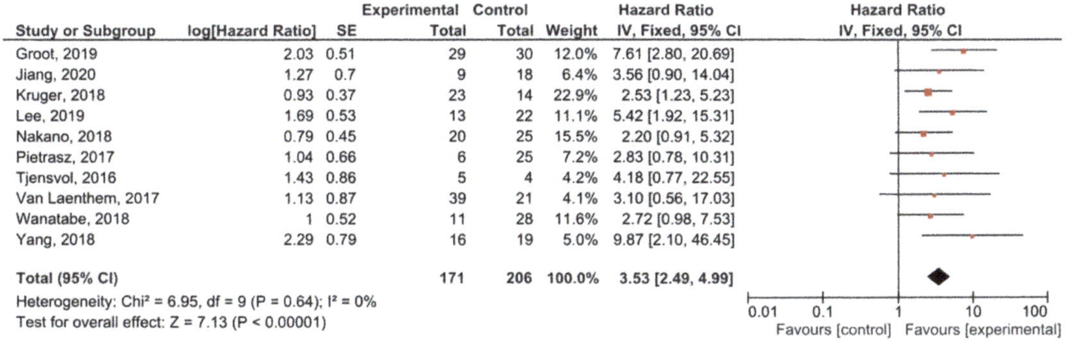

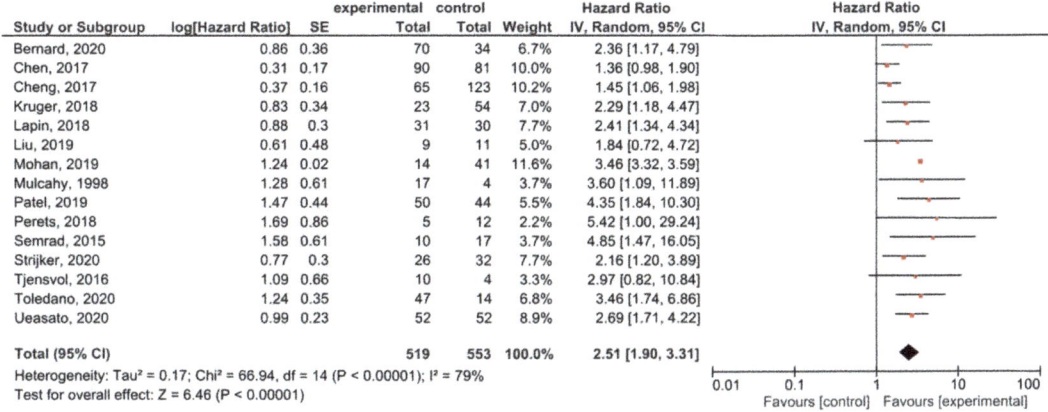

Figure 6. Forest plot presenting the relationship between the presence of *KRAS* mutations after treatment in PDAC patients and PFS.

Changes in cfDNA positivity during the treatment with PFS as an outcome were examined in three studies. The responders (patients who were *KRAS* positive before treatment and *KRAS* negative after treatment) had a better prognosis than the non-responders (patients who were *KRAS* positive before treatment and remained *KRAS* positive after the treatment) (HR = 5.30, 95% CI: 1.02–27.63, n = 3) (Supplemental Figure S7).

3.4. Analysis of the Locally-Advanced and Metastatic Disease

A subgroup analysis of the studies examining the locally advanced and metastatic PDAC showed that *KRAS* mutations had significant prognostic value for OS (HR = 2.51, 95% CI: 1.90–3.31, n = 15) (Figure 7). There was a high degree of heterogeneity in the OS analysis (I^2 = 79%) but no publication bias (p = 0.061) (Supplemental Figure S8). In the analysis examining only the metastatic disease, the effect was similar (HR = 1.90, 95% CI: 1.39–2.61, n = 6) (Supplemental Figure S9).

Figure 7. Forest plot presenting the relationship between the presence of *KRAS* mutations before treatment in locally-advanced and metastatic PDAC patients and OS.

A subgroup analysis of the studies examining locally-advanced and metastatic PDAC showed that *KRAS* mutations demonstrated significant prognostic value for PFS (HR = 2.51, 95% CI: 1.98–3.19, n = 7) (Figure 8). There was not enough data to perform a separate analysis of metastatic disease with PFS as an outcome, or to test the funnel plot asymmetry (Supplemental Figure S10).

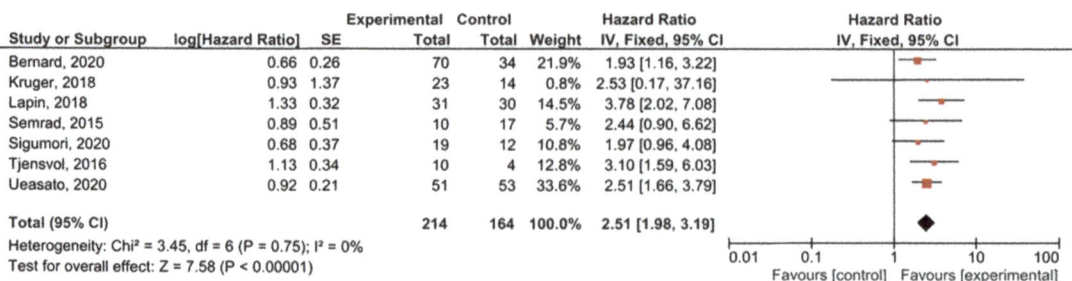

Figure 8. Forest plot presenting the relationship between the presence of *KRAS* mutations before treatment in locally-advanced and metastatic PDAC patients and PFS.

4. Discussion

In this study, we found an overall negative impact of *KRAS* mutations on OS and PFS in PDAC (HR = 2.42, 95% CI: 1.95–2.99 and HR = 2.46, 95% CI: 2.01–3.00, respectively). The subgroup analysis of locally-advanced and metastatic disease presented similar results (HR = 2.51, 95% CI: 1.90–3.31). In studies assessing the pre-treatment presence of *KRAS* mutations, there was a high degree of heterogeneity in OS (I^2 = 87%) and a moderate level of heterogeneity in the PFS analysis (I^2 = 48%), which was remarkably decreased in the analysis of studies measuring post-treatment *KRAS* mutations (I^2 = 24% and I^2 = 0%, for OS and PFS, respectively).

There is a constant effort to find novel biomarkers which could improve the diagnosis, follow-up and therapeutic approaches in pancreatic cancer. The discovery that nucleic acids originating from cancer cells can be found in the peripheral circulation of cancer patients has had a major impact towards the development of non-invasive techniques, such as liquid-biopsy methodology, for the detection of tumor biomarkers. The analysis of cell-free DNA (cfDNA) for genetic abnormalities is a new promising research area for the diagnosis and prognosis of pancreatic cancer patients. CfDNA is also found in the blood of healthy individuals due to the continuous apoptosis/necrosis of hematopoietic cell line cells [6,68]. It usually consists of short fragments of less than 1000 base pairs (bp), with most being under 200bp [69]. When cell-free DNA originates from cancer cells, it is denoted as circulated tumor DNA (ctDNA). CtDNA is released into circulation primarily by the apoptosis of tumor cells and/or as a result of tumor necrosis [70,71]. Due to CtDNA's extremely low concentration (as low as 0.01% of total cfDNA) and its fragmented and short-sized nature, the detection of the mutational status of ctDNA is very challenging, and highly sensitive techniques have to be utilized for its detection.

Different techniques are available for cfDNA/ctDNA detection: NGS, ddPCR, BEAMing, RFLP-PCR, and nested PCR, etc. For the mutational screening of cfDNA/ctDNA, the next-generation sequencing method (NGS) has been usually applied (both targeted and whole-genome sequencing). As the quantification of tumor-specific mutations in ctDNA has been shown to be more relevant for studying tumors, DdPCR was the most common technique used in the published studies due to its high sensitivity in the detection of rare mutations, its ability to quantify copy number variations and specific genomic loci, as well as its relatively simple workflow, in contrast to other methods [71]. Similar to the conventional PCR, this technology uses Taq-polymerase and primers/probes, but before the amplification reaction itself, the sample is divided into particles ("partitioning")—tens of thousands of droplets—and the PCR reaction takes place in each of them. Another difference from conventional or real-time (qPCR) is that it is possible to perform the direct quantification of the PCR product, without using a standard curve. The primary applications for ddPCR are rare allele detection in heterogeneous samples like liquid biopsies or FFPE samples of solid tumors, non-invasive prenatal diagnostics, viral load detection, gene expression and copy number variation, single cell gene expression profiling, and the validation of low-frequency mutations identified by sequencing analysis. Moreover, epigenomic markers originating from tumor cells could be analyzed (methylation sites, circulating regulatory RNAs) [72]. A good agreement between BEAMing and ddPCR has been shown, with a kappa value of 0.91 (95% CI: 0.85–0.95) [73]. Recent advances in NGS technology have enabled similar sensitivity to the detection of ctDNA by ddPCR [74]. As each presented molecular platform has advantages and disadvantages, without evidence of a clear advantage for all of the purposes [28], the choice of platform should be determined to best meet the scientific and clinical questions being posed.

Most studies included measurements of ct/cf DNA in plasma, as plasma has been the preferred source for the extraction of circulating DNA. Even though serum contains a much higher amount (approximately a 2–24-times higher amount) of cfDNA than plasma, serum is not favored due to the possibility of contamination from white blood cells during clotting [75,76]. In this study, the sensitivity analysis excluding studies which used serum for cfDNA/ctDNA detection demonstrated similar results to those including only plasma measurements (HR = 2.49, 95% CI: 2.00–3.10).

Previous research has shown that the decrease in the levels of ctDNA during the treatment of PDAC patients may be a result of a significant reduction in the tumor burden. In contrast, the increase of the postoperative ctDNA levels may be due to a ctDNA release caused by tissue damage during surgery. Levy et al. showed that, in patients with PDAC, an endoscopic ultrasound fine-needle aspiration may be associated with increased an plasma concentration of cfDNA and the increased detection of mutant *KRAS* after the procedure [28]. Another reason for the increase in postoperative ctDNA levels may be a recurrence or tumor metastasis [47]. Lee et al. [42] suggested the importance of the post-operative analysis of ctDNA. Several of the studies included in this systematic review had pre/post treatment measurements of ctDNA, but only a few reported the survival between pre-positive/post-positive, pre-positive/post-negative, pre-negative/post-negative and pre-negative/post-positive patients. A meta-analysis of three studies that reported the survival between responders (pre-positive/post-negative) and non-responders (pre-positive/post-positive) presented poorer survival for persistently positive *KRAS* patients (HR = 5.30, 95% CI: 1.02–27.63, n = 3). Based on the main results of this meta-analysis, in terms of their survival prognosis, PDAC patients may be grouped in two categories: those who are ctDNA positive with worse outcomes, and those who are ctDNA negative with better outcomes [42,47,59]. In cases where the ctDNA is detectable at diagnosis but becomes undetectable post-treatment, a reduction in the relapse risk is present in comparison with those in whom the ctDNA remains detectable. CtDNA can provide valuable information to determine the treatment decisions stratifying patients at low and high risk of the progression and recurrence of the disease. Prospective research should be conducted based on standardized protocols in order to evaluate further treatment strategies. It was observed previously that, in the subset of patients with resectable PDAC, ctDNA may assist the clinician in the timely detection of recurrence and the concordant introduction/addition of therapeutic measures [42,77]. It should be noted that most of the studies from this systematic review included patients with varying disease stages, thus limiting the interpretation of the prognostic role of ctDNA in resectable disease, or as a marker of disease recurrence. The data collected was utilized to determine the ways in which ctDNA's presence impacts the prognosis, rather than how specific ctDNA subtypes impact the prognosis or at what stage in the disease/treatment course these prognostic predictors are valid. Wild-type alternative and other onco-drivers present in cfDNA in specific patient cohorts (ex. *KRAS* G12C) are known to be highly actionable, allowing for precision medicine [78].

RAS genes (*HRAS*, *KRAS*, and *NRAS*) comprise the most frequently mutated oncogene family in human cancer. *KRAS* is mutated in 25% of all of the cancer cases, and is associated with poor disease prognosis [77]. Given that *KRAS* mutations are found in nearly all of the PDAC, this cancer type is arguably the most RAS-addicted cancer. Its roles in pancreatic cancer cell processes, such as increased proliferation, survival, migration and invasion, are well known [78]. An activating point mutation of the *KRAS* oncogene on codon 12 (exon 2) is the initiating event in the majority of PDAC cases (70–95%). $KRAS^{G12D}$ and

$KRAS^{G12V}$ mutations constitute about 80% of the *KRAS* mutations in PDAC [79]. For decades, *KRAS* oncoprotein was classified as undruggable cancer target [77]. According to growing evidence linking *KRAS* mutations to increased PDAC growth, the National Cancer Institute identified the targeting of *KRAS* as one of four major priorities for pancreatic cancer research. Targeted therapies and *KRAS* inhibitors appear to be very promising. A recent review investigating small-molecule *KRAS* inhibitors suggested that combining the antitumor effects from innovative new *KRAS* inhibitors like AMG510 with other agents, nanoparticles, or other auxiliary processes that can overcome the PDAC biochemical and tissue delivery issues offers hope for a new therapeutic way forward in PDAC [80].

Recently, the significance of a multigene approach based on liquid biopsy was highlighted to guide individual tailored therapy for PDAC patients. Alterations in other driver genes such as *CDKN2A*, *BRCA1/2*, *ERB2* and *NTRK*, etc. have been shown to be associated with PDAC, and they are also relevant to targeted treatments. In the recent study by Pishvaian et al. presenting 1856 patients with PDAC, 58% of the patients had molecular testing, actionable molecular alterations were identified in 26%, out of which 46 patients received a matched therapy as a second- or later-line therapy and presented a better OS [81]. In a study including 259 PDAC patients with varying disease stages, a potentially actionable mutation was detected in 29% [82], while in a study including patients with advanced PDAC, therapeutically relevant alterations were observed in 48% of the samples [83]. Given the difficulties that exist in obtaining a tumor sample in PDAC, the results of these studies highlight the importance of performing molecular profiling based on liquid biopsy, due to its simplicity and accessibility, and the importance of finding actionable early mutations in a tumor with limited therapeutic options. In addition, given that mutations may vary during the course of the disease, it is important to monitor these molecular changes [84]. With the ongoing debate regarding the use of neoadjuvant therapy in purely resectable PDAC patients, it should be also noted that ctDNA detection may play a relevant role in answering a key question: who, from these particular groups of patients, is a candidate for neoadjuvant therapy?

A strength of this study was the broad sensitive search strategy used across multiple bibliographic databases that resulted in 3997 articles screened and 48 studies included in the systematic review. The most recent meta-analysis of similar scope started with an initial set of 724 articles, with the inclusion of 18 articles due to its narrow specific search strategy [10]. The greatest number of patients (n = 3524) included in this analysis generated the most comprehensive meta-analysis of the assessment of the prognostic utility of cfDNA/ctDNA's in PDAC, while the meta-analysis assessing *KRAS* mutations included a total 2400 patients. In addition, in order to increase the utility of the data with were not directly shown, but were available in figures or as individual data, we used several recommended techniques to obtain HRs.

This study had several limitations, related to the clarification of liquid biopsy results in general, and those related to the proper understanding of the meta-analyses' results. The accurate interpretation of liquid biopsy results is rather challenging because of the presence of somatic mosaicism in plasma. One of the most common sources of the biological background noise of blood liquid biopsy is somatic mutation in blood cells [85]. The accumulation of somatic mutations in hematopoietic stem cells leads to their clonal expansion. This process, called clonal hematopoiesis (CH) is common in an aging healthy population [86]. Interestingly, not only mutations related to hematological malignancies, but also mutations in genes characteristic for solid tumors are detected as a result of CH. Mutations in the *KRAS* gene are also found as CH-mutations [87]. It is very important to exclude these non-tumor derived CH-mutations, in order to avoid the incorrect interpretation and inappropriate therapeutic management of solid tumors. CH mutations can be determined by performing the paired sequencing of plasma cfDNA and DNA from white blood cells. It is expected that artificial intelligence tools, such as machine learning, will enable the distinction between CH mutations and tumor-derived molecular alterations in liquid biopsy [85].

A relatively large number of studies were included, resulting in a wide range of initial tumor burdens, mixed-size patient groups and various methods of ctDNA detection, all of which contributed to increased heterogeneity. Different therapies, study designs and a range of follow up times also contributed to this high value of heterogeneity. Specific conclusions based on tumor stage, ctDNA concentration and mutations other than *KRAS* were not possible to derive. The studies included in our meta-analyses encompassed, predominantly, patients from European and Asian populations (Figure 2). Given that the misclassification of the variants coming from data that did not include dissimilar subpopulations could potentially lead to the inadequate treatments of individuals from underrepresented populations [88], the conclusions derived here should be treated cautiously. Large-scale population studies indicated that there are more significant numbers of population-specific variations than we believed previously [89,90]. Thus, the potential of ctDNA to improve the health outcomes for PDAC patients should be evaluated in the context of various populations. The results of the meta-analysis presenting the relationship between the presence of *KRAS* mutations before treatment and the survival of PDAC patients should be interpreted with caution due to the presence of significant publication bias.

5. Conclusions

The assessment of *KRAS* mutation by liquid biopsy can be considered as an additional tool for the estimation of the disease course and outcome in PDAC patients. While ddPCR was utilized in most studies to detect the *KRAS* mutations, due to greater test sensitivity, other technologies in the era of NGS may also be useful in clinical practice. The choice of the molecular platform should be determined in order to best meet the scientific and clinical questions being posed.

Supplementary Materials: The following are available online at https://www.mdpi.com/article/10.3390/cancers13143378/s1, Figure S1: Funnel plot of the meta-analysis presented in Figure 3, Figure S2: Forest plot presenting the relationship between presence of KRAS mutations before treatment in PDAC patients and OS: sensitivity analysis excluding samples from serum, Figure S3: Funnel plot of the meta-analysis presented in Figure 4, Figure S4: Forest plot presenting the relationship between presence of KRAS mutations before treatment in PDAC patients and PFS: sensitivity analysis including only PFS but not DFS and DSS, Figure S5: Funnel plot of the meta-analysis presented in Figure 5, Figure S6: Funnel plot of the meta-analysis presented in Figure 6, Figure S7: Forest plot comparing PFS between responders (patients who were KRAS positive before treatment and KRAS negative after treatment) and non-responders (patients who were KRAS positive before treatment and remained KRAS positive after the treatment), Figure S8: Funnel plot of the meta-analysis presented in Figure 7, Figure S9: Forest plot presenting the relationship between presence of KRAS mutations before treatment in metastatic PDAC patients and OS, Figure S10: Funnel plot of the meta-analysis presented in Figure 8.

Author Contributions: Conceptualization, J.M.-L., P.M., N.M.M., D.R.; methodology, J.M.-L., P.M., S.P., N.V., N.M.M., D.R.; software, J.M.-L., P.M., N.R., N.M.M.; validation, N.R., V.D., N.M., S.P., N.V.; formal analysis, J.M.-L., P.M., N.R., N.M., N.M.M., D.R.; investigation, J.M.-L., P.M., N.R., V.D., N.M., S.P., N.V., N.M.M., D.R.; resources, S.P., N.V., N.M.M., D.R.; data curation, J.M.-L., P.M., N.R., V.D., N.M., N.M.M.; writing—original draft preparation, J.M.-L., P.M., N.R., N.M., N.M.M., D.R.; writing—review and editing, J.M.-L., P.M., N.R., V.D., N.M., S.P., N.V., N.M.M., D.R.; visualization, J.M.-L., P.M., N.V., N.M.M.; supervision, S.P., N.V., N.M.M., D.R.; project administration, J.M.-L., P.M., N.M.M., D.R.; funding acquisition, J.M.-L., P.M., V.D., N.M.M., D.R. All authors have read and agreed to the published version of the manuscript.

Funding: This research received no external funding.

Institutional Review Board Statement: Not applicable.

Informed Consent Statement: Not applicable.

Data Availability Statement: All of the data generated in this research are in the manuscript or its supplemental files.

Acknowledgments: We would like to thank our colleagues from Heliant Ltd., Belgrade, Serbia, for creating a geographical overview of patient cases included in the meta-analyses.

Conflicts of Interest: The authors declare no conflict of interest.

References

1. Van Cutsem, E.; Hidalgo, M.; Canon, J.L.; Macarulla, T.; Bazin, I.; Poddubskaya, E.; Manojlovic, N.; Radenkovic, D.; Verslype, C.; Raymond, E.; et al. Phase I/II trial of pimasertib plus gemcitabine in patients with metastatic pancreatic cancer. *Int. J. Cancer* **2018**, *143*, 2053–2064. [CrossRef]
2. American Cancer Society. *Cancer Facts & Figures 2020*; American Cancer Society: Atlanta, GA, USA, 2020.
3. Paulson, A.S.; Tran Cao, H.S.; Tempero, M.A.; Lowy, A.M. Therapeutic Advances in Pancreatic Cancer. *Gastroenterology* **2013**, *144*, 1316–1326. [CrossRef]
4. GBD 2017 Disease and Injury Incidence and Prevalence Collaborators. Global, regional, and national incidence, prevalence, and years lived with disability for 354 diseases and injuries for 195 countries and territories, 1990–2017: A systematic analysis for the Global Burden of Disease Study 2017. *Lancet* **2018**, *392*, 1789–1858. [CrossRef]
5. Institute for Health Metrics and Evaluation. Available online: http://ghdx.healthdata.org/gbd-results-tool (accessed on 26 August 2020).
6. Bronkhorst, A.J.; Ungerer, V.; Holdenrieder, S. The emerging role of cell-free DNA as a molecular marker for cancer management. *Biomol. Detect Quantif.* **2019**, *17*, 100087. [CrossRef]
7. Kato, S.; Janku, F. Cell-free DNA as a novel marker in cancer therapy. *Biomark Med.* **2015**, *9*, 703–712. [CrossRef]
8. Gall, T.M.H.; Belete, S.; Khanderia, E.; Frampton, A.E.; Jiao, L.R. Circulating Tumor Cells and Cell-Free DNA in Pancreatic Ductal Adenocarcinoma. *Am. J. Pathol.* **2019**, *189*, 71–81. [CrossRef]
9. Mohan, S.; Ayub, M.; Rothwell, D.G.; Gulati, S.; Kilerci, B.; Hollebecque, A.; Sun Leong, H.; Smith, N.K.; Sahoo, S.; Descamps, T.; et al. Analysis of circulating cell-free DNA identifies KRAS copy number gain and mutation as a novel prognostic marker in Pancreatic cancer. *Sci. Rep.* **2019**, *9*, 11610. [CrossRef] [PubMed]
10. Chen, L.; Zhang, Y.; Cheng, Y.; Zhang, D.; Zhu, S.; Ma, X. Prognostic value of circulating cell-free DNA in patients with pancreatic cancer: A systemic review and meta-analysis. *Gene* **2018**, *679*, 328–334. [CrossRef] [PubMed]
11. Nygaard, A.D.; Holdgaard, P.C.; Spindler, K.L.; Pallisgaard, N.; Jakobsen, A. The correlation between cell-free DNA and tumour burden was estimated by PET/CT in patients with advanced NSCLC. *Br. J. Cancer* **2014**, *110*, 363–368. [CrossRef] [PubMed]
12. Hindson, B.J.; Ness, K.D.; Masquelier, D.A.; Belgrader, P.; Heredia, N.J.; Makarewicz, A.J.; Bright, I.J.; Lucero, M.Y.; Hiddessen, A.L.; Legler, T.C.; et al. High-throughput droplet digital PCR system for absolute quantitation of DNA copy number. *Anal. Chem.* **2011**, *83*, 8604–8610. [CrossRef] [PubMed]
13. Lapin, M.; Oltedal, S.; Tjensvoll, K.; Buhl, T.; Smaaland, R.; Garresori, H.; Javle, M.; Glenjen, N.I.; Abelseth, B.K.; Gilje, B.; et al. Fragment size and level of cell-free DNA provide prognostic information in patients with advanced pancreatic cancer. *J. Transl. Med.* **2018**, *16*, 300. [CrossRef] [PubMed]
14. Liberati, A.; Altman, D.G.; Tetzlaff, J.; Mulrow, C.; Gøtzsche, P.C.; Ioannidis, J.P.; Clarke, M.; Devereaux, P.J.; Kleijnen, J.; Moher, D. The PRISMA statement for reporting systematic reviews and meta-analyses of studies that evaluate healthcare interventions: Explanation and elaboration. *BMJ* **2009**, *339*, b2700. [CrossRef] [PubMed]
15. Stroup, D.F.; Berlin, J.A.; Morton, S.C.; Olkin, I.; Williamson, G.D.; Rennie, D.; Moher, D.; Becker, B.J.; Sipe, T.A.; Thacker, S.B. Meta-analysis of observational studies in epidemiology: A proposal for reporting. Meta-analysis of Observational Studies in Epidemiology (MOOSE) group. *JAMA* **2000**, *283*, 2008–2012. [CrossRef] [PubMed]
16. Higgins, J.P.T.; Thomas, J.; Chandler, J.; Cumpston, M.; Li, T.; Page, M.J.; Welch, V.A. (Eds.) *Cochrane Handbook for Systematic Reviews of Interventions*, 2nd ed.; John Wiley & Sons: Hoboken, NJ, USA; Chichester, UK, 2019.
17. Wells, G.A.; Shea, B.; O'Connell, D.; Peterson, J.; Welch, V.; Losos, M.; Tugwell, P. *The Newcastle–Ottawa Scale (NOS) for Assessing the Quality of Nonrandomisedstudies in Meta-Analysis*; Ottawa Hospital Research Institute: Ottawa, ON, Canada, 2014; Available online: http://www.ohri.ca/programs/clinical_epidemiology/oxford.asp (accessed on 26 June 2021).
18. Cramond, F.; O'Mara-Eves, A.; Doran-Constant, L.; Rice, A.S.; Macleod, M.; Thomas, J. The development and evaluation of an online application to assist in the extraction of data from graphs for use in systematic reviews. *Wellcome Open Res.* **2018**, *3*, 157. [CrossRef]
19. Tierney, J.F.; Stewart, L.A.; Ghersi, D.; Burdett, S.; Sydes, M.R. Practical methods for incorporating summary time-to-event data into meta-analysis. *Trials* **2007**, *8*, 16. [CrossRef]
20. Nomoto, S.; Nakao, A.; Kasai, Y.; Harada, A.; Nonami, T.; Takagi, H. Detection of ras gene mutations in perioperative peripheral blood with pancreatic adenocarcinoma. *Jpn. J. Cancer Res.* **1996**, *87*, 793–797. [CrossRef]
21. Semrad, T.; Barzi, A.; Lenz, H.J.; Hutchins, I.M.; Kim, E.J.; Gong, I.Y.; Tanaka, M.; Beckett, L.; Holland, W.; Burich, R.A.; et al. Pharmacodynamic separation of gemcitabine and erlotinib in locally advanced or metastatic pancreatic cancer: Therapeutic and biomarker results. *Int. J. Clin. Oncol.* **2015**, *20*, 518–524. [CrossRef] [PubMed]
22. Tjensvoll, K.; Lapin, M.; Buhl, T.; Oltedal, S.; Steen-Ottosen Berry, K.; Gilje, B.; Søreide, J.A.; Javle, M.; Nordgård, O.; Smaaland, R. Clinical relevance of circulating KRAS mutated DNA in plasma from patients with advanced pancreatic cancer. *Mol. Oncol.* **2016**, *10*, 635–643. [CrossRef]

23. Ako, S.; Nouso, K.; Kinugasa, H.; Dohi, C.; Matushita, H.; Mizukawa, S.; Muro, S.; Akimoto, Y.; Uchida, D.; Tomoda, T.; et al. Utility of serum DNA as a marker for KRAS mutations in pancreatic cancer tissue. *Pancreatology* **2017**, *17*, 285–290. [CrossRef]
24. Allenson, K.; Castillo, J.; San Lucas, F.A.; Scelo, G.; Kim, D.U.; Bernard, V.; Davis, G.; Kumar, T.; Katz, M.; Overman, M.J.; et al. High prevalence of mutant KRAS in circulating exosome-derived DNA from early-stage pancreatic cancer patients. *Ann. Oncol.* **2017**, *28*, 741–747. [CrossRef]
25. Del Re, M.; Vivaldi, C.; Rofi, E.; Vasile, E.; Miccoli, M.; Caparello, C.; d'Arienzo, P.D.; Fornaro, L.; Falcone, A.; Danesi, R. Early changes in plasma DNA levels of mutant KRAS as a sensitive marker of response to chemotherapy in pancreatic cancer. *Sci. Rep.* **2017**, *7*, 7931. [CrossRef] [PubMed]
26. Sefrioui, D.; Blanchard, F.; Toure, E.; Basile, P.; Beaussire, L.; Dolfus, C.; Perdrix, A.; Paresy, M.; Antonietti, M.; Iwanicki-Caron, I.; et al. Diagnostic value of CA19.9, circulating tumour DNA and circulating tumour cells in patients with solid pancreatic tumours. *Br. J. Cancer* **2017**, *117*, 1017–1025. [CrossRef]
27. Kruger, S.; Heinemann, V.; Ross, C.; Diehl, F.; Nagel, D.; Ormanns, S.; Liebmann, S.; Prinz-Bravin, I.; Westphalen, C.B.; Haas, M.; et al. Repeated mutKRASctDNA measurements represent a novel and promising tool for early response prediction and therapy monitoring in advanced pancreatic cancer. *Ann. Oncol.* **2018**, *29*, 2348–2355. [CrossRef]
28. Levy, M.J.; Kipp, B.R.; Milosevic, D.; Schneider, A.R.; Voss, J.S.; Avula, R.; Kerr, S.E.; Henry, M.R.; Highsmith, E., Jr.; Liu, M.C.; et al. Analysis of Cell-Free DNA to Assess Risk of Tumoremia Following Endoscopic Ultrasound Fine-Needle Aspiration of Pancreatic Adenocarcinomas. *Clin. Gastroenterol. Hepatol.* **2018**, *16*, 1632–1640.e1. [CrossRef]
29. Perets, R.; Greenberg, O.; Shentzer, T.; Semenisty, V.; Epelbaum, R.; Bick, T.; Sarji, S.; Ben-Izhak, O.; Sabo, E.; Hershkovitz, D. Mutant KRAS Circulating Tumor DNA Is an Accurate Tool for Pancreatic Cancer Monitoring. *Oncologist* **2018**, *23*, 566–572. [CrossRef] [PubMed]
30. Groot, V.P.; Mosier, S.; Javed, A.A.; Teinor, J.A.; Gemenetzis, G.; Ding, D.; Haley, L.M.; Yu, J.; Burkhart, R.A.; Hasanain, A.; et al. Circulating Tumor DNA as a Clinical Test in Resected Pancreatic Cancer. *Clin. Cancer Res.* **2019**, *25*, 4973–4984. [CrossRef] [PubMed]
31. Okada, T.; Mizukami, Y.; Ono, Y.; Sato, H.; Hayashi, A.; Kawabata, H.; Koizumi, K.; Masuda, S.; Teshima, S.; Takahashi, K.; et al. Digital PCR-based plasma cell-free DNA mutation analysis for early-stage pancreatic tumor diagnosis and surveillance. *J. Gastroenterol.* **2020**, *55*, 1183–1193. [CrossRef]
32. IBM Corp. *Released 2017. IBM SPSS Statistics for Windows, Version 25.0*; IBM Corp: Armonk, NY, USA, 2017.
33. Higgins, J.P.T.; Thompson, S.G. Quantifying heterogeneity in a meta-analysis. *Stat Med.* **2002**, *21*, 1539–1558. [CrossRef]
34. Cheng, H.; Luo, G.; Jin, K.; Fan, Z.; Huang, Q.; Gong, Y.; Xu, J.; Yu, X.; Liu, C. Kras mutation correlating with circulating regulatory T cells predicts the prognosis of advanced pancreatic cancer patients. *Cancer Med.* **2020**, *9*, 2153–2159. [CrossRef] [PubMed]
35. Yamada, T.; Nakamori, S.; Ohzato, H.; Oshima, S.; Aoki, T.; Higaki, N.; Sugimoto, K.; Akagi, K.; Fujiwara, Y.; Nishisho, I.; et al. Detection of K-ras gene mutations in plasma DNA of patients with pancreatic adenocarcinoma: Correlation with clinicopathological features. *Clin. Cancer Res.* **1998**, *4*, 1527–1532.
36. Castells, A.; Puig, P.; Móra, J.; Boadas, J.; Boix, L.; Urgell, E.; Solé, M.; Capellà, G.; Lluís, F.; Fernández-Cruz, L.; et al. K-ras mutations in DNA extracted from the plasma of patients with pancreatic carcinoma: Diagnostic utility and prognostic significance. *J. Clin. Oncol.* **1999**, *17*, 578–584. [CrossRef]
37. Kinugasa, H.; Nouso, K.; Miyahara, K.; Morimoto, Y.; Dohi, C.; Tsutsumi, K.; Kato, H.; Matsubara, T.; Okada, H.; Yamamoto, K. Detection of K-ras gene mutation by liquid biopsy in patients with pancreatic cancer. *Cancer* **2015**, *121*, 2271–2280. [CrossRef]
38. Hadano, N.; Murakami, Y.; Uemura, K.; Hashimoto, Y.; Kondo, N.; Nakagawa, N.; Sueda, T.; Hiyama, E. Prognostic value of circulating tumour DNA in patients undergoing curative resection for pancreatic cancer. *Br. J. Cancer* **2016**, *115*, 59–65. [CrossRef] [PubMed]
39. Chen, I.; Raymond, V.M.; Geis, J.A.; Collisson, E.A.; Jensen, B.V.; Hermann, K.L.; Erlander, M.G.; Tempero, M.; Johansen, J.S. Ultrasensitive plasma ctDNA KRAS assay for detection, prognosis, and assessment of therapeutic response in patients with unresectable pancreatic ductal adenocarcinoma. *Oncotarget* **2017**, *8*, 97769–97786. [CrossRef] [PubMed]
40. Henriksen, S.D.; Madsen, P.H.; Larsen, A.C.; Johansen, M.B.; Pedersen, I.S.; Krarup, H.; Thorlacius-Ussing, O. Cell-free DNA promoter hypermethylation in plasma as a predictive marker for survival of patients with pancreatic adenocarcinoma. *Oncotarget* **2017**, *8*, 93942–93956. [CrossRef] [PubMed]
41. Yang, X.; Xu, W.; Tian, X.; Wu, J.; Lv, A.; Li, C.; Guan, X.; Qian, H.; Hao, C. Diagnostic and prognostic value of KRAS mutations in circulating pancreatic ductal adenocarcinoma tumor DNA. *Transl. Cancer Res.* **2018**, *7*, 622–633. [CrossRef]
42. Lee, B.; Lipton, L.; Cohen, J.; Tie, J.; Javed, A.A.; Li, L.; Goldstein, D.; Burge, M.; Cooray, P.; Nagrial, A.; et al. Circulating tumor DNA as a potential marker of adjuvant chemotherapy benefit following surgery for localized pancreatic cancer. *Ann. Oncol.* **2019**, *30*, 1472–1478. [CrossRef] [PubMed]
43. Liu, X.; Liu, L.; Ji, Y.; Li, C.; Wei, T.; Yang, X.; Zhang, Y.; Cai, X.; Gao, Y.; Xu, W.; et al. Enrichment of short mutant cell-free DNA fragments enhanced detection of pancreatic cancer. *EBioMedicine* **2019**, *41*, 345–356. [CrossRef] [PubMed]
44. Guo, S.; Shi, X.; Shen, J.; Gao, S.; Wang, H.; Shen, S.; Pan, Y.; Li, B.; Xu, X.; Shao, Z.; et al. Preoperative detection of KRAS G12D mutation in ctDNA is a powerful predictor for early recurrence of resectable PDAC patients. *Br. J. Cancer* **2020**, *122*, 857–867. [CrossRef]

45. Watanabe, F.; Suzuki, K.; Tamaki, S.; Abe, I.; Endo, Y.; Takayama, Y.; Ishikawa, H.; Kakizawa, N.; Saito, M.; Futsuhara, K.; et al. Longitudinal monitoring of KRAS-mutated circulating tumor DNA enables the prediction of prognosis and therapeutic responses in patients with pancreatic cancer. *PLoS ONE* **2019**, *14*, e0227366. [CrossRef] [PubMed]
46. Lin, M.; Alnaggar, M.; Liang, S.; Chen, J.; Xu, K.; Dong, S.; Du, D.; Niu, L. Circulating Tumor DNA as a Sensitive Marker in Patients Undergoing Irreversible Electroporation for Pancreatic Cancer. *Cell Physiol. Biochem.* **2018**, *47*, 1556–1564. [CrossRef]
47. Nakano, Y.; Kitago, M.; Matsuda, S.; Nakamura, Y.; Fujita, Y.; Imai, S.; Shinoda, M.; Yagi, H.; Abe, Y.; Hibi, T.; et al. KRAS mutations in cell-free DNA from preoperative and postoperative sera as a pancreatic cancer marker: A retrospective study. *Br. J. Cancer* **2018**, *118*, 662–669. [CrossRef] [PubMed]
48. Jiang, J.; Ye, S.; Xu, Y.; Chang, L.; Hu, X.; Ru, G.; Guo, Y.; Yi, X.; Yang, L.; Huang, D. Circulating Tumor DNA as a Potential Marker to Detect Minimal Residual Disease and Predict Recurrence in Pancreatic Cancer. *Front. Oncol.* **2020**, *10*, 1220. [CrossRef] [PubMed]
49. Sausen, M.; Phallen, J.; Adleff, V.; Jones, S.; Leary, R.J.; Barrett, M.T.; Anagnostou, V.; Parpart-Li, S.; Murphy, D.; Kay Li, Q.; et al. Clinical implications of genomic alterations in the tumour and circulation of pancreatic cancer patients. *Nat. Commun.* **2015**, *6*, 7686. [CrossRef]
50. Van Laethem, J.L.; Riess, H.; Jassem, J.; Haas, M.; Martens, U.M.; Weekes, C.; Peeters, M.; Ross, P.; Bridgewater, J.; Melichar, B.; et al. Phase I/II Study of Refametinib (BAY 86-9766) in Combination with Gemcitabine in Advanced Pancreatic cancer. *Target Oncol.* **2017**, *12*, 97–109. [CrossRef] [PubMed]
51. Singh, N.; Rashid, S.; Dash, N.R.; Gupta, S.; Saraya, A. Clinical significance of promoter methylation status of tumor suppressor genes in circulating DNA of pancreatic cancer patients. *J. Cancer Res. Clin. Oncol.* **2020**, *146*, 897–907. [CrossRef]
52. Bernard, V.; Kim, D.U.; San Lucas, F.A.; Castillo, J.; Allenson, K.; Mulu, F.C.; Stephens, B.M.; Huang, J.; Semaan, A.; Guerrero, P.A.; et al. Circulating Nucleic Acids Are Associated With Outcomes of Patients With Pancreatic Cancer. *Gastroenterology* **2019**, *156*, 108–118.e4. [CrossRef]
53. Chen, H.; Tu, H.; Meng, Z.Q.; Chen, Z.; Wang, P.; Liu, L.M. K-ras mutational status predicts poor prognosis in unresectable pancreatic cancer. *Eur. J. Surg. Oncol.* **2010**, *36*, 657–662. [CrossRef]
54. Mulcahy, H.E.; Lyautey, J.; Lederrey, C.; qi Chen, X.; Anker, P.; Alstead, E.M.; Ballinger, A.; Farthing, M.J.; Stroun, M. A prospective study of K-ras mutations in the plasma of pancreatic cancer patients. *Clin. Cancer Res.* **1998**, *4*, 271–275.
55. Earl, J.; Garcia-Nieto, S.; Martinez-Avila, J.C.; Montans, J.; Sanjuanbenito, A.; Rodríguez-Garrote, M.; Lisa, E.; Mendía, E.; Lobo, E.; Malats, N.; et al. Circulating tumor cells (Ctc) and kras mutant circulating free Dna (cfdna) detection in peripheral blood as biomarkers in patients diagnosed with exocrine pancreatic cancer. *BMC Cancer* **2015**, *15*, 797. [CrossRef]
56. Singh, N.; Gupta, S.; Pandey, R.M.; Chauhan, S.S.; Saraya, A. High levels of cell-free circulating nucleic acids in pancreatic cancer are associated with vascular encasement, metastasis and poor survival. *Cancer Investig.* **2015**, *33*, 78–85. [CrossRef]
57. Adamo, P.; Cowley, C.M.; Neal, C.P.; Mistry, V.; Page, K.; Dennison, A.R.; Isherwood, J.; Hastings, R.; Luo, J.; Moore, D.A.; et al. Profiling tumour heterogeneity through circulating tumour DNA in patients with pancreatic cancer. *Oncotarget* **2017**, *8*, 87221–87233. [CrossRef]
58. Cheng, H.; Liu, C.; Jiang, J.; Luo, G.; Lu, Y.; Jin, K.; Guo, M.; Zhang, Z.; Xu, J.; Liu, L.; et al. Analysis of ctDNA to predict prognosis and monitor treatment responses in metastatic pancreatic cancer patients. *Int. J. Cancer* **2017**, *140*, 2344–2350. [CrossRef]
59. Pietrasz, D.; Pécuchet, N.; Garlan, F.; Didelot, A.; Dubreuil, O.; Doat, S.; Imbert-Bismut, F.; Karoui, M.; Vaillant, J.C.; Taly, V.; et al. Plasma Circulating Tumor DNA in Pancreatic Cancer Patients Is a Prognostic Marker. *Clin. Cancer Res.* **2017**, *23*, 116–123. [CrossRef]
60. Kim, M.K.; Woo, S.M.; Park, B.; Yoon, K.A.; Kim, Y.H.; Joo, J.; Lee, W.J.; Han, S.S.; Park, S.J.; Kong, S.Y. Prognostic Implications of Multiplex Detection of KRAS Mutations in Cell-Free DNA from Patients with Pancreatic Ductal Adenocarcinoma. *Clin. Chem.* **2018**, *64*, 726–734. [CrossRef] [PubMed]
61. Patel, H.; Okamura, R.; Fanta, P.; Patel, C.; Lanman, R.B.; Raymond, V.M.; Kato, S.; Kurzrock, R. Clinical correlates of blood-derived circulating tumor DNA in pancreatic cancer. *J. Hematol. Oncol.* **2019**, *12*, 130. [CrossRef] [PubMed]
62. Bachet, J.B.; Blons, H.; Hammel, P.; Hariry, I.E.; Portales, F.; Mineur, L.; Metges, J.P.; Mulot, C.; Bourreau, C.; Cain, J.; et al. Circulating Tumor DNA is Prognostic and Potentially Predictive of Eryaspase Efficacy in Second-line in Patients with Advanced Pancreatic Adenocarcinoma. *Clin. Cancer Res.* **2020**, *26*, 5208–5216. [CrossRef] [PubMed]
63. Strijker, M.; Soer, E.C.; de Pastena, M.; Creemers, A.; Balduzzi, A.; Beagan, J.J.; Busch, O.R.; van Delden, O.M.; Halfwerk, H.; van Hooft, J.E.; et al. Circulating tumor DNA quantity is related to tumor volume and both predict survival in metastatic pancreatic ductal adenocarcinoma. *Int. J. Cancer* **2020**, *146*, 1445–1456. [CrossRef] [PubMed]
64. Toledano-Fonseca, M.; Cano, M.T.; Inga, E.; Rodríguez-Alonso, R.; Gómez-España, M.A.; Guil-Luna, S.; Mena-Osuna, R.; de la Haba-Rodríguez, J.R.; Rodríguez-Ariza, A.; Aranda, E. Circulating Cell-Free DNA-Based Liquid Biopsy Markers for the Non-Invasive Prognosis and Monitoring of Metastatic Pancreatic Cancer. *Cancers* **2020**, *12*, 1754. [CrossRef]
65. Uesato, Y.; Sasahira, N.; Ozaka, M.; Sasaki, T.; Takatsuki, M.; Zembutsu, H. Evaluation of circulating tumor DNA as a biomarker in pancreatic cancer with liver metastasis. *PLoS ONE* **2020**, *15*, e0235623. [CrossRef]
66. Wei, T.; Zhang, J.; Li, J.; Chen, Q.; Zhi, X.; Tao, W.; Ma, J.; Yang, L.; Lou, Y.; Ma, T.; et al. Genome-wide profiling of circulating tumor DNA depicts landscape of copy number alterations in pancreatic cancer with liver metastasis. *Mol. Oncol.* **2020**, *14*, 1966–1977. [CrossRef]

67. Sugimori, M.; Sugimori, K.; Tsuchiya, H.; Suzuki, Y.; Tsuyuki, S.; Kaneta, Y.; Hirotani, A.; Sanga, K.; Tozuka, Y.; Komiyama, S.; et al. Quantitative monitoring of circulating tumor DNA in patients with advanced pancreatic cancer undergoing chemotherapy. *Cancer Sci.* **2020**, *111*, 266–278. [CrossRef] [PubMed]
68. Snyder, M.; Kircher, M.; Hill, A.; Daza, R.; Shendure, J. Cell-free DNA Comprises an In Vivo Nucleosome Footprint that Informs Its Tissues-Of-Origin. *Cell* **2016**, *164*, 57–68. [CrossRef]
69. Fernando, M.R.; Jiang, C.; Krzyzanowski, G.D.; Ryan, W.L. Analysis of human blood plasma cell-free DNA fragment size distribution using EvaGreen chemistry based droplet digital PCR assays. *Clin. Chim. Acta* **2018**, *483*, 39–47. [CrossRef] [PubMed]
70. Li, H.; Jing, C.; Wu, J.; Ni, J.; Sha, H.; Xu, X.; Du, Y.; Lou, R.; Dong, S.; Feng, J. Circulating tumor DNA detection: A potential tool for colorectal cancer management. *Oncol. Lett.* **2019**, *17*, 1409–1416. [CrossRef] [PubMed]
71. Lee, J.S.; Rhee, T.M.; Pietrasz, D.; Bachet, J.B.; Laurent-Puig, P.; Kong, S.Y.; Takai, E.; Yachida, S.; Shibata, T.; Lee, J.W.; et al. Circulating tumor DNA as a prognostic indicator in resectable pancreatic ductal adenocarcinoma: A systematic review and meta-analysis. *Sci. Rep.* **2019**, *18*, 16971. [CrossRef] [PubMed]
72. Vesovic, N.; Tosic, N.; Djurasevic, T.K.; Andric, Z.; Zdravkovic, D.; Pavlovic, S.; Jovanovic, D. Expression pattern of circulating long non-coding RNA GAS5 as a novel biomarker in non-small cell lung cancer patients. *Arch. Med. Sci.* **2020**. [CrossRef]
73. O'Leary, B.; Hrebien, S.; Beaney, M.; Fribbens, C.; Garcia-Murillas, I.; Jiang, J.; Li, Y.; Huang Bartlett, C.; André, F.; Loibl, S.; et al. Comparison of BEAMing and Droplet Digital PCR for Circulating Tumor DNA Analysis. *Clin. Chem.* **2019**, *65*, 1405–1413. [CrossRef]
74. Pécuchet, N.; Rozenholc, Y.; Zonta, E.; Pietrasz, D.; Didelot, A.; Combe, P.; Gibault, L.; Bachet, J.B.; Taly, V.; Fabre, E.; et al. Analysis of Base-Position Error Rate of Next-Generation Sequencing to Detect Tumor Mutations in Circulating DNA. *Clin. Chem.* **2016**, *62*, 1492–1503. [CrossRef]
75. Heitzer, E.; Ulz, P.; Geigl, J.B. Circulating tumor DNA as a liquid biopsy for cancer. *Clin Chem.* **2015**, *61*, 112–123. [CrossRef]
76. Trigg, R.M.; Martinson, L.J.; Parpart-Li, S.; Shaw, J.A. Factors that influence quality and yield of circulating-free DNA: A systematic review of the methodology literature. *Heliyon* **2018**, *4*, e00699. [CrossRef]
77. Mullard, A. Cracking KRAS. *Nat. Rev. Drug Discov.* **2019**, *18*, 887–891. [CrossRef]
78. Waters, A.M.; Der, C.J. KRAS: The Critical Driver and Therapeutic Target for Pancreatic Cancer. *Cold Spring Harb. Perspect Med.* **2018**, *8*, a031435. [CrossRef]
79. Haigis, K.M. KRAS Alleles: The Devil Is in the Detail. *Trends Cancer* **2017**, *3*, 686–697. [CrossRef]
80. Gillson, J.; Ramaswamy, Y.; Singh, G.; Gorfe, A.A.; Pavlakis, N.; Samra, J.; Mittal, A.; Sahni, S. Small Molecule KRAS Inhibitors: The Future for Targeted Pancreatic Cancer Therapy? *Cancers* **2020**, *12*, 1341. [CrossRef] [PubMed]
81. Pishvaian, M.J.; Blais, E.M.; Brody, J.R.; Lyons, E.; DeArbeloa, P.; Hendifar, A.; Mikhail, S.; Chung, V.; Sahai, V.; Sohal, D.P.S.; et al. Overall survival in patients with pancreatic cancer receiving matched therapies following molecular profiling: A retrospective analysis of the Know Your Tumor registry trial. *Lancet Oncol.* **2020**, *21*, 508–518. [CrossRef]
82. Takai, E.; Totoki, Y.; Nakamura, H.; Morizane, C.; Nara, S.; Hama, N.; Suzuki, M.; Furukawa, E.; Kato, M.; Hayashi, H.; et al. Clinical utility of circulating tumor DNA for molecular assessment in pancreatic cancer. *Sci. Rep.* **2015**, *5*, 18425. [CrossRef]
83. Botrus, G.; Kosirorek, H.; Sonbol, M.B.; Kusne, Y.; Uson Junior, P.L.S.; Borad, M.J.; Ahn, D.H.; Kasi, P.M.; Drusbosky, L.M.; Dada, H.; et al. Circulating Tumor DNA-Based Testing and Actionable Findings in Patients with Advanced and Metastatic Pancreatic Adenocarcinoma. *Oncologist* **2021**. [CrossRef]
84. Heredia-Soto, V.; Rodríguez-Salas, N.; Feliu, J. Liquid Biopsy in Pancreatic Cancer: Are We Ready to Apply It in the Clinical Practice? *Cancers* **2021**, *13*, 1986. [CrossRef]
85. Chan, H.T.; Chin, Y.M.; Nakamura, Y.; Low, S.K. Clonal Hematopoiesis in Liquid Biopsy: From Biological Noise to Valuable Clinical Implications. *Cancers* **2020**, *12*, 2277. [CrossRef]
86. Jaiswal, S.; Fontanillas, P.; Flannick, J.; Manning, A.; Grauman, P.V.; Mar, B.G.; Lindsley, R.C.; Mermel, C.H.; Burtt, N.; Chavez, A.; et al. Age-related clonal hematopoiesis associated with adverse outcomes. *N. Engl. J. Med.* **2014**, *371*, 2488–2498. [CrossRef]
87. Ptashkin, R.N.; Mandelker, D.L.; Coombs, C.C.; Bolton, K.; Yelskaya, Z.; Hyman, D.M.; Solit, D.B.; Baselga, J.; Arcila, M.E.; Ladanyi, M.; et al. Prevalence of Clonal Hematopoiesis Mutations in Tumor-Only Clinical Genomic Profiling of Solid Tumors. *JAMA Oncol.* **2018**, *4*, 1589–1593. [CrossRef]
88. Manrai, A.K.; Funke, B.H.; Rehm, H.L.; Olesen, M.S.; Maron, B.A.; Szolovits, P.; Margulies, D.M.; Loscalzo, J.; Kohane, I.S. Genetic Misdiagnoses and the Potential for Health Disparities. *N. Engl. J. Med.* **2016**, *375*, 655–665. [CrossRef]
89. Lek, M.; Karczewski, K.J.; Minikel, E.V.; Samocha, K.E.; Banks, E.; Fennell, T.; O'Donnell-Luria, A.H.; Ware, J.S.; Hill, A.J.; Cummings, B.B.; et al. Analysis of protein-coding genetic variation in 60,706 humans. *Nature* **2016**, *536*, 285–291. [CrossRef]
90. Karczewski, K.J.; Francioli, L.C.; Tiao, G.; Cummings, B.B.; Alföldi, J.; Wang, Q.; Collins, R.L.; Laricchia, K.M.; Ganna, A.; Birnbaum, D.P.; et al. The mutational constraint spectrum quantified from variation in 141,456 humans. *Nature* **2020**, *581*, 434–443. [CrossRef]

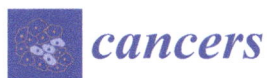 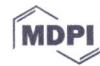

Review

Is Laparoscopic Pancreaticoduodenectomy Feasible for Pancreatic Ductal Adenocarcinoma?

Chang Moo Kang [1,2,*] and **Woo Jung Lee** [1,2]

1. Division of Hepatobiliary and Pancreatic Surgery, Department of Surgery, Yonsei University College of Medicine, Seoul 03772, Korea; wjlee@yuhs.ac
2. Pancreatobiliary Cancer Center, Yonsei Cancer Center, Severance Hospital, Seoul 03772, Korea
* Correspondence: cmkang@yuhs.ac; Tel.: +82-2-2228-2135

Received: 20 October 2020; Accepted: 14 November 2020; Published: 18 November 2020

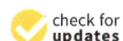

Simple Summary: Pancreatic cancer is known to be one of the most lethal malignant diseases in gastrointestinal tract. Margin-negative pancreatectomy followed by postoperative adjuvant chemotherapy is essential treatment for long-term survival. Due to anatomical complexity and technical difficulty, laparoscopic pancreaticoduodenectomy is still controversial. However, with the advance of laparoscopic surgery, laparoscopic pancreatic resection of pancreatic head cancer has been carefully applied in well selected patients. The accumulating data are suggesting its technical feasibility, safety, and potential equivalent long-term oncologic outcome. In this review, the current status of laparoscopic pancreaticoduodenectomy for pancreatic head cancer is summarized. In addition, potential surgical indications and future perspectives of laparoscopic pancreaticoduodenectomy for pancreatic cancer are discussed for safe implementation in our clinical practice.

Abstract: Margin-negative radical pancreatectomy is the essential condition to obtain long-term survival of patients with pancreatic cancer. With the investigation for early diagnosis, introduction of potent chemotherapeutic agents, application of neoadjuvnat chemotherapy, advancement of open and laparoscopic surgical techniques, mature perioperative management, and patients' improved general conditions, survival of the resected pancreatic cancer is expected to be further improved. According to the literatures, laparoscopic pancreaticoduodenectomy (LPD) is also thought to be good alternative strategy in managing well-selected resectable pancreatic cancer. LPD with combined vascular resection is also feasible, but only expert surgeons should handle these challenging cases. LPD for pancreatic cancer should be determined based on surgeons' proficiency to fulfil the goals of the patient's safety and oncologic principles.

Keywords: laparoscopic; pancreaticoduodenectomy; pancreatic cancer

---

1. Introduction

Pancreatic cancer is one of the most lethal malignant tumors in the human gastrointestinal tract. Its overall survival is reported to be around 5%. Until now, margin-negative pancreatectomy and postoperative adjuvant chemotherapy is known as the standard treatment option for cure of the disease [1,2]. However, most pancreatic cancer patients are found in the advanced cancer stage. Only about 15% of the patients are eligible for resection and more than half of the patients usually develop local or systemic recurrence within 2 years after surgery. The 5-year survival of the patients who underwent radical pancreatectomy is known to be around 20%. Recent statistical perspectives estimated that pancreatic cancer will be one of the top 3 cancers killing humans in 2030 [3].

The pancreas is a difficult internal organ to be accessed by minimally invasive surgery. It is located in retroperitoneal space, and major vascular structures are near the pancreas. Therefore, laparoscopic exposure and dissection of the pancreas are difficult and even small breakage of tributary vessels will result in massive bleeding to obscure a clear surgical field. In addition, in the case of pancreatic head lesions, laparoscopic management of remnant pancreas and resected bile duct is still a great hurdle to overcome for safe surgical procedure [4]. However, with the advance of laparoscopic technique and experiences, laparoscopic distal pancreatectomy (LDP) is regarded as a safe and standard approach in well-selected left-sided pancreatic tumor [5], and even laparoscopic pancreaticoduodenectomy (LPD) is carefully thought to be an appropriate surgical option to treat periampullary lesions [6].

In the past, the Yonsei criteria was suggested as appropriate tumor conditions for oncologically safe laparoscopic radical distal pancreatectomy (LDP) [7]. According to our experience, the Yonsei criteria was found to be not only selection criteria for LDP, but also a clinically detectable parameter to predict long-term survival of left-sided pancreatic cancer [8]. Carefully expanding indications for LDP is quite acceptable as long as patients' safety and oncologic principles are maintained [9]. In the absence of randomized trials, uncertainty regarding the oncologic efficacy of LDP still exists. However, accumulating experience shows that LDP is associated with comparable survival, R0 resection, and use of adjuvant chemotherapy when comparing to open distal pancreatectomy (ODP) [10,11].

On the other hand, the current status of LPD has a long way to go in terms of technical and oncological safety. Unlike LDP, many surgeons are still within their learning curve period. Nickel et al. [12] performed a meta-analysis of randomized controlled trials comparing LPD and open pancreaticoduodenectomy (OPD) [13–15]. They concluded that at the current level of evidence, LPD shows no advantage over OPD except lower estimated intraoperative blood loss. Even though three currently available randomized control trials (RCT) were included for meta-analysis, lack of blinding of the patients and personnel assessing the main outcomes, and the learning curve issue should be considered when interpreting the results. Especially, pancreatic head cancer requires not only for skillful laparoscopic techniques but also wisdom to select appropriate patients for safe and effective margin-negative LPD, because curative resection is known to be basis for long-term survival of pancreatic cancer. Due to aggressive tumor biology and anatomical intimacy between the pancreas and major vascular structures, LPD for pancreatic cancer should be performed by expert surgeons who have already overcome of their learning-curve period [16–18]. It should be the last stage of LPD application in periampullary cancers after acquisition of full technical maturation.

It might be too early to generalize the potential oncological role of LPD in managing pancreatic head cancer, however several emerging articles from expert surgeons are providing future insight that LPD can be safe and effective in well-selected pancreatic cancer patients [19–21]. In fact, recent NCCN guideline version 1. 2020 pancreatic adenocarcinoma recommended surgical treatment by laparotomy or minimally invasive surgery as treatment for resectable pancreatic cancer [22]. LPD is no longer just a debatable issue in treating pancreatic cancer, but already regarded as one of the recommendable options in clinical oncology of pancreatic cancer. However, the articles presented as the basis for such a guideline were thought to be limited; they were published a long time ago, and were not focused on pancreatic cancer [23,24]. More detailed concerns about indications and understanding the current status of LPD in treating pancreatic cancer will be a strong background to increase the justification of clinical practice of LPD for pancreatic cancer.

2. Rationale of Minimally Invasive Pancreaticoduodenectomy for Pancreatic Cancer

2.1. Technical Feasibility

2.1.1. Surgical Extent

Lymph node (LN) involvement is analyzed to be a very important prognostic factor in pancreatic cancer. Indeed, more than half of the resected pancreatic cancer showed LN metastasis and poor survival outcomes [25]. Then, for potentially clearing metastatic LNs, can extended pancreaticoduodenectomy (PD), clearing LNs around celiac, superior mesenteric artery (SMA), paraaortic, and hepatoduodenal ligament, as well as nerve plexus dissection around celiac, hepatic artery, and SMA, improve oncologic outcome in patients with resectable pancreatic cancer (Table 1)? Due to frequent recurrence and poor long-term oncologic outcomes following curative resection of pancreatic cancer, extended dissection was once advocated in surgical management of pancreatic cancer [26–28]. However, these are all retrospective observational studies, and selection bias should be considered when interpreting surgical outcomes. To optimize the surgical extent of PD in treating pancreatic cancer, researchers performed several important prospective randomized control studies to determine the optimal extent of surgical resection in treating resectable pancreatic cancer (Table 2).

Table 1. Topographic differences in extent of lymph node dissection between standard pancreaticoduodenectomy (PD) and extended PD.

Surgical Extent	Standard	Extended
LN station *	13, 17, 12b	13,17, 12b, 12a,12p, 8a, 8p, 5, 6, 9, 16, 14a, 14b,14c
Circumferential Nerve plexus dissection (Celiac/HA/SMA)	-/-/-	±/±/±

* Mentioned in more than 3 RCTs [29]; HA, hepatic artery; SMA, superior mesenteric artery.

Table 2. Literature review of randomized control trials (RCTs) comparing standard PD and extended PD in treating pancreatic cancer.

Author, Year	Surgical Extent	N	Op-Time, Hr/Min.	EBL, mL	#LNs	R0, %	LOH, Day	Cx., %	POPF, %	DGE, %	Mx., %	5YOS, %
Pedrazzoli, 1998 [30]	STD	40	371.9	2671	13.3	NA	22.7	47.5	12.5	NA	5	552d √
	EXT	41	396.7	3149	19.8 *	NA	19.3	48.5	7.5	NA	4.9	589d √
Yeo, 2005 [31]	STD	146(84)	5.9	740	17.0	88	11.3	29	6	6	4	10
	EXT	148(83)	6.4 *	800	28.5 *	93	14.3 *	43 *	13 *	16 *	2	25
Farnell, 2005 [32]	STD	40	6.2	NA	15	76	13	62.5	8	28	0	16
	EXT	39	7.6 *	NA $	34 *	82	16	34.1	13	36	3	17
Nimura, 2012 [33]	STD	51	426	NA	13.3	94.1	43.8	19.6	NA	NA	0	15.7
	EXT	50	547	NA	40.1 *	90	42.4	22.0	NA	NA	2	6.0
Jang, 2014 [34]	STD	83	355.5	372	17.3	85.5	19.7	32.0	9.6	9.6	0	18.8m √
	EXT	86	419.6 *	563 *	33.7 *	90.7	22.8	43.0	12.8	5.8	2.3	16.5m √

STD, standard dissection; EXT, extended dissection; EBL, estimated blood loss; LN, lymph node; LOH, length of hospital stay; POPF, postoperative pancreatic fistula; DGE, delayed gastric emptying; Mx, mortality; 5YOS, 5-year overall survival; *, p < 0.05; √, median survival time; $, incidence of transfusion 5% vs. 23%, p = 0.01.

When looking at the number of retrieved LNs, extended PD shows a higher number of retrieved LNs than standard PD (Table 2). However, a recent meta-analysis [29] to review oncologic outcomes of five randomized controlled trials comparing extended and standard lymphadenectomy in patients with PD for pancreatic cancer demonstrated that PD with standard dissection was safe (shorter operation time, less transfusion, less overall postoperative complications, and similar R0) and showed similar long-term survival outcomes to that of extended dissection (HR = 1.01 [95% CI: 0.77–1.34], p = 0.923). It is known that intraoperative transfusion [35] and postoperative complications [36,37] have an adverse impact on survival of resected pancreatic cancer, suggesting potential benefit of standard dissection in treating pancreatic cancer. Although the number of retrieved lymph nodes is reported to be one of the important prognostic factors in treating pancreatic cancer [38,39], recently lymph node ratio, and number of positive lymph nodes, "NOT total nodes examined", were associated with overall survival in resected pancreatic cancer [40].

In summary, standard PD is not inferior and has comparable oncologic outcomes in treating resectable pancreatic cancer. Therefore, PD with routine extended lymph node dissection is not recommended due to higher morbidity and comparable long-term survival. According to the current technical availability of LPD, at least the extent of standard dissection is thought to be well achieved by current laparoscopic surgical technique (Figure 1).

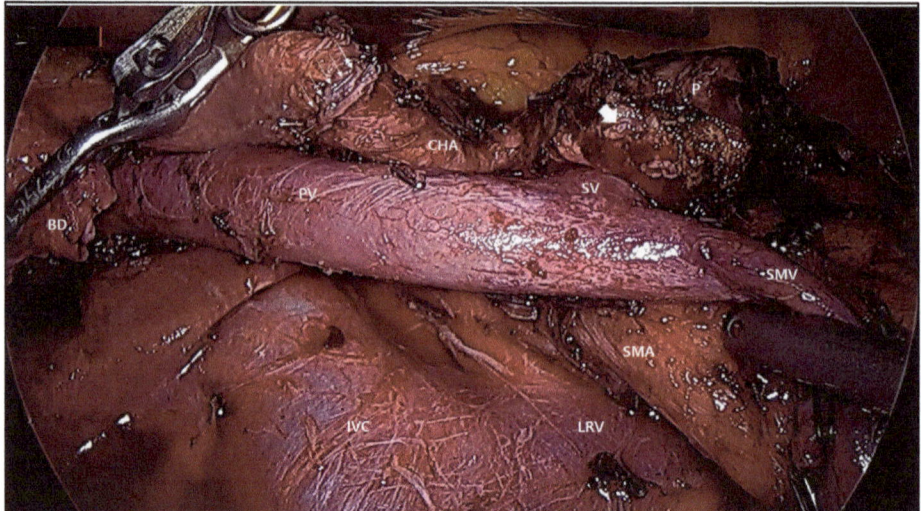

Figure 1. Laparoscopic view after resection of pancreatic head cancer. BD; bile duct, PV; portal vein, CHA; common hepatic artery. P; pancreas, SV; splenic vein, SMV; superior mesenteric vein, SMA; superior mesenteric artery, LRV; left renal vein, IVC; inferior vena cava, gastroduodenal artery stump (white arrows), pancreatic duct (thick white arrow).

2.1.2. Retroperitoneal Margin

Cancer cell involvement in the resection margin is known to be associated with early tumor recurrence and poor long-term oncologic outcomes [41]. The pancreatic neck and head wrap the superior mesenteric vein (SMV)/portal vein (PV), and the uncinate process of the pancreas is elongated from the pancreatic head and extends behind the SMV/PV to contact the right lateral aspect of the SMA. There are abundant lymphatics and neural tissues around this area. Surgeons need to consider not only the pancreatic neck margin, but also the retroperitoneal margin, the so called SMA lateral margin, when performing radical PD for pancreatic cancer, because pancreatic cancer cells can invade and infiltrate along the nerve tissue in the pancreas toward major arterial systems (the SMA, common hepatic artery, and celiac axis) [42–44]. Therefore, even in case of pancreatic cancer that is very separated from the SMA, pancreatic cancer cells can invade SMA through this nerve tissue. The oncologic significance of retroperitoneal margin clearance has been reported [45,46]. Butler et al. [47] recently performed systemic review on the oncologic role of periadventitial dissection of SMA in affecting margin status after PD for pancreatic cancer. According to this review, it was suggested that positive margin was associated with decreased survival and SMA margin involvement was the most often, which ranged 15–45% of resected pancreatic cancer.

Surgical dissection of nerve tissue (retroperitoneal margin) around SMA is not that simple. Not uncommonly, it is usually difficult to exactly differentiate from pancreatic uncinated process and SMA due to abundant lymphatic tissue, inflammatory changes associated with pancreatitis, and neural tissue around SMA. These tissues are all intermingled altogether. In addition, it is difficult to expose the right lateral aspect of SMA because this area is behind the SMV-SV confluence. Lastly, there are abundant lymphovascular structures and even small breakage of tributary vessels around SMA and SMV usually give rise massive bleeding to prevent from further safe dissection for margin-negative resection.

Therefore, considering oncologic significance of retroperitoneal margin in treating pancreatic cancer, surgical design and plan to obtain cancer-free retroperitoneal margin is very important. There are several surgical techniques to secure retroperitoneal margin during LPD (Table 3). Rho et al. [48] introduced the potential application of indocyanine green (ICG) to facilitate the securement of the SMA lateral margin in laparoscopic PD, which is based on the idea that the pancreas is a well perfused organ and near infra-red light can detect ICG location through fluorescent illumination. When ICG is accumulated in the pancreatic head, near-infrared light can show visual differentiation between the uncinated process and surrounding soft tissues along the SMA (Figure 2), helping surgeons to obtain a negative retroperitoneal margin. The impact of long-term oncologic outcome of ICG-based SMA lateral border dissection remains to be investigated further, however it is thought to be a useful technique when performing LPD in resectable pancreatic cancer. Nagakawa et al. [49] introduced the technique to expose the inferior pancreaticoduodenal artery and SMA lateral border by proximal-dorsal jejunal vein (PDPV) pre-isolation, which is thought to be one of the approaches for standard PD. Moreover, Morales et al. [50] and Zimmitti et al. [51] demonstrate the surgical method to obtain the clear SMA margin by applying the SMA artery first approach. Despite requiring advanced laparoscopic skills, these methods are thought to be useful for margin-negative resection in selected cases of relatively advanced pancreatic cancer. Kuroki et al. [52] also introduced the concept of the pancreas-hanging maneuver by Penrose drain in managing SMA margin during LDP, however, they did not describe the R0 resection rate among the patients with this technique, and no patients with pancreatic head cancer were involved.

Table 3. Several approaches to obtain clear SMA lateral margin.

Author, Year	Concept	N	Op-Time	EBL, mL	R0, %	LOH, Day	Cx, %	Mx., %
Kuroki, 2010 [52] #	Pancreas-hanging maneuver	9	NA	642	NA	19	NA	NA
Zimmitti, 2016 [51]	Periadventitial dissection of SMA	16	590	150	100	16	3	NA
Rho, 2018 [48]	ICG-guided differentiation of uncinate process from SMA lateral border	10	432	166	100	16.7	2	0
Nagakawa, 2018 [49]	PDJV preisolation method	21	489.38	183	NA	22.43	5	NA
Morales, 2019 [50]	Periadventitial dissection of for SMA TMpE	59	NA	NA	86	NA	NA *	NA

Pancreatic cancer was not included, * intraoperative massive bleeding in 3 cases, PDJV; proximal-dorsal jejunal vein, TMpE; total mesopancreas excision, SMA; superior mesenteric artery.

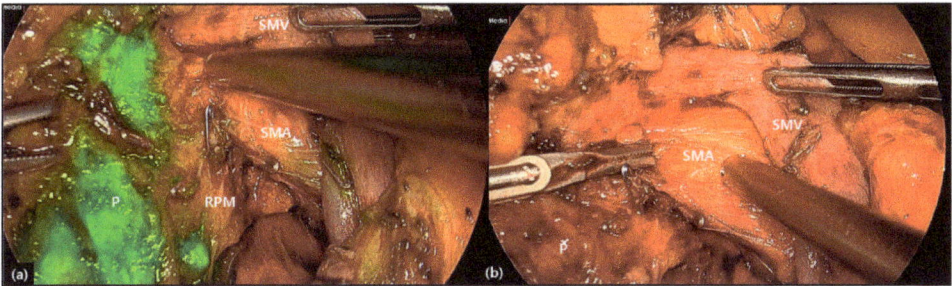

Figure 2. Intraoperative usage of indocyanine green (ICG) during obtaining the retroperitoneal margin of the pancreas. The ICG stained area is part of the uncinated process (**a**), which can be differentiated from the SMA to obtain the retroperitoneal margin (**b**). It can help the surgeon design surgical dissection. Note soft tissue around the SMA (retroperitoneal margin) is not stained by ICG. P; uncinated process of the pancreas, SMA; superior mesenteric artery, SMV; superior mesenteric vein, RPM; retroperitoneal margin.

2.1.3. Combined Vascular Resection

Pancreatic cancer usually is found at an advanced stage of cancer. In spite of resectable pancreatic cancer, due to anatomic intimacy between the pancreas and surrounding major venous vascular structures, unexpected portal vein (PV) and superior mesenteric vein invasion (SMV) is often encountered during the operation. In the past, several articles [53,54] concluded that the oncologic outcome of PD with combined venous vascular resection (PD-VR) is not favorable, however some others showed that PD-VR did not increase the complication rate and postoperative mortality [55,56]. PD-VR is no longer considered an absolute contraindication in pancreatic head cancer. It is regarded as a safe and feasible option to improve the resection rate of pancreatic cancer. Especially, the oncologic role of combined venous vascular resection became highlighted as the concept of neoadjuvant chemotherapy was introduced in managing borderline or locally advanced pancreatic cancer. However, Peng et al. [57] recently evaluated the value of PD with combine vascular resection (PD-VR) for pancreatic head cancer. In this meta-analysis, a total of 12,031 patients (2186 patients with PD-VR, 22.2%) from 30 published articles were investigated. In comparison with the PD group, it was analyzed that the PD-VR group had a lower R0 resection rate and higher rates of complications such as biliary fistula, reoperation rate, delayed gastric emptying, cardiopulmonary abnormalities, hemorrhage, in-hospital mortality, and 30-day mortality. In addition, the blood loss, operation time, and total length of hospital stay were higher in the PD-VR group, concluding that PD-VR for pancreatic cancer should be carefully considered by selected pancreatic surgeons.

Until now, only a few case reports [58–62] and case series [19,63–65] have been reported on the technical feasibility and safety of LPD with combined venous vascular resection (LPD-VR, Table 4). Tangential resection with stapler or hand suture or patch reconstruction appears to be common among the patients with LPD-VR (Figure 3), which is also confirmed when comparing with OPD-VR [19]. As shown above, postoperative morbidity and mortality related to combined vascular resection are not ignorable, and segmental resection and end-to-end anastomosis or artificial graft, or renal vein graft must be a challenging procedure. Therefore, LPD-VR also needs to be performed in well-selected patients and by highly selected expert surgeons.

Table 4. Summary of articles reporting more than 5 cases of LPD-venous vascular resection (LPD-VR) for pancreatic cancer.

Author, Year	N	Op-Time, min	EBL, mL	Cx, %	Mx, %	LOH, Day	Survival
Cai, 2018 [63]	18(14) T: 8 E-E: 6 AG: 4	448	213	6(33.3)	None	13	Mean FU; 11 mo., 2 death (1 renal failure, 1 tumor metastasis)
Khatkov, 2017 [64]	8(5) T: 4 T+Patch:1 E-E: 3	560	450	2(25)	1(12.5) Due to heart failure	15	FU (4–12 mo.) 6 death due to tumor progression
Kendrick, 2011 [65]	11(9) T: 6 T+Patch: 4 RVG: 1	413	500	6	None	7	Median FU:7.2 mo. N/A
Croome, 2015 [19]	31(25) T: 12 T+Patch: 10 E-E: 7 RVG: 1 AG: 1	465	841.8	11(35)/2(6.4 *)	1(3.2)	6	Median FU : 15.2 mo. * no survival differences between OPD group ($p = 0.14$)

T, tangential resection; E-E, end-to-end anastomosis; RVG, renal vein graft; AG, artificial graft.

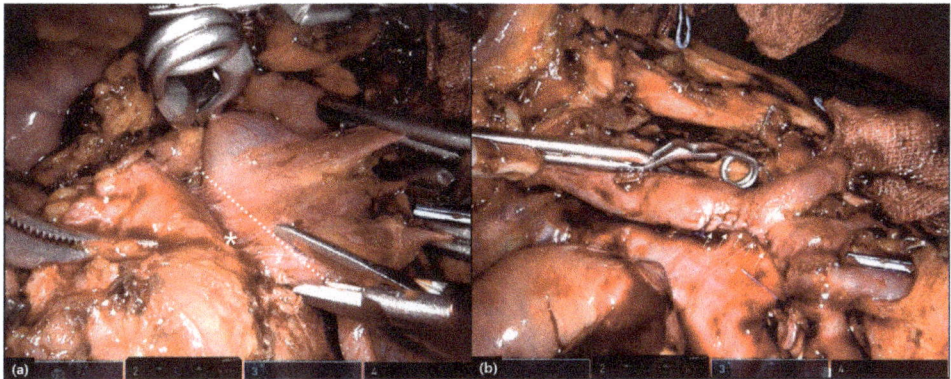

Figure 3. Combined venous vascular resection during laparoscopic pancreaticoduodenectomy (LPD). Tangential wedge resection of SMV is performed after transient clamping venous system (**a**). Primary repair of resected venous system (**b**). Tangential resection line (white dotted line), tumor invasion (white *), primary repair (white arrows).

The long-term oncologic efficacy of LPD-VR is lacking, but Croome et al. [19] demonstrated no statistical significance between LPD-VR and OPD-VR in terms of overall survival, leaving some room to be further investigated. In addition, there are other modified techniques for reconstruction following LPD-VR, using falciform ligament [66], parietal peritoneum [67], and hepatic ligament teres [68], suggesting further potential applications of laparoscopic technique remain to be studied.

2.1.4. Repeated Pancreatectomy for Pancreatic Cancer in Remnant Pancreas

Even after R0 radical resection, patients with PC often experience local recurrence. However, it has been reported that about 0.5–4.6% of pancreatic cancers develop in remnant pancreas [69,70]. Since 1995, re-resection of pancreatic cancer in remnant pancreas has been proposed for improving oncologic outcome [71]. The first case series reporting 30 patients with surgery for recurred pancreatic cancer also suggested that resection for recurrent pancreatic cancer can be performed safely, and questioned a potential subgroup who might actually benefit form re-resection of recurred pancreatic cancer [72].

As experience of resected remnant pancreatic cancer accumulated, Yamada et al. [73] published the results of resection of recurrent remnant pancreatic cancer in Japanese society of hepato-biliary-pancreatic surgery. Clinical data from 114 patients with remnant pancreatic cancer after initial pancreatectomy were analyzed. It was found that median survival of the resected remnant pancreatic cancer was superior to the non-resected group (26 and 14 months, respectively [hazard ratio: 0.56, $p = 0.012$]), showing that re-resection of remnant pancreatic cancer could offer a favorable outcome and chance for cure. Similarly, the recent literature [69] reviewing 49 reported patients with resected remnant pancreatic cancer following resection of the primary pancreatic cancer demonstrated that median disease-free survival was 44.4 months (12–143 months), and median survival time was 32 months after repeated pancreatectomy. In addition, another systemic review demonstrated that re-resection of isolated local recurrent pancreatic cancer showed the most favorable survival outcomes (median, 32 months) comparing with chemoradiation therapy (19 months), stereotactic body radiation therapy (16 months) [74], suggesting the role of aggressive surgical extirpation of recurred remnant pancreatic cancer for improving prognosis. Table 5 summarized recent review articles reporting oncologic benefit of repeated pancreatectomy for pancreatic cancer. It was found that completion total pancreatectomy is the most common procedure for treating recurred pancreatic cancer in remnant pancreas and nearly no postoperative mortality is reported. Reported median survival time (14–32 months), and 5-year overall survival (40.6%) following repeated pancreatectomy are much longer than unresectable pancreatic cancer in recent RCTs [75].

Then, is laparoscopic repeated pancreatectomy feasible and does it provide a potential oncologic role in treating recurrent pancreatic cancer in remnant pancreas? Until now, very few reports have been published showing the technical feasibility of laparoscopic completion of total pancreatectomy for remnant recurrent pancreatic cancer following LPD for primary pancreatic cancer. Recently, Kang et al. (accepted in Ann Hepatobiliary Pancreat Surg 2020, and in process) successfully demonstrated the technical feasibility of laparoscopic repeated pancreatectomy for recurrent pancreatic cancer following initial laparoscopic radical pancreatectomy. In addition, Nagakawa et al. [76] and Sunagawa et al. [77] also showed the technical feasibility of laparoscopic resection of remnant pancreatic cancer after LPD for other primary cancer. All these reports are suggesting the technical feasibility and potential role of a minimally invasive approach even in recurrent pancreatic cancer in remnant pancreas. Further study is mandatory.

Table 5. Summary of review articles of repeated pancreatectomy for recurred pancreatic cancer in remnant pancreas.

Author, Year	$N_{Literatures}$	$N_{Patients}$	Initial Px (PP)PD/DP/ect)	Repeated Px TP/TP+PV/ect	Time Interval	Cx	Mx	Survival (From Initial Px/From Repeated Px)
Suzuki, 2019 [69]	17	49	31/17/1 (DPPHR)	44/4/1 (Segmentectomy)	12–143 month	NA	NA	114 months/ 32 months
Hashimoto, 2017 [78]	12	88	NA	78/5/5 (DP)	13–49 month	0–27%	0%	NA /14–27.5 months
Zhou, 2016 [79]	19	55	33/21/1 (DPPHR)	52/0/1 (DPPHR)	7–143 month	NA	0%	NA 5YOS, 40.6%
Choi, 2020 [80]	17	50	32/17/1	46/0/4 (partial)	18–88 month	NA	2%	107 months/ 60 months

Px, pancreatectomy; DP, distal pancreatectomy; NA, not available.

3. Current Literature

Recently, three meta-analyses have been published, comparing the oncologic outcomes of LPD and OPD. Jiang et al. [81] systematically reviewed the articles comparing LPD and OPD for the treatment of pancreatic cancer. They found 8 studies involving 15,278 patients and performed meta-analysis. It is thought that this meta-analysis was the first to evaluate clinical efficacy of LPD for the treatment of pancreatic cancer with long-term survival outcomes. It was found that there was no significant difference in the 5-year overall survival (HR: 0.97, 95% CI: 0.82–1.15, $p = 0.76$). In addition, LPD resulted in a higher rate of R0 resection, more harvested lymph nodes, shorter hospital stays, and less estimated blood loss, concluding that LPD is not inferior to OPD with respect to long-term oncologic outcomes, as well as better short-term surgical outcomes in patients with pancreatic cancer.

Chen et al. [82] also evaluated 1507 patients from 6 comparative cohort studies, comparing LPD with OPD for pancreatic cancer. Similar short-term oncologic outcomes were identified, such as lymph nodes harvested, R0 rate, number of positive lymph nodes, adjuvant treatment, and time to adjuvant treatment. Interestingly, in spite of comparable 1-year and 2-year survival, the following 3-year (OR 1.50, $p = 0.007$), 4-year (OR 1.73, $p = 0.04$), and 5-year survivals (OR 2.11, $p = 0.001$) were significantly longer in LPD group.

Yin et al. [83] identified 6 studies including 9144 pancreatic cancer patients and evaluated short-term and long-term oncological outcomes. They noted that fewer postoperative complications ($p = 0.005$), better trend of performance in R0 resection ($p = 0.07$), retrieved number of lymph nodes ($p = 0.07$), and comparable long-term survival ($p = 0.49$) were associated with LPD, concluding that LPD can be a suitable alternative to OPD in selected PDAC patients with respect to both surgical and oncological outcomes.

In addition, there are several articles analyzing the national cancer data base (NCDB) to overview the safety and effectiveness of LPD in treating pancreatic cancer. Sharpe et al. (study period: 2010–2011) [84] showed that, among the 4421 patients, a very limited number of patients (384 patients, 9%) underwent LPD for pancreatic cancer, and about one third of cases (118 patients, 30%) were performed in high volume centers (5 institutions, 3.8%). They demonstrated that LPD was equivalent to OPD in length of stay, R0-resection, lymph node count, and readmission rate, however a higher 30-day mortality rate in LPD group was noted in lower volume centers (7.5% vs. 3.4%, $p = 0.003$), raising concerns about the safety of LPD in treating pancreatic cancer due to a surmountable learning curve for the procedure. Kantor et al. (study period: 2010–2013) [85] analyzed 8213 patients with pancreatic cancer to show short-term and long-term oncologic outcomes of LPD and OPD. They found that LPD (828 patients, 10%) provides comparable short-term oncologic and long-term overall survival outcomes with OPD (20.7 months vs. 20.9 months, $p = 0.68$). In addition, decreased incidence of prolonged length of hospital stay (OR = 0.79), decreased rate of readmission and decrease in incidence of delay to adjuvant chemotherapy for LPD (OR 0.71, $p = 0.11$) were noted in LPD, suggesting a trend towards accelerated recovery. Higher 30-day mortality was still noted in LPD performed by lower volume centers (<20 LPDs, 5.6% vs. 0%, $p < 0.01$), however no significant differences of 30-day and 90-day mortality in high volume centers (≥20 LPDs) between LPD and OPD (0% vs. 1.3%, $p = 0.08$, and 0.6% vs. 3.4% $p = 0.08$, respectively). Chapman et al. (study period: 2010–2013) [86] evaluated the safety of LPD in elderly patients (≥75 years old, 1768 patients). Although it was found that more than 60% of the patients with LPD was performed in low volume centers (<5 LPDs), no significant differences were found in R0-status, number of lymph nodes examined, lymph node, status, receipt of adjuvant chemotherapy, days to initiation of adjuvant chemotherapy, readmission rates, or 30-day mortality between two groups ($p > 0.05$). Ninety-day mortality was significantly lower in LP (7.2 vs. 12.2%, $p = 0.049$). It was observed that there was a trend towards improved OS (HR = 0.85, $p > 0.05$) in the LPD group compared to the OPD group after adjusting for patient and tumor-related characteristics. Lastly, Torphy et al. (study period: 2010–2015) [87] also compared short-term and oncologic outcome of minimally invasive PD (MIPD) with those of OPD across low and high-volume centers. Among the patients with pancreatic cancer who underwent PD, 3754 patients (17.1%) were found to be performed minimally invasively. It was found that patients with MIPD for pancreatic cancer were less likely to stay in the hospital (OR, 0.75; 95% CI, 0.68–0.82). Thirty-day mortality, 90-day mortality, unplanned readmissions, margins, lymph nodes harvested, and receipt of adjuvant chemotherapy were equivalent between two groups.

Table 6 shows the recent significant articles comparing LPD and OPD in treating pancreatic cancer. When looking at the individual data, they are all pointing out that LPD can provide equivalent or superior short-term oncologic outcomes with comparable long-term survival outcome, suggesting that LPD is technically feasible and even oncologically safe in treating pancreatic cancer. It is interesting to note that every reported article demonstrates a smaller amount of intraoperative blood loss comparing with OPD. This observation is very important to improve the long-term oncologic outcomes of resected pancreatic cancer, because a lower volume of intraoperative estimated blood loss can lead to a lower chance of unnecessary intraoperative blood transfusion. Potential deleterious effects of blood transfusion on oncologic outcomes have been explained by several hypothesized mechanisms, primarily via the induction of immunosuppression [88,89]. In several studies, intraoperative transfusion was found to be one of the independent prognostic factors in resected pancreatic cancer [90–92]. In addition, a recent meta-analysis [35] to evaluate potential relationship between perioperative blood transfusion and prognosis of pancreatic cancer surgery also demonstrated detrimental effect of blood transfusion on survival in univariate (68.4%, 13 out of 19 studies) and multivariate analysis (47.4%, 9 out of 19 studies) respectively, showing overall blood transfusion associated with pancreatic cancer surgery can be related to shorter overall survival (pooled odds ratio 2.43, 95% confidence interval 1.90–3.10). Considering poor long-term oncologic outcomes of pancreatic cancer, intraoperative transfusion must be an attractive issue for pancreatic surgeons, because it is thought to be a surgeon-controllable factor by reducing intraoperative blood loss. In the near future, appropriate transfusion guidelines including strict transfusion threshold and active investigation on alternative to allogenic blood transfusion are necessary in managing pancreatic cancer patients.

Table 6. Summarized recent articles investigating oncologic outcomes comparing between LPD and open pancreaticoduodenectomy (OPD) for pancreatic cancer.

Author, Years	Approach	N	Age	Gender (Male)	Op-Time	EBL	TF	Retrieved LNs	R0	Cx. (≥Clavien IIIB)	POPF	DGE	Mx.	LOH	Adjuvant CTx	Time to Adjuvant CTx	Survival	Anastomosis Technique
Croome, 2014 [19]	OPD	214	65.4	131	387.6	866.7	71	20.1	17	29	Grade B/C: 29(13.6)	Grade B/C: 26 (12)	4	9	164	59	25.3	
	LPD	108	66.6	51*	379.4	492.4*	21*	21.4	84	6	6(5.6)	39(18)	1	6*	82	48*	21.8	Robot: 5, open: 7, lapa: 96. No detail description
Conard, 2017 [92]	OPD	25	66	18	NA	NA	10	17	21	III(A+B):11 IV:4 V:2	Yes: 10 No: 15	NA		27	11	NA	29.6	
	LPD	40	68	26	NA	NA	14	18	35	III(A+B):12 IV:10 V:2	Yes: 12 No: 28	NA		24.5	14	NA	35.5	ALL Laparoscopic reconstruction, E-to-S DTM internal stent PJ
Stauffer, 2017 [93]	OPD	193	68.9	96	375	600	90	17	154	58	Total:20 A:6 B:9 C:5	Total:28 A:12 B:6 C:10	10	9	122	55	20.3	
	LPD	58	69.9	32	518*	250*	20*	27*	49	13	Total:6 A:2 B:4 C:0	Total:10 A:4 B:3 C:3	2	6	41	54	18.5	Open conversion: 14, Lapa: 44, Two-layer DTM PJ
Kuesters, 2018 [94]	OPD	278	68	137	428	NA	65	16	195	107	NA	NA	6	16	NA	NA	18	
	LPD	62	71	31	477*	NA	9	17	54*	25	NA	NA	3	14*	NA	NA	22	All Open reconstruction No detail description
Choi, 2020 [21]	OPD	34	63.3	18	471.2	448.8	2	20.6	24	NA	None:24 BL:6 B:3 C:1	None:30 A:2 B:2 C:0		19.9	27	55.1	44.6	
	LPD	27	63.3	12	477.7	232.5*	0	13.3	25	NA	None:17 BL:8 B:1 C:1	None:23 A:3 B:0 C:1		21.1	21	59.5	45.2	All Laparoscopic reconstruction, E-to-S DTM internal stent PJ
Zhou, 2019 [95]	OPD	93	64	68	260	200	7	11	88	13	Total:86 BL:74 B/C:12	Total:66 A:27 B/C:39	2	14	47	43.5	20	
	LPD	55	63	40	330*	150*	16*	18*	55	6	Total:20 BL:13 B/C:7	Total:1 A:0 B/C:1	0	13	26	39	18.7	All laparoscopic reconstruction, E-to-S DTM internal stent PJ

* $p < 0.05$, TF; transfusion; LNs; lymph nodes, POPF; postoperative pancreatic fistula, DGE; delayed gastric emptying, CD; Clavien-Dindo Classification, CTx; chemotherapy, DTM; duct-to-mucosa anastomosis, PJ; pancreaticojejunostomy.

However, all these articles showing comparable oncologic outcomes between LPD and OPD are based on retrospective studies, where unavoidable selection bias should be always concerned. Therefore, the advantages of laparoscopic PD on short-term surgical outcomes and comparable long-term survival rates should be regarded with careful interpretation.

However, unfortunately there is no randomized control trial (RCT) comparing LPD and OPD for pancreatic cancer. All conclusions were based on retrospective observational studies. Therefore, the interpretation of above these articles should be careful because there are unavoidable limitations, such as small sample size, selection bias, learning-curve issue, and heterogeneity in reported data.

Which approach, laparoscopic vs. open, is better regarding surgical approach to pancreatic cancer? An RCT is still needed to actually elucidate the true oncologic value of LPD, and to suggest standard care in treating pancreatic cancer. However, an RCT regarding this issue is not that easy to conduct because most pancreatic cancers are found to be at an advanced stage at diagnosis, and the surgical technique of LPD is not fully matured in the present surgical society. In fact, three RCTs comparing LPD and OPD were reported [13–15], but their study population included not only pancreatic cancer but also other periampullary cancer, benign and low-grade malignant tumors of the pancreas. Overall, they demonstrated no statistical differences, except less blood loss in LPD, and shorter operative time in OPD.

However, when looking at the last study recently performed by Hilst et al. [15], nine surgeons who had experienced more than 20 cases of LPD or OPD were involved. This clinical trial was prematurely terminated due to safety concerns of LPD. This phenomenon is thought to be a part of reflection to previous NCDB-based studies showing LPDs done in low volume centers were associated with higher mortality rate [84,85]. Taking the tumor biology of pancreatic cancer and its clinical presentations into consideration, associated pancreatitis, cholangitis, and potential risk of vascular involvements usually make laparoscopic oncologic dissection much more difficult and even dangerous. Therefore, LPD for treating pancreatic cancer should be a more challenging issue. All recent studies agree with the fact that many cases are required to overcome the learning curve for safe LPDs [16,17]. Therefore, under reasonable inclusion criteria, it is highly demanded that expert surgeons with good experience in both LPD and OPD should collaborate for a well-designed RCT to answer this question (ClinicalTrials.gov Identifier: NCT03870698). For a while, the currently accumulated expert surgeons' experiences might be regarded as the highest level of evidence that we can take in current clinical situation of pancreatic cancer.

4. Proposal Potential Indications

Previously, we suggested a model for determining the indications of minimally invasive radical distal pancreatectomy for left-sided pancreatic cancer [7]. A similar approach will be possible in LPD for pancreatic cancer. Technical feasibility, procedural safety (or surgical risk), and surgical extent for margin-negative resection (oncologic clearance) should be considered in defining potential indication of LPD. A surgeon's capacity of technical feasibility should cover the surgical extent requiring for curative resection. Figure 4 shows the dynamic relationships between these factors.

As the surgical extent for curative resection increases, the following will happen: First, the potential surgical risk may increase. Second, advanced surgical technique is highly required to ensure surgical extent for obtaining margin-negative resection. However, at some point, an appropriate surgical procedure for curative resection cannot be maintained by the laparoscopic approach due to surgeons' own technical issues and patients' co-morbidities. Therefore, there must be an optimum surgical extent that can be obtained by individual surgeons' own surgical techniques for margin-negative resection.

From that point of view, three types of surgical extent of LPD can be available. *Type 0* LPD is PD with standard dissection. It does not require any type of combined vascular resection. *Type I* LPD requires combined venous vascular resection. In this surgical extent, most cases need tangential (wedge) resection of PV, or SMV with primary repair (*Type Ia* LPD). *Type Ib* LPD requires more complicated procedures for margin-negative resection, such as tangential resection with patch repair, segmental resection with end-to-end anastomosis or reconstruction using artificial graft (venous resection 2). In selected cases, combined arterial resection (*Type II* LPD) will be required, but quite limited [93].

For example, (A) surgeons' technique for LPD is not enough to achieve curative resection in resectable pancreatic cancer. This group of surgeons need to do open PD for curative resection of the pancreatic cancer. However, (B) surgeons' technique for LPD is good enough for obtaining margin-negative radical resection. They may perform LPD in well-selected cases expecting no combined vascular resection (Type 0 LPD). Only a few surgeons can perform LPD even with combined venous vascular resection (tangential or segmental) or even combined arterial resection in well-selected patients (Type I and II LPD). Therefore, considering the present technical feasibility to maintain patient's safety, and margin-negative curative pancreatectomy, tumor conditions that could be removed by standard PD without combined vascular resection (Type 0 LPD) will be the primary indication for LPD. Others (Type I and II) can be performed in selected cases by only expert surgeons.

When looking at the anatomic relationship between pancreatic cancer and major vascular structures at diagnostic stage, anatomically *"resectable"* pancreatic cancer includes potential candidates who can undergo LPD for curative intent in clinical practice [94]. However, unexpected involvement of adjacent venous systems, such as superior mesenteric vein (SMV), or portal vein (PV) because of severe pancreatitis or tumor invasion, can be encountered during LPD for resectable pancreatic cancers, and this situation might be necessary for combined vascular resection. Only expert surgeons are responsible for this advanced stage of the pancreatic cancer. These cases mostly will result in elective conversion to open for procedural safety and curative resection [95].

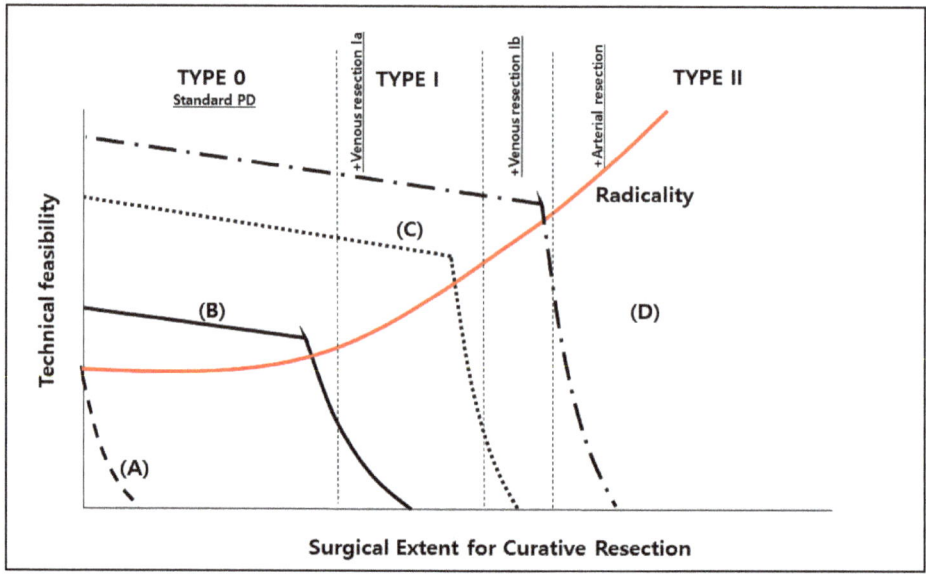

Figure 4. Model for determining surgical indication of LPD for pancreatic cancer. Regardless of laparoscopic or open PD for pancreatic cancer, surgical approach should be allowed only when surgeons' technical feasibility can obtain the appropriate surgical extent for margin-negative resection. Therefore, indication of LPD can vary according to surgeons' techniques and disease extent. OPD will be recommended in surgeon (**A**). Type 0 LPD can be done in surgeon (**B**). Type Ia LPD and Type Ib LPD can be allowed for surgeon (**C**) and surgeon (**D**), respectively. Anatomically *resectable* pancreatic cancer with intact fat plane between pancreas and major vascular structures is thought to be the ideal tumor conditions for LPD (Tumor conditions controlled by Type 0 LPD). Note: This author follows Fortner's initial classification of regional pancreatectomy [96].

Therefore, in the beginning stage, it is thought that only a small proportion of resectable pancreatic cancer without contact with the SMV-PV complex could be a potential indication for LPD (Type 0 LPD) for generalizing concept of LPD for pancreatic cancer (Figure 5). However, in the near future, with the advance of a diagnostic strategy for early detection and surgical techniques, potential candidates for LPD are certain to increase

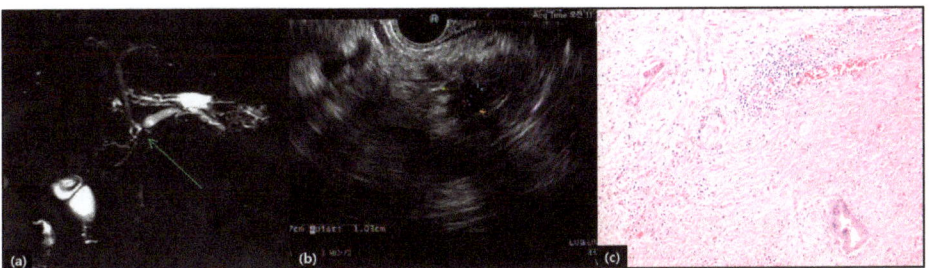

Figure 5. A case with extremely appropriate pancreatic cancer for LPD. A case of early pancreatic cancer in a 71-year-old, male patient, incidental finding of pancreatic duct dilatation during routine medical check-up. Preoperative image studies showed less than 1 cm sized pancreatic mass with secondary pancreatic duct dilatation (**a**,**b**). Type 0 LPD was performed on 24 October 2019, and discharged 9 days postoperatively. Pathological examination reported 3.0 mm-sized pancreatic ductal adenocarcinoma with good differentiation (×100, **c**). resected margins were free from malignant cells (safety margin ≥ 1 cm). No lymph node metastasis was noted among 23 retrieved lymph nodes.

5. Conclusions

It is worthy to emphasize that margin-negative radical pancreatectomy is the essential condition to obtain long-term survival of patients with pancreatic cancer. With the investigation for early diagnosis, introduction of potent chemotherapeutic agents, application of neoadjuvant chemotherapy, advancement of open and laparoscopic surgical techniques, mature perioperative management, and improved patients' general conditions, survival of resected pancreatic cancer is expected to be further improved. OPD will still be mainstream in treating resectable pancreatic cancer. Particularly, OPD with anatomy-driven extended dissection will play significant role in treating advanced pancreatic cancer following neoadjuvant chemotherapy, which harbors the potential risk of combined major venous or arterial resection.

On the other hand, the technical and oncological feasibility of LPD for pancreatic cancer is still controversial. Considering difficult clinical circumstances to perform RCT, the currently reported experiences are thought to be the highest level of evidence that we can consider in managing pancreatic cancer. According to the literature, it can be carefully concluded that LPD is thought to be a good alternative strategy in managing well-selected resectable pancreatic cancer. LPD with combined vascular resection is also feasible, but only expert surgeons should handle these challenging cases.

In spite of potential advantages of the laparoscopic approach, it provides surgeons with fundamental limitations during surgical procedures, such as 2-D operative view, fulcrum-effect, limited motion of the instruments, attenuated touch sensation, and enhancing tremor. Theoretically, the robotic surgical system was introduced to overcome these hurdles. However, it is also true that many laparoscopic surgeons had already overcome these limitations. Therefore, surgical approach should be determined according to the surgeon's expertise, patients' general condition, and tumor biology. As long as surgical principles for pancreatic cancer are kept in mind, open, laparoscopic or robotic approach to PD for pancreatic cancer are expected to provide meaningful short- and long-term oncologic outcomes of resected pancreatic cancer.

Finally, in application of minimally invasive pancreatectomy for pancreatic cancer, patients' safety and principles of surgical oncology should be kept in mind [97]. In fact, these two principles should be considered not only in LPD but also in OPD. Whether PD is performed by laparoscopic or open approach, surgical approach should be determined by a surgeon's own technical expertise to fulfil these two goals.

Funding: This research was funded by a Faculty Research Grant of Yonsei University College of Medicine for 6-2015-0053.

Conflicts of Interest: The authors declare no conflict of interest.

References

1. Stocken, D.D.; Büchler, M.W.; Dervenis, C.; Bassi, C.; Jeekel, H.; Klinkenbijl, J.H.; Bakkevold, K.E.; Takada, T.; Amano, H.; Neoptolemos, J.P. Meta-analysis of randomised adjuvant therapy trials for pancreatic cancer. *Br. J. Cancer* **2005**, *92*, 1372–1381. [CrossRef] [PubMed]
2. Parmar, A.; Chaves-Porras, J.; Saluja, R.; Perry, K.; Rahmadian, A.P.; Santos, S.D.; Ko, Y.J.; Berry, S.; Doherty, M.; Chan, K.K.W. Adjuvant treatment for resected pancreatic adenocarcinoma: A systematic review and network meta-analysis. *Crit. Rev. Oncol. Hematol.* **2020**, *145*, 102817. [CrossRef] [PubMed]
3. Rahib, L.; Smith, B.D.; Aizenberg, R.; Rosenzweig, A.B.; Fleshman, J.M.; Matrisian, L.M. Projecting Cancer Incidence and Deaths to 2030: The Unexpected Burden of Thyroid, Liver, and Pancreas Cancers in the United States. *Cancer Res.* **2014**, *74*, 2913. [CrossRef] [PubMed]
4. Kang, C.M.; Lee, S.H.; Chung, M.J.; Hwang, H.K.; Lee, W.J. Laparoscopic pancreatic reconstruction technique following laparoscopic pancreaticoduodenectomy. *J. Hepatobiliary Pancreat. Sci* **2015**, *22*, 202–210. [CrossRef]
5. De Rooij, T.; van Hilst, J.; van Santvoort, H.; Boerma, D.; van den Boezem, P.; Daams, F.; van Dam, R.; Dejong, C.; van Duyn, E.; Dijkgraaf, M.; et al. Minimally Invasive Versus Open Distal Pancreatectomy (LEOPARD): A Multicenter Patient-blinded Randomized Controlled Trial. *Ann. Surg.* **2019**, *269*, 2–9. [CrossRef]
6. Zhang, H.; Lan, X.; Peng, B.; Li, B. Is total laparoscopic pancreaticoduodenectomy superior to open procedure? A meta-analysis. *World J. Gastroenterol.* **2019**, *25*, 5711–5731. [CrossRef]
7. Kang, C.M.; Lee, S.H.; Lee, W.J. Minimally invasive radical pancreatectomy for left-sided pancreatic cancer: Current status and future perspectives. *World J. Gastroenterol.* **2014**, *20*, 2343–2351. [CrossRef]
8. Lee, S.H.; Hwang, H.K.; Kang, C.M.; Lee, W.J. The Yonsei criteria as a clinically detectable parameter for excellent prognosis in resected left-sided pancreatic cancer: Outcomes of a propensity score-matched analysis. *Surg. Endosc.* **2017**, *31*, 4656–4664. [CrossRef]
9. Hong, S.S.; Hwang, H.K.; Lee, W.J.; Kang, C.M. Feasibility and Safety of Laparoscopic Radical Distal Pancreatosplenectomy with Adrenalectomy in Advanced Pancreatic Cancer. *Ann. Surg. Oncol.* **2020**. [CrossRef]
10. Van Hilst, J.; Korrel, M.; de Rooij, T.; Lof, S.; Busch, O.R.; Groot Koerkamp, B.; Kooby, D.A.; van Dieren, S.; Abu Hilal, M.; Besselink, M.G. Oncologic outcomes of minimally invasive versus open distal pancreatectomy for pancreatic ductal adenocarcinoma: A systematic review and meta-analysis. *Eur. J. Surg. Oncol.* **2019**, *45*, 719–727. [CrossRef]
11. Van Hilst, J.; de Rooij, T.; Klompmaker, S.; Rawashdeh, M.; Aleotti, F.; Al-Sarireh, B.; Alseidi, A.; Ateeb, Z.; Balzano, G.; Berrevoet, F.; et al. Minimally Invasive versus Open Distal Pancreatectomy for Ductal Adenocarcinoma (DIPLOMA): A Pan-European Propensity Score Matched Study. *Ann. Surg.* **2019**, *269*, 10–17. [CrossRef] [PubMed]
12. Nickel, F.; Haney, C.M.; Kowalewski, K.F.; Probst, P.; Limen, E.F.; Kalkum, E.; Diener, M.K.; Strobel, O.; Müller-Stich, B.P.; Hackert, T. Laparoscopic Versus Open Pancreaticoduodenectomy: A Systematic Review and Meta-analysis of Randomized Controlled Trials. *Ann. Surg.* **2020**, *271*, 54–66. [CrossRef] [PubMed]
13. Palanivelu, C.; Senthilnathan, P.; Sabnis, S.C.; Babu, N.S.; Srivatsan Gurumurthy, S.; Anand Vijai, N.; Nalankilli, V.P.; Praveen Raj, P.; Parthasarathy, R.; Rajapandian, S. Randomized clinical trial of laparoscopic versus open pancreatoduodenectomy for periampullary tumours. *Br. J. Surg.* **2017**, *104*, 1443–1450. [CrossRef] [PubMed]
14. Poves, I.; Burdío, F.; Morató, O.; Iglesias, M.; Radosevic, A.; Ilzarbe, L.; Visa, L.; Grande, L. Comparison of Perioperative Outcomes Between Laparoscopic and Open Approach for Pancreatoduodenectomy: The PADULAP Randomized Controlled Trial. *Ann. Surg.* **2018**, *268*, 731–739. [CrossRef]

15. Van Hilst, J.; de Rooij, T.; Bosscha, K.; Brinkman, D.J.; van Dieren, S.; Dijkgraaf, M.G.; Gerhards, M.F.; de Hingh, I.H.; Karsten, T.M.; Lips, D.J.; et al. Laparoscopic versus open pancreatoduodenectomy for pancreatic or periampullary tumours (LEOPARD-2): A multicentre, patient-blinded, randomised controlled phase 2/3 trial. *Lancet Gastroenterol. Hepatol.* **2019**, *4*, 199–207. [CrossRef]
16. Song, K.B.; Kim, S.C.; Lee, W.; Hwang, D.W.; Lee, J.H.; Kwon, J.; Park, Y.; Lee, S.J.; Park, G. Laparoscopic pancreaticoduodenectomy for periampullary tumors: Lessons learned from 500 consecutive patients in a single center. *Surg Endosc.* **2020**, *34*, 1343–1352. [CrossRef]
17. Choi, M.; Hwang, H.K.; Lee, W.J.; Kang, C.M. Total laparoscopic pancreaticoduodenectomy in patients with periampullary tumors: A learning curve analysis. *Surg. Endosc.* **2020**. [CrossRef]
18. Wang, M.; Peng, B.; Liu, J.; Yin, X.; Tan, Z.; Liu, R.; Hong, D.; Zhao, W.; Wu, H.; Chen, R.; et al. Practice Patterns and Perioperative Outcomes of Laparoscopic Pancreaticoduodenectomy in China: A Retrospective Multicenter Analysis of 1029 Patients. *Ann. Surg.* **2019**. [CrossRef]
19. Croome, K.P.; Farnell, M.B.; Que, F.G.; Reid-Lombardo, K.M.; Truty, M.J.; Nagorney, D.M.; Kendrick, M.L. Pancreaticoduodenectomy with major vascular resection: A comparison of laparoscopic versus open approaches. *J. Gastrointest. Surg.* **2015**, *19*, 189–194. [CrossRef]
20. Kuesters, S.; Chikhladze, S.; Makowiec, F.; Sick, O.; Fichtner-Feigl, S.; Hopt, U.T.; Wittel, U.A. Oncological outcome of laparoscopically assisted pancreatoduodenectomy for ductal adenocarcinoma in a retrospective cohort study. *Int. J. Surg.* **2018**, *55*, 162–166. [CrossRef]
21. Choi, M.; Hwang, H.K.; Rho, S.Y.; Lee, W.J.; Kang, C.M. Comparing laparoscopic and open pancreaticoduodenectomy in patients with pancreatic head cancer: Oncologic outcomes and inflammatory scores. *J. Hepato-Biliary Pancreat. Sci.* **2020**, *27*, 124–131. [CrossRef] [PubMed]
22. National Comprehensive Cancer, N. NCCN Clinical Practice Guidelines in Oncology (NCCN Guidelines®). Pancreatic Adenocarcinoma. Version 1. 2020. Available online: https://www.nccn.org/professionals/physician_gls/pdf/pancreatic.pdf (accessed on 12 June 2020).
23. Gumbs, A.A.; Rodriguez Rivera, A.M.; Milone, L.; Hoffman, J.P. Laparoscopic pancreatoduodenectomy: A review of 285 published cases. *Ann. Surg. Oncol.* **2011**, *18*, 1335–1341. [CrossRef] [PubMed]
24. Venkat, R.; Edil, B.H.; Schulick, R.D.; Lidor, A.O.; Makary, M.A.; Wolfgang, C.L. Laparoscopic distal pancreatectomy is associated with significantly less overall morbidity compared to the open technique: A systematic review and meta-analysis. *Ann. Surg.* **2012**, *255*, 1048–1059. [CrossRef] [PubMed]
25. Morales-Oyarvide, V.; Rubinson, D.A.; Dunne, R.F.; Kozak, M.M.; Bui, J.L.; Yuan, C.; Qian, Z.R.; Babic, A.; Da Silva, A.; Nowak, J.A.; et al. Lymph node metastases in resected pancreatic ductal adenocarcinoma: Predictors of disease recurrence and survival. *Br. J. Cancer* **2017**, *117*, 1874–1882. [CrossRef]
26. Takao, S.; Shinchi, H.; Maemura, K.; Kurahara, H.; Natsugoe, S.; Aikou, T. Survival benefit of pancreaticoduodenectomy in a Japanese fashion for a limited group of patients with pancreatic head cancer. *Hepato-Gastroenterology* **2008**, *55*, 1789–1795.
27. Iacono, C.; Accordini, S.; Bortolasi, L.; Facci, E.; Zamboni, G.; Montresor, E.; Marinello, P.D.; Serio, G. Results of pancreaticoduodenectomy for pancreatic cancer: Extended versus standard procedure. *World J. Surg.* **2002**, *26*, 1309–1314. [CrossRef]
28. Yang, Y.M.; Wan, Y.L.; Tian, X.D.; Zhuang, Y.; Huang, Y.T. Outcome of pancreaticoduodenectomy with extended retroperitoneal lymphadenectomy for adenocarcinoma of the head of the pancreas. *Chin. Med. J.* **2005**, *118*, 1863–1869.
29. Orci, L.A.; Meyer, J.; Combescure, C.; Bühler, L.; Berney, T.; Morel, P.; Toso, C. A meta-analysis of extended versus standard lymphadenectomy in patients undergoing pancreatoduodenectomy for pancreatic adenocarcinoma. *HPB* **2015**, *17*, 565–572. [CrossRef]
30. Pedrazzoli, S.; DiCarlo, V.; Dionigi, R.; Mosca, F.; Pederzoli, P.; Pasquali, C.; Klöppel, G.; Dhaene, K.; Michelassi, F. Standard versus extended lymphadenectomy associated with pancreatoduodenectomy in the surgical treatment of adenocarcinoma of the head of the pancreas: A multicenter, prospective, randomized study. Lymphadenectomy Study Group. *Ann. Surg.* **1998**, *228*, 508–517. [CrossRef]
31. Yeo, C.J.; Cameron, J.L.; Sohn, T.A.; Coleman, J.; Sauter, P.K.; Hruban, R.H.; Pitt, H.A.; Lillemoe, K.D. Pancreaticoduodenectomy with or without extended retroperitoneal lymphadenectomy for periampullary adenocarcinoma: Comparison of morbidity and mortality and short-term outcome. *Ann. Surg.* **1999**, *229*, 613–622. [CrossRef]

32. Farnell, M.B.; Pearson, R.K.; Sarr, M.G.; DiMagno, E.P.; Burgart, L.J.; Dahl, T.R.; Foster, N.; Sargent, D.J. A prospective randomized trial comparing standard pancreatoduodenectomy with pancreatoduodenectomy with extended lymphadenectomy in resectable pancreatic head adenocarcinoma. *Surgery* **2005**, *138*, 618–628. [CrossRef] [PubMed]
33. Nimura, Y.; Nagino, M.; Takao, S.; Takada, T.; Miyazaki, K.; Kawarada, Y.; Miyagawa, S.; Yamaguchi, A.; Ishiyama, S.; Takeda, Y.; et al. Standard versus extended lymphadenectomy in radical pancreatoduodenectomy for ductal adenocarcinoma of the head of the pancreas: Long-term results of a Japanese multicenter randomized controlled trial. *J. Hepatobiliary Pancreat. Sci.* **2012**, *19*, 230–241. [CrossRef] [PubMed]
34. Jang, J.Y.; Kang, M.J.; Heo, J.S.; Choi, S.H.; Choi, D.W.; Park, S.J.; Han, S.S.; Yoon, D.S.; Yu, H.C.; Kang, K.J.; et al. A prospective randomized controlled study comparing outcomes of standard resection and extended resection, including dissection of the nerve plexus and various lymph nodes, in patients with pancreatic head cancer. *Ann. Surg.* **2014**, *259*, 656–664. [CrossRef] [PubMed]
35. Mavros, M.N.; Xu, L.; Maqsood, H.; Gani, F.; Ejaz, A.; Spolverato, G.; Al-Refaie, W.B.; Frank, S.M.; Pawlik, T.M. Perioperative Blood Transfusion and the Prognosis of Pancreatic Cancer Surgery: Systematic Review and Meta-analysis. *Ann. Surg. Oncol.* **2015**, *22*, 4382–4391. [CrossRef] [PubMed]
36. Kang, C.M.; Kim, D.H.; Choi, G.H.; Kim, K.S.; Choi, J.S.; Lee, W.J. Detrimental effect of postoperative complications on oncologic efficacy of R0 pancreatectomy in ductal adenocarcinoma of the pancreas. *J. Gastrointest. Surg.* **2009**, *13*, 907–914. [CrossRef] [PubMed]
37. Kasahara, N.; Noda, H.; Kakizawa, N.; Kato, T.; Watanabe, F.; Ichida, K.; Endo, Y.; Aizawa, H.; Rikiyama, T. A lack of postoperative complications after pancreatectomy contributes to the long-term survival of patients with pancreatic cancer. *Pancreatology* **2019**, *19*, 686–694. [CrossRef] [PubMed]
38. La Torre, M.; Nigri, G.; Petrucciani, N.; Cavallini, M.; Aurello, P.; Cosenza, G.; Balducci, G.; Ziparo, V.; Ramacciato, G. Prognostic assessment of different lymph node staging methods for pancreatic cancer with R0 resection: pN staging, lymph node ratio, log odds of positive lymph nodes. *Pancreatology* **2014**, *14*, 289–294. [CrossRef]
39. Strobel, O.; Hinz, U.; Gluth, A.; Hank, T.; Hackert, T.; Bergmann, F.; Werner, J.; Büchler, M.W. Pancreatic adenocarcinoma: Number of positive nodes allows to distinguish several N categories. *Ann. Surg.* **2015**, *261*, 961–969. [CrossRef]
40. Elshaer, M.; Gravante, G.; Kosmin, M.; Riaz, A.; Al-Bahrani, A. A systematic review of the prognostic value of lymph node ratio, number of positive nodes and total nodes examined in pancreatic ductal adenocarcinoma. *Ann. R. Coll. Surg. Engl.* **2017**, *99*, 101–106. [CrossRef]
41. Rau, B.M.; Moritz, K.; Schuschan, S.; Alsfasser, G.; Prall, F.; Klar, E. R1 resection in pancreatic cancer has significant impact on long-term outcome in standardized pathology modified for routine use. *Surgery* **2012**, *152*, S103–S111. [CrossRef]
42. Yi, S.Q.; Miwa, K.; Ohta, T.; Kayahara, M.; Kitagawa, H.; Tanaka, A.; Shimokawa, T.; Akita, K.; Tanaka, S. Innervation of the pancreas from the perspective of perineural invasion of pancreatic cancer. *Pancreas* **2003**, *27*, 225–229. [CrossRef] [PubMed]
43. Jin, G.; Sugiyama, M.; Tuo, H.; Oki, A.; Abe, N.; Mori, T.; Masaki, T.; Fujioka, Y.; Atomi, Y. Distribution of lymphatic vessels in the neural plexuses surrounding the superior mesenteric artery. *Pancreas* **2006**, *32*, 62–66. [CrossRef] [PubMed]
44. Makino, I.; Kitagawa, H.; Ohta, T.; Nakagawara, H.; Tajima, H.; Ohnishi, I.; Takamura, H.; Tani, T.; Kayahara, M. Nerve plexus invasion in pancreatic cancer: Spread patterns on histopathologic and embryological analyses. *Pancreas* **2008**, *37*, 358–365. [CrossRef] [PubMed]
45. Westgaard, A.; Tafjord, S.; Farstad, I.N.; Cvancarova, M.; Eide, T.J.; Mathisen, O.; Clausen, O.P.; Gladhaug, I.P. Resectable adenocarcinomas in the pancreatic head: The retroperitoneal resection margin is an independent prognostic factor. *BMC Cancer* **2008**, *8*, 5. [CrossRef] [PubMed]
46. Lüttges, J.; Vogel, I.; Menke, M.; Henne-Bruns, D.; Kremer, B.; Klöppel, G. The retroperitoneal resection margin and vessel involvement are important factors determining survival after pancreaticoduodenectomy for ductal adenocarcinoma of the head of the pancreas. *Virchows Arch.* **1998**, *433*, 237–242. [CrossRef]

47. Butler, J.R.; Ahmad, S.A.; Katz, M.H.; Cioffi, J.L.; Zyromski, N.J. A systematic review of the role of periadventitial dissection of the superior mesenteric artery in affecting margin status after pancreatoduodenectomy for pancreatic adenocarcinoma. *HPB* **2016**, *18*, 305–311. [CrossRef]
48. Rho, S.Y.; Kim, J.S.; Chong, J.U.; Hwang, H.K.; Yoon, D.S.; Lee, W.J.; Kang, C.M. Indocyanine Green Perfusion Imaging-Guided Laparoscopic Pancreaticoduodenectomy: Potential Application in Retroperitoneal Margin Dissection. *J. Gastrointest. Surg.* **2018**, *22*, 1470–1474. [CrossRef]
49. Nagakawa, Y.; Hosokawa, Y.; Sahara, Y.; Takishita, C.; Hijikata, Y.; Osakabe, H.; Nakajima, T.; Shirota, T.; Katsumata, K.; Nakamura, M.; et al. Approaching the superior mesenteric artery from the right side using the proximal-dorsal jejunal vein preisolation method during laparoscopic pancreaticoduodenectomy. *Surg. Endosc.* **2018**, *32*, 4044–4051. [CrossRef]
50. Morales, E.; Zimmitti, G.; Codignola, C.; Manzoni, A.; Garatti, M.; Sega, V.; Rosso, E. Follow "the superior mesenteric artery": Laparoscopic approach for total mesopancreas excision during pancreaticoduodenectomy. *Surg. Endosc.* **2019**, *33*, 4186–4191. [CrossRef]
51. Zimmitti, G.; Manzoni, A.; Addeo, P.; Garatti, M.; Zaniboni, A.; Bachellier, P.; Rosso, E. Laparoscopic pancreatoduodenectomy with superior mesenteric artery-first approach and pancreatogastrostomy assisted by mini-laparotomy. *Surg. Endosc.* **2016**, *30*, 1670–1671. [CrossRef]
52. Kuroki, T.; Tajima, Y.; Kitasato, A.; Adachi, T.; Kanematsu, T. Pancreas-hanging maneuver in laparoscopic pancreaticoduodenectomy: A new technique for the safe resection of the pancreas head. *Surg. Endosc.* **2010**, *24*, 1781–1783. [CrossRef] [PubMed]
53. Nakagohri, T.; Kinoshita, T.; Konishi, M.; Inoue, K.; Takahashi, S. Survival benefits of portal vein resection for pancreatic cancer. *Am. J. Surg.* **2003**, *186*, 149–153. [CrossRef]
54. Shibata, C.; Kobari, M.; Tsuchiya, T.; Arai, K.; Anzai, R.; Takahashi, M.; Uzuki, M.; Sawai, T.; Yamazaki, T. Pancreatectomy combined with superior mesenteric-portal vein resection for adenocarcinoma in pancreas. *World J. Surg.* **2001**, *25*, 1002–1005. [CrossRef] [PubMed]
55. Fuhrman, G.M.; Leach, S.D.; Staley, C.A.; Cusack, J.C.; Charnsangavej, C.; Cleary, K.R.; El-Naggar, A.K.; Fenoglio, C.J.; Lee, J.E.; Evans, D.B. Rationale for en bloc vein resection in the treatment of pancreatic adenocarcinoma adherent to the superior mesenteric-portal vein confluence. Pancreatic Tumor Study Group. *Ann. Surg.* **1996**, *223*, 154–162. [CrossRef] [PubMed]
56. Leach, S.D.; Lee, J.E.; Charnsangavej, C.; Cleary, K.R.; Lowy, A.M.; Fenoglio, C.J.; Pisters, P.W.; Evans, D.B. Survival following pancreaticoduodenectomy with resection of the superior mesenteric-portal vein confluence for adenocarcinoma of the pancreatic head. *Br. J. Surg.* **1998**, *85*, 611–617. [CrossRef] [PubMed]
57. Peng, C.; Zhou, D.; Meng, L.; Cao, Y.; Zhang, H.; Pan, Z.; Lin, C. The value of combined vein resection in pancreaticoduodenectomy for pancreatic head carcinoma: A meta-analysis. *BMC Surg.* **2019**, *19*, 84. [CrossRef]
58. Park, H.; Kang, I.; Kang, C.M. Laparoscopic pancreaticoduodenectomy with segmental resection of superior mesenteric vein-splenic vein-portal vein confluence in pancreatic head cancer: Can it be a standard procedure? *Ann. Hepatobiliary Pancreat. Surg.* **2018**, *22*, 419–424. [CrossRef]
59. Awad, Z.T. Totally laparoscopic pancreaticoduodenectomy for pancreatic head cancer with involvement of the superior mesenteric vein-portal vein confluence. *Ann. Surg. Oncol.* **2014**, *21*, 3439. [CrossRef]
60. Garbarino, G.M.; Fuks, D.; Cowan, J.; Ward, M.; Moisan, F.; Donatelli, G.; Beaussier, M.; Gayet, B. Total Laparoscopic Pancreaticoduodenectomy with Venous Reconstruction for Pancreatic Head Cancer with Involvement of the Superior Mesenteric Vein-Portal Vein Confluence. *Ann. Surg. Oncol.* **2018**, *25*, 4035–4036. [CrossRef]
61. Palanisamy, S.; Deuri, B.; Naidu, S.B.; Vaiyapurigoundar Palanisamy, N.; Natesan, A.V.; Palanivelu, P.R.; Parthasarathy, R.; Palanivelu, C. Major venous resection and reconstruction using a minimally invasive approach during laparoscopic pancreaticoduodenectomy: One step forward. *Asian J. Endosc. Surg.* **2015**, *8*, 468–472. [CrossRef]
62. Rosso, E.; Zimmitti, G.; Iannelli, A.; Garatti, M. The 'TRIANGLE Operation' by Laparoscopy: Radical Pancreaticoduodenectomy with Major Vascular Resection for Borderline Resectable Pancreatic Head Cancer. *Ann. Surg. Oncol.* **2019**. [CrossRef]

63. Cai, Y.; Gao, P.; Li, Y.; Wang, X.; Peng, B. Laparoscopic pancreaticoduodenectomy with major venous resection and reconstruction: Anterior superior mesenteric artery first approach. *Surg. Endosc.* **2018**, *32*, 4209–4215. [CrossRef] [PubMed]
64. Khatkov, I.E.; Izrailov, R.E.; Khisamov, A.A.; Tyutyunnik, P.S.; Fingerhut, A. Superior mesenteric-portal vein resection during laparoscopic pancreatoduodenectomy. *Surg. Endosc.* **2017**, *31*, 1488–1495. [CrossRef] [PubMed]
65. Kendrick, M.L.; Sclabas, G.M. Major venous resection during total laparoscopic pancreaticoduodenectomy. *HPB* **2011**, *13*, 454–458. [CrossRef] [PubMed]
66. Dokmak, S.; Aussilhou, B.; Calmels, M.; Maghrebi, H.; Ftériche, F.S.; Soubrane, O.; Sauvanet, A. Laparoscopic pancreaticoduodenectomy with reconstruction of the mesentericoportal vein with the parietal peritoneum and the falciform ligament. *Surg. Endosc.* **2018**, *32*, 3256–3261. [CrossRef] [PubMed]
67. Dokmak, S.; Chérif, R.; Duquesne, I.; Delattre, R.; Aussilhou, B.; Soubrane, O.; Sauvanet, A. Laparoscopic Pancreaticoduodenectomy with Reconstruction of the Portal Vein with the Parietal Peritoneum. *Ann. Surg. Oncol.* **2016**, *23*, 2664. [CrossRef] [PubMed]
68. Wei, Q.; Chen, Q.P.; Guan, Q.H.; Zhu, W.T. Repair of the portal vein using a hepatic ligamentum teres patch for laparoscopic pancreatoduodenectomy: A case report. *World J. Clin. Cases* **2019**, *7*, 2879–2887. [CrossRef]
69. Suzuki, S.; Shimoda, M.; Shimazaki, J.; Maruyama, T.; Nishida, K. Clinical Outcome of Resected Remnant Pancreatic Cancer After Resection of the Primary Pancreatic Cancer. *J. Investig. Surg.* **2019**, *32*, 670–678. [CrossRef]
70. Ishida, J.; Toyama, H.; Matsumoto, I.; Asari, S.; Goto, T.; Terai, S.; Nanno, Y.; Yamashita, A.; Mizumoto, T.; Ueda, Y.; et al. Second primary pancreatic ductal carcinoma in the remnant pancreas after pancreatectomy for pancreatic ductal carcinoma: High cumulative incidence rates at 5 years after pancreatectomy. *Pancreatology* **2016**, *16*, 615–620. [CrossRef]
71. Inoue, K.; Kosuge, T.; Shimada, K.; Yamamoto, J.; Takayama, T.; Ozaki, H.; Nose, H. Repeated radical resection and intraoperative irradiation for recurrent pancreatic ductal adenocarcinoma after pancreatoduodenectomy. *Surgery* **1995**, *118*, 909–911. [CrossRef]
72. Kleeff, J.; Reiser, C.; Hinz, U.; Bachmann, J.; Debus, J.; Jaeger, D.; Friess, H.; Büchler, M.W. Surgery for recurrent pancreatic ductal adenocarcinoma. *Ann. Surg.* **2007**, *245*, 566–572. [CrossRef] [PubMed]
73. Yamada, S.; Kobayashi, A.; Nakamori, S.; Baba, H.; Yamamoto, M.; Yamaue, H.; Fujii, T. Resection for recurrent pancreatic cancer in the remnant pancreas after pancreatectomy is clinically promising: Results of a project study for pancreatic surgery by the Japanese Society of Hepato-Biliary-Pancreatic Surgery. *Surgery* **2018**, *164*, 1049–1056. [CrossRef] [PubMed]
74. Groot, V.P.; van Santvoort, H.C.; Rombouts, S.J.; Hagendoorn, J.; Borel Rinkes, I.H.; van Vulpen, M.; Herman, J.M.; Wolfgang, C.L.; Besselink, M.G.; Molenaar, I.Q. Systematic review on the treatment of isolated local recurrence of pancreatic cancer after surgery; re-resection, chemoradiotherapy and SBRT. *HPB* **2017**, *19*, 83–92. [CrossRef] [PubMed]
75. Karasic, T.B.; O'Hara, M.H.; Loaiza-Bonilla, A.; Reiss, K.A.; Teitelbaum, U.R.; Borazanci, E.; De Jesus-Acosta, A.; Redlinger, C.; Burrell, J.A.; Laheru, D.A.; et al. Effect of Gemcitabine and nab-Paclitaxel With or Without Hydroxychloroquine on Patients With Advanced Pancreatic Cancer: A Phase 2 Randomized Clinical Trial. *JAMA Oncol.* **2019**, *5*, 993–998. [CrossRef] [PubMed]
76. Nakagawa, Y.; Fukami, Y.; Harada, T.; Maeda, A.; Takayama, Y.; Takahashi, T.; Uji, M.; Kaneoka, Y. Laparoscopic pancreaticoduodenectomy for remnant pancreatic recurrence after laparoscopic distal pancreatectomy and hepatectomy for greater omentum leiomyosarcoma. *Asian J. Endosc. Surg.* **2020**, *13*, 117–120. [CrossRef]
77. Sunagawa, H.; Mayama, Y.; Orokawa, T.; Oshiro, N. Laparoscopic total remnant pancreatectomy after laparoscopic pancreaticoduodenectomy. *Asian J. Endosc. Surg.* **2014**, *7*, 71–74. [CrossRef]
78. Hashimoto, D.; Chikamoto, A.; Masuda, T.; Nakagawa, S.; Imai, K.; Yamashita, Y.I.; Reber, H.A.; Baba, H. Pancreatic Cancer Arising From the Remnant Pancreas: Is It a Local Recurrence or New Primary Lesion? *Pancreas* **2017**, *46*, 1083–1090. [CrossRef]
79. Zhou, Y.; Song, A.; Wu, L.; Si, X.; Li, Y. Second pancreatectomy for recurrent pancreatic ductal adenocarcinoma in the remnant pancreas: A pooled analysis. *Pancreatology* **2016**, *16*, 1124–1128. [CrossRef]

80. Choi, M.; Lee, S.J.; Shin, D.M.; Hwang, H.K.; Lee, W.J.; Kang, C.M. Laparoscopic repeated pancreatectomy for isolated local recurrence in remnant pancreas following laparoscopic radical pancreatectomy for pancreatic ductal adenocarcinoma: Two cases report. *Ann. Hepatobiliary Pancreat Surg.* **2020**. Forthcoming.
81. Jiang, Y.L.; Zhang, R.C.; Zhou, Y.C. Comparison of overall survival and perioperative outcomes of laparoscopic pancreaticoduodenectomy and open pancreaticoduodenectomy for pancreatic ductal adenocarcinoma: A systematic review and meta-analysis. *BMC Cancer* **2019**, *19*, 781. [CrossRef]
82. Chen, K.; Zhou, Y.; Jin, W.; Zhu, Q.; Lu, C.; Niu, N.; Wang, Y.; Mou, Y.; Chen, Z. Laparoscopic pancreaticoduodenectomy versus open pancreaticoduodenectomy for pancreatic ductal adenocarcinoma: Oncologic outcomes and long-term survival. *Surg. Endosc.* **2020**, *34*, 1948–1958. [CrossRef] [PubMed]
83. Yin, Z.; Jian, Z.; Hou, B.; Jin, H. Surgical and Oncological Outcomes of Laparoscopic Versus Open Pancreaticoduodenectomy in Patients With Pancreatic Duct Adenocarcinoma. *Pancreas* **2019**, *48*, 861–867. [CrossRef] [PubMed]
84. Sharpe, S.M.; Talamonti, M.S.; Wang, C.E.; Prinz, R.A.; Roggin, K.K.; Bentrem, D.J.; Winchester, D.J.; Marsh, R.D.; Stocker, S.J.; Baker, M.S. Early National Experience with Laparoscopic Pancreaticoduodenectomy for Ductal Adenocarcinoma: A Comparison of Laparoscopic Pancreaticoduodenectomy and Open Pancreaticoduodenectomy from the National Cancer Data Base. *J. Am. Coll. Surg.* **2015**, *221*, 175–184. [CrossRef]
85. Kantor, O.; Talamonti, M.S.; Sharpe, S.; Lutfi, W.; Winchester, D.J.; Roggin, K.K.; Bentrem, D.J.; Prinz, R.A.; Baker, M.S. Laparoscopic pancreaticoduodenectomy for adenocarcinoma provides short-term oncologic outcomes and long-term overall survival rates similar to those for open pancreaticoduodenectomy. *Am. J. Surg.* **2017**, *213*, 512–515. [CrossRef] [PubMed]
86. Chapman, B.C.; Gajdos, C.; Hosokawa, P.; Henderson, W.; Paniccia, A.; Overbey, D.M.; Gleisner, A.; Schulick, R.D.; McCarter, M.D.; Edil, B.H. Comparison of laparoscopic to open pancreaticoduodenectomy in elderly patients with pancreatic adenocarcinoma. *Surg. Endosc.* **2018**, *32*, 2239–2248. [CrossRef]
87. Torphy, R.J.; Friedman, C.; Halpern, A.; Chapman, B.C.; Ahrendt, S.S.; McCarter, M.M.; Edil, B.H.; Schulick, R.D.; Gleisner, A. Comparing Short-term and Oncologic Outcomes of Minimally Invasive Versus Open Pancreaticoduodenectomy Across Low and High Volume Centers. *Ann. Surg.* **2019**, *270*, 1147–1155. [CrossRef]
88. Blajchman, M.A.; Bardossy, L.; Carmen, R.; Sastry, A.; Singal, D.P. Allogeneic blood transfusion-induced enhancement of tumor growth: Two animal models showing amelioration by leukodepletion and passive transfer using spleen cells. *Blood* **1993**, *81*, 1880–1882. [CrossRef]
89. Kaplan, J.; Sarnaik, S.; Gitlin, J.; Lusher, J. Diminished helper/suppressor lymphocyte ratios and natural killer activity in recipients of repeated blood transfusions. *Blood* **1984**, *64*, 308–310. [CrossRef]
90. Yao, H.S.; Wang, Q.; Wang, W.J.; Hu, Z.Q. Intraoperative allogeneic red blood cell transfusion in ampullary cancer outcome after curative pancreatoduodenectomy: A clinical study and meta-analysis. *World J. Surg.* **2008**, *32*, 2038–2046. [CrossRef]
91. Kim, S.Y.; Choi, M.; Hwang, H.K.; Rho, S.Y.; Lee, W.J.; Kang, C.M. Intraoperative Transfusion is Independently Associated with a Worse Prognosis in Resected Pancreatic Cancer-a Retrospective Cohort Analysis. *J. Clin. Med.* **2020**, *9*, 689. [CrossRef]
92. Kneuertz, P.J.; Patel, S.H.; Chu, C.K.; Maithel, S.K.; Sarmiento, J.M.; Delman, K.A.; Staley, C.A., 3rd; Kooby, D.A. Effects of perioperative red blood cell transfusion on disease recurrence and survival after pancreaticoduodenectomy for ductal adenocarcinoma. *Ann. Surg. Oncol.* **2011**, *18*, 1327–1334. [CrossRef] [PubMed]
93. Kauffmann, E.F.; Napoli, N.; Cacace, C.; Menonna, F.; Vistoli, F.; Amorese, G.; Boggi, U. Resection or repair of large peripancreatic arteries during robotic pancreatectomy. *Updates Surg.* **2020**, *72*, 145–153. [CrossRef] [PubMed]
94. Tempero, M.A. NCCN Guidelines Updates: Pancreatic Cancer. *J. Natl. Compr. Canc. Netw.* **2019**, *17*, 603–605. [CrossRef] [PubMed]
95. Stiles, Z.E.; Dickson, P.V.; Deneve, J.L.; Glazer, E.S.; Dong, L.; Wan, J.Y.; Behrman, S.W. The impact of unplanned conversion to an open procedure during minimally invasive pancreatectomy. *J. Surg. Res.* **2018**, *227*, 168–177. [CrossRef] [PubMed]

96. Fortner, J.G.; Klimstra, D.S.; Senie, R.T.; Maclean, B.J. Tumor size is the primary prognosticator for pancreatic cancer after regional pancreatectomy. *Ann. Surg.* **1996**, *223*, 147–153. [CrossRef]
97. Kang, C.M. ASO Author Reflections: From Concept to Real Clinical Practice of Laparoscopic Distal Pancreatectomy for Left-Sided Pancreatic Cancer. *Ann. Surg. Oncol.* **2020**. [CrossRef]

Publisher's Note: MDPI stays neutral with regard to jurisdictional claims in published maps and institutional affiliations.

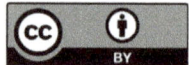 © 2020 by the authors. Licensee MDPI, Basel, Switzerland. This article is an open access article distributed under the terms and conditions of the Creative Commons Attribution (CC BY) license (http://creativecommons.org/licenses/by/4.0/).

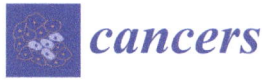

Review

Achieving 'Marginal Gains' to Optimise Outcomes in Resectable Pancreatic Cancer

Sarah Powell-Brett [1,*], Rupaly Pande [1,†] and Keith J. Roberts [1,2]

1. Department of Hepatopancreatobiliary Surgery and Liver Transplantation, University Hospitals Birmingham NHS Foundation Trust, Birmingham B15 2GW, UK; rpande@nhs.net (R.P.); Keith.Roberts@uhb.nhs.uk (K.J.R.)
2. Institute of Immunology and Immunotherapy, University of Birmingham, Birmingham B15 2TT, UK
* Correspondence: sarah.powell-brett1@nhs.net; Tel.: +44-(0)788-775-4856
† Joint 1st authors.

Simple Summary: Improving outcomes in pancreatic cancer is achievable through the accumulation of marginal gains. There exists evidence of variation and undertreatment in many areas of the care pathway. By fully realising the existing opportunities, there is the potential for immediate improvements in outcomes and quality of life.

Abstract: Improving outcomes among patients with resectable pancreatic cancer is one of the greatest challenges of modern medicine. Major improvements in survival will result from the development of novel therapies. However, optimising existing pathways, so that patients realise benefits of already proven treatments, presents a clear opportunity to improve outcomes in the short term. This narrative review will focus on treatments and interventions where there is a clear evidence base to improve outcomes in pancreatic cancer, and where there is also evidence of variation and under-treatment. Avoidance of preoperative biliary drainage, treatment of pancreatic exocrine insufficiency, prehabiliation and enhanced recovery after surgery, reducing perioperative complications, optimising opportunities for elderly patients to receive therapy, optimising adjuvant chemotherapy and regular surveillance after surgery are some of the strategies discussed. Each treatment or pathway change represents an opportunity for marginal gain. Accumulation of marginal gains can result in considerable benefit to patients. Given that these interventions already have evidence base, they can be realised quickly and economically.

Keywords: pancreatic cancer; pancreatic exocrine insufficiency; adjuvant chemotherapy; biliary drainage; prehabilitation; ERAS

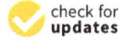

Citation: Powell-Brett, S.; Pande, R.; Roberts, K.J. Achieving 'Marginal Gains' to Optimise Outcomes in Resectable Pancreatic Cancer. *Cancers* 2021, 13, 1669. https://doi.org/10.3390/cancers13071669

Academic Editor: Tsutomu Fujii

Received: 4 February 2021
Accepted: 24 March 2021
Published: 1 April 2021

Publisher's Note: MDPI stays neutral with regard to jurisdictional claims in published maps and institutional affiliations.

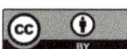

Copyright: © 2021 by the authors. Licensee MDPI, Basel, Switzerland. This article is an open access article distributed under the terms and conditions of the Creative Commons Attribution (CC BY) license (https://creativecommons.org/licenses/by/4.0/).

1. Introduction

Pancreatic cancer is projected to become the second leading cause of all cancer-related deaths by 2030 [1,2]. Although surgical resection is the foundation of 'resectable' pancreatic cancer management, alone it is associated with a less than 10% chance of cure [3]. High rates of perioperative morbidity and mortality, slow or poorly organised pathways to surgery, suboptimal preoperative management of jaundice, suboptimal use of (neo)adjuvant therapy and failure to address malnutrition all contribute to poor outcomes. It is therefore unsurprising that there can be a negative attitude and feelings of nihilism when considering the outlook for these patients.

Wide variations in care and a lack of standardised practice, however, offer an easy way to improve outcomes in the near future. Pathways to expedite surgery, prescribing of enzyme therapy, access to adjuvant chemotherapy and tackling frailty are just a few examples of how care has the potential to be optimised. Optimising an individual aspect of care represents an opportunity for a marginal gain. Individually, each gain realised may be relatively minor when observed across an entire patient cohort, but when multiple, the effect of aggregated marginal gains can be considerable. The aggregation of marginal gains was popularised in elite level cycling where its success was clear to see at Olympic level and major events such as the Tour de France. The principals have been adopted in healthcare among various patient populations from cancer surgery, stroke recovery, prehabilitation, cardiac surgery and anaesthesia [4–6]. This narrative review highlights common failings in the care of pancreatic cancer patients and describes where gains can be made. The aggregation of these marginal gains could improve outcomes and experience for a great many patients with resectable pancreatic cancer.

2. Pre-Operative Pathways

At presentation, resectable pancreatic cancer is in an exponential phase of growth and most primary tumours harbour cells that can metastasise [7]. Enhancing pre-operative pathways to ensure that patients are treated as quickly as possible and their functional status is optimised is essential to enabling the delivery of the highest standard of care. This section will focus on avoidance of pre-operative biliary drainage, prehabilitation, and optimisation of nutritional status.

2.1. Preoperative Biliary Drainage in Resectable Pancreatic Cancer

The majority of patients with resectable pancreatic cancer present with jaundice. Historically reluctance to operate in the presence of jaundice was related to concerns over renal, cardiac and liver dysfunction, coagulopathy and, at the time, high rates of perioperative morbidity and mortality associated with pancreatic surgery in the absence of jaundice [8].

Hence, in theory, relief of jaundice by preoperative biliary drainage (PBD) is perceived to improve these disturbances and prevent postoperative complications, though in practice, the role and propriety of PBD must be challenged.

The concept of correcting jaundice prior to resection was introduced by A.O. Whipple through staged PD, initially a cholecystogastrostomy to relieve jaundice followed by resection once the jaundice was within 'safe' limits. This further developed into nonoperative approaches through percutaneous transhepatic cholangiopathy (PTC) and biliary drainage in the 1960s and later followed by endoscopic retrograde cholangiopancreatography (ERCP) in the 1970s [9,10].

For many decades ERCP served both diagnostic and therapeutic purposes. However, the sensitivity and specificity of CT to diagnose pancreatic cancer has made ERCP, as a diagnostic tool, obsolete.

The main drawback of PBD is the associated rate of complications. These complications impair quality of life, can delay or prevent future surgery and are occasionally fatal. PBD itself requires resource and invariably delays treatment pathways [11,12].

The DROP trial randomised patients to upfront early surgery within 7 days or PBD- and plastic stent and delayed surgery between 4–6 weeks [13]. This landmark RCT showed the rate of serious complications at 120 days postoperatively to be far higher in the PBD group (74 vs. 39%, $p < 0.001$). This was largely due to drainage-related complications, cholangitis (26 vs. 2%), pancreatitis (7 vs. 0%) along with the need for change of stent in 30% of patients. There are also higher rates of perioperative infections, associated with changes in the biliary microbiome related to PBD [14,15] It is therefore advised that intraoperative bile cultures are taken and appropriate antibiotic administered to address this higher rate of complications [16].

Self-expanding metal stents (SEMS) have gained in popularity over plastic stents based on significantly greater patency and reduction in infectious complications [13,17,18]. The experience of patients undergoing PBD with fully covered SEMS, with a prospective study which mirrored the protocol of the DROP trial, superimposed the complication rates of PBD-SEMS over the cohorts within the DROP trial [19]. Though SEMS were associated with lower rates of complications than plastic stents, the rate remained significantly greater than upfront surgery (51 vs. 39%). Subsequent meta-analysis confirms advantages of metal over plastic stents with reduced rates of need for endoscopic reintervention (OR0.3), preoperative complications (OR 0.42) and cholangitis (OR 0.09) [20]. However, pancreatitis is more common (OR 3.6) and, though not reported, post hoc analysis of resection rates demonstrates a lower resection rate among patients with metal stents (plastic, 147/190 vs. metal 93/139; Chi square p = 0.04) [19,20]. A more recent network meta-analysis demonstrated a remarkably high rate of complications with plastic stents (38–93%), a much lower rate with SEMS (0–15%) whilst data regarding outcomes from percutaneous drainage is not at extensively reported (31%) [21]. This study also concluded that avoidance of PBD was associated with the best outcome.

The association between PBD and reduced resection rates was not observed in individual randomised trials. However, it is logical to associate complications such as pancreatitis or pathway delays with a reduction in resection rate. Many high-volume centres have reported that increasing time to surgery reduces resection rates, data confirmed within a recent systematic review and meta-analysis [22–25]. It may be that this higher resection rate and avoidance of complications translates into increased survival benefit, when analysed on an intention to treat basis [26]. This is controversial as some authors have associated hyperbilirbuinaemia at the time of resection with worse cancer outcomes [27].

Given the many benefits of avoiding PBD, the National Institute for Health and Care Excellence (NICE) in the United Kingdom, now recommend upfront surgery without PBD where possible [28].

What remains to be defined is a safe upper limit of bilirubin in terms of safety and oncologic outcomes and why PBD remains so widely used despite the evidence of harm. Associated venous resection appears safe in the presence of jaundice, even when levels of bilirubin exceed 300 µmol/L (>17.5 mg/dL) [29]. It may be assumed that elderly patients are safer to undergo PBD and surgery rather than upfront surgery but elderly patients are less likely to tolerate complications of PBD and remain on a surgical pathway than younger patients.

Numerous studies have established seemingly arbitrary upper limits of bilirubin at which PBD is indicated [27,30–35]. A common threshold of >250 umol/L is used and cited by The Guidelines for Perioperative Care for Pancreaticoduodenectomy: Enhanced Recovery After Surgery (ERAS®) Society Recommendations [36]; Both Sauvanet and Li et al. reported higher complication rates when surgery was performed with a bilirubin of >300 µmol/L [27,37]. However, contrary to this, van der Gaag, quoted a bilirubin level of ≤300 µmol/L at surgery and demonstrated significantly lower infective complications, whilst Pamecha et al. showed that a bilirubin level of ≥15 mg/dL (≥265 µmol/L) was not an independent risk factor for complications [13,38,39].

As stated above, it is the authors experience that surgery, even with venous resection, can be performed with no difference in complications with bilirubin in excess of 300 µmol/L. To summarise, there is no clear data that defines an upper limit of bilirubin at which PBD is indicated. The authors recommend an approach with prospective evaluation of outcomes and a step wise increase in threshold of bilirubin at which to undertake PBD. Variation in the rate of increase of bilirubin, the difficulty/time needed to complete staging tests and other factors such as renal function or evidence of biliary sepsis mean that there is unlikely to be a single value which can be applied to all patients.

It is useful to consider when PBD is indicated. Jaundiced patients undergoing neoadjuvant therapy clearly require PBD; if there are major diagnostic delays, though an assessment of risk of cancer progression must be weighed up against potential risks of surgery in such cases or if the patient is too frail to undergo surgery. Such patients, however, in our experience rarely improve significantly after PBD. Cholangitis has been considered a contraindication for PBD, though in our practice we frequently employ external biliary drainage, antibiotics, fluid replacement therapy and surgery within the same week if markers of infection are improving. This has controlled sepsis, avoided complications of PBD and kept patients within an early surgery pathway. See Table 1. For a summary of potential indications for PBD and Table 2 for optimizing care should PBD be undertaken.

Table 1. Absolute and relative indications for Percutaneous biliary drainage (PBD).

	Indication for PDB	Comment
Absolute	Neoadjuvant therapy	
	Renal dysfunction	If mild, percutaneous external drainage and fluid replacement may permit early surgery with trans-sphincteric drainage to reduce the risk of pancreatitis
	Cholangitis with organ dysfunction	If mild, percutaneous external drainage and fluid replacement may permit early surgery with trans-sphincteric drainage to reduce the risk of pancreatitis
Relative	Bilirubin level	Exact cut off leve currently unclear, see text.
	Delay to surgery	Need to consider daily rate if increase in bilirubin as this may vary from patient to patient
	Malnutrition	Ensure exocrine insufficiency corrected and balance delays to surgery, cancer progression against severity of malnutrition
	Frailty	Frail patients are less likely to tolerate complications of PBD so a difficult discussion or choice often needs to be made. For some frail patients, direct to surgery may be there best chance to have surgery as delays or complications of PBD can exacerbate frailty

Table 2. Tips for optimising care in the event of PBD requirement.

Indication for PDB	Comment
Initial attempt at PBD	ERCP with self-expanding metal stent
Position of stent	The stent should be short and ideally not occlude the cystic duct origin as this can lead to cholecystitis which can delay surgery or chemotherapy
Periprocedural care	Antibiotics before and after the procedure Regular observations with escalation to medical team in event of abdominal pain and/or hypotension. Consideration of CT in event to exclude pancreatitis or perforation.
Options if initial PBD fails	Maximum of two attempts at ERCP. If unsuccessful for PTC with stent placement as a rescue option (referral to specialist centre may be optimal depending on local experience)
Definition of successful PBD	Biliary drainage is defined as successful if the serum bilirubin level decreased by 50% or more within 2 weeks after the procedure.

Malnutrition associated with obstructive jaundice and its effects on outcomes following surgery is a further area of controversy. In studies by Padillo et al., malnutrition was more commonly associated with patients older than 68 years and those with high levels of bilirubin with the suggestion that PBD should be considered to allow alleviation of these modifiable factors preoperatively [40,41]. However, evidence for the optimal duration of PBD to improve nutritional status is experimental and its role in malnutrition must be considered in the broader context of pancreatic exocrine insufficiency [42–45]. Exocrine insufficiency is prevalent at diagnosis, and although not the sole cause of malnutrition, it is a major driver of malnutrition and is poorly treated; thus, delays to surgery can exacerbate malnutrition if PEI is not addressed. A balance must be struck between early surgery and better treatment of PEI versus correcting jaundice and improving nutrition. A proposed optimal pathway would be to provide PERT for all patients and provide early surgery where possible; where a patient has a poor performance status with malnutrition, a pathway of PBD, PERT, and dietician input would be advocated.

2.2. Pancreatic Exocrine Insufficiency and Overcoming Malnutrition to Improve Outcomes

Pancreatic exocrine insufficiency (PEI) and pancreatic enzyme replacement therapy (PERT) should be considered at all stages of management of pancreatic cancer, it is included in this section on pre-operative pathways as correct treatment is essential as early in the care pathway as possible. PEI is far from trivial and should be considered as organ failure. Untreated failure of other organ systems can be rapidly fatal (for example, renal, cardiac or respiratory failure or even diabetes) and withholding treatment in these settings is reserved only for those patients who are on end-of-life pathways. Consequently, it is remarkable that PEI is underdiagnosed and undertreated. *In the authors view, this single issue represents the simplest pathway improvement in this review and also the intervention with the chance to achieve most gain.*

Addressing pancreatic exocrine insufficiency (PEI) can have an effect upon survival as strong as that as surgery or chemotherapy and yet many patients remains untreated [46]. A 2016 systematic review of PEI demonstrated a pre-operative prevalence of 44% and a post-operative prevalence of 74% (for those undergoing pancreatico-duodenectomy for malignancy). This is likely a conservative estimate owing to the frequent use of faecal elastase (FE-1) to diagnose PEI (FE-1 has been shown to underestimate PEI following resection) [47,48]. Furthermore, there is a gradual reduction of exocrine function at a median value of 10% per month [49]. With the gold standard of testing and longer term follow up, Lemaire et al. found the post-operative incidence of PEI to be 94% [50]. In resectable disease the mechanisms underlying PEI are complex and multifactorial. Almost all physiologic control is lost after pancreatoduodenectomy, and together with other factors result in insufficient enzymes arriving at the wrong time, to the wrong place and at the wrong pH for effective function [51,52] (see Figure 1).

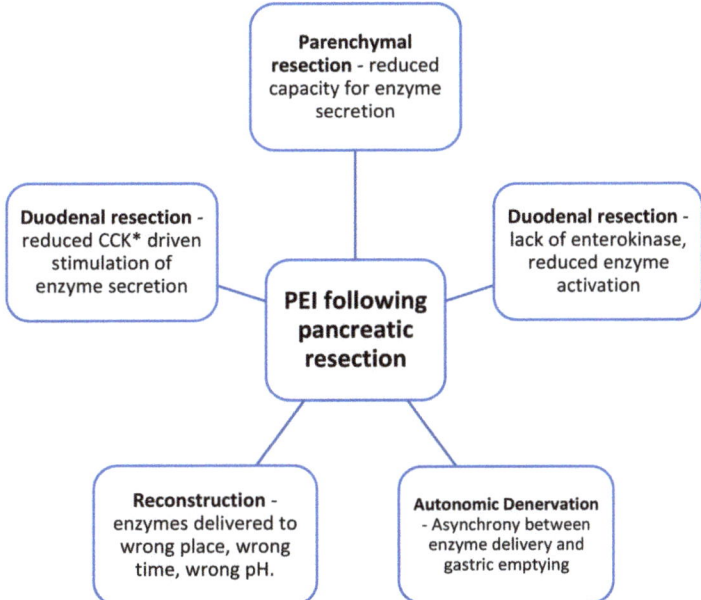

Figure 1. Factors contributing to PEI following pancreatico-duodenectomy. *CCK = cholecystokinin.

Symptoms of PEI include pain, bloating, frequency, urgency, diarrhoea, fatty stool, flatulence, loss of appetite, nausea and vomiting and are physically and mentally distressing. The 'classical' sign of steathorrhoea is often absent, either because PEI is not severe enough or because the patient may have unconsciously adopted behaviours to avoid fat intake [53–55]. PEI is frequently untreated or undertreated worldwide. Studies from the UK, Europe and Australia demonstrate that only a minority of patients receive PERT [56–59]. Reasons for under prescribing are multifactorial and may relate to the lack of an acceptable or accurate routine diagnostic test that can yield results in near real time [47,60–62]. Confusing symptoms of cancer, weight loss and abdominal discomfort, further complicate diagnosis.

The consequences of PEI must not be underestimated, these include: weight loss, malnutrition, micronutrient deficiency, cardiovascular events, osteoporosis, fractures and sarcopenia [63]. The effect of PEI on operative outcomes is considerable, being associated with higher rates of post-operative complications, longer hospital stays and increased costs [64–67].

Pancreatic enzyme replacement therapy (PERT) is cheap, mitigates against weight loss and improves quality of life. The most compelling argument for PERT is emerging evidence that it improves survival [46,58,68–71]. Given the failings of diagnostic tests for PEI and the evident benefits of PERT, it is recommended for all patients with pancreatic cancer by NICE in the United Kingdom [28].

A healthy pancreas is estimated to produce 900,000 United States Pharmacopeia (USP) of lipase in response to a meal. Sufficient absorption of fat can be maintained at around 10% of normal capacity, there is thus a need for around 90,000 USP per meal. Given that in the majority of pancreatic disease some function remains an appropriate starting dose in resected pancreatic cancer is 75,000 USP with a main meal and 25,000 with a snack [69], most effective when given across the course of, or just after, a meal rather than before [72]. Co-prescription of a proton pump inhibitor is often required after pancreatoduodenectomy as a failure to neutralise gastric acid leads to enzymes remaining inactive [73].

Pre-operative malnutrition is associated with significantly poorer post-operative outcomes for pancreatic resection, addressing this extends beyond just the prescribing of PERT [74,75]. The international Study Group on Pancreatic Surgery (ISGPS) released a position paper on nutritional support and therapy in pancreatic surgery, this emphasizes the importance of pre-operative assessment of nutritional status and recommends nutritional supplements in those who have, or are at risk of developing, moderate malnutrition [76]. Those with, or at risk of severe malnutrition may benefit from formal nutritional support with enteral or parenteral feeding [76]. Regular dietician input to asses response, compliance, diet, diabetic optimization, and the potential need for nutritional supplements is required [77].

Although outside the scope of this article to describe in detail, immunonutrition is worthy of note. Immunonutrition aims to influence the systemic immune system using nutritional supplements with immune modulating contents such as arginine, omega-3 fatty acid and RNA. This is not yet part of routine clinical practice, however, there is evidence that initiation in the pre-operative period could improve post-operative outcomes [78–81]. The most recent systematic review and meta-analysis of immunonutrition in pancreatic resection, concluded that immunonutrition reduces infectious complications (especially wound infection) and length of stay [82].

2.3. Benefits of and Access to Surgical Resection of Pancreatic Cancer in the Elderly

Benefits of resection do not diminish with increasing age [83,84]. Yet, many elderly patients are considered too frail for surgery and there is significant age-related disparity in access to surgery. Ageism is a major problem faced by elderly cancer patients; elderly patients without comorbidity are less likely to receive cancer therapy than younger patients with comorbidity. Advanced age, in the absence of comorbidity, is mistakenly considered a more significant barrier to surgery than comorbidity [85]. Elderly patients are less likely to undergo standard resection, less likely to undergo resection with concomitant venous resection and less likely to achieve negative margins [86–88]. An American population based study of over 45,000 patients with pancreatic adenocarcinoma observed that the rate of surgery decreased with increasing age: 21% of those under 50, 19% between the age of 50 and 70 and only 13% of those over 70 received surgery [87].

Concerns over risk and perceived lack of benefit of surgery are prohibitive and account for the discrepancies in care. However, a systematic review of surgery among elderly patients with pancreatic cancer demonstrated that over time, perioperative mortality has improved for elderly patients following pancreatic resection when compared to non-elderly patients, with mortality preceding the year 2000 being significantly higher in elderly patients, but similar from 2000 onwards [86]. Major surgical complications (post-operative pancreatic fistula, delayed gastric emptying, post pancreatectomy haemorrhage and surgical site infections) were similar between the elderly and the non-elderly; however, respiratory complications did occur more frequently in the elderly population. Prehabilitation can improve physical functioning and prevent deterioration among patients whilst waiting for cancer surgery [89–94]. The benefits of surgery are not diminished by age and therefore older patients with appropriate performance status should not be denied access based on chronological age alone. Treatment decisions for the elderly should be made in a multidisciplinary setting, should ideally include the use of a tool such as the comprehensive geriatric assessment and the input of a geriatrician to avoid discrepancies in treatment based on chronological age [95,96].

2.4. Prehabilitation

Resection is the only curative option for pancreatic cancer, however, the majority of patients with a new diagnosis are not suitable for operative management [97]. Baseline functional status influences receipt of curative resection, receipt of adjuvant chemotherapy, the rate and severity of post-operative complications and long term quality of life [89,98–100]. Functional status is often poor in patients with pancreatic cancer, this is contributed to by older age at diagnosis, pre-operative sarcopenia, malnutrition and obstructive jaundice [101]. Prehabilitation refers to any interventions, prior to definitive treatment that are aimed at improving patient health and lifestyle [102]. The concept centres around pre-operative conditioning to improve nutritional status and aerobic capacity. Studies of prehabilitation in other types of major surgery have suggested that these programmes can improve both access to definitive treatment, and post-operative outcomes [103] (See Table 3). A recent trial randomised patients to standard of care versus standard of care plus prehabilitation in patients having major abdominal surgery found that the prehabilitation cohort had improved aerobic capacity and a reduction in 30-day readmissions [104]. Unfortunately, systematic reviews and meta-analysis have determined that although prehabilitation programmes can potentially improve surgical outcomes, the evidence is weak, this is most likely do to the variation in prehabilitation regimens and study heterogeneity [102,103,105–108].

The majority of evidence for prehabilitation is limited to those undergoing colorectal resection, hepatic resection or major cardio-thoracic surgery, few studies look specifically at the impact of prehabilitation in pancreatic resection [109–114] (Table 1). Two studies have reported on the association between prehabilitation and post-operative outcomes in pancreatic cancer; Ausania et al. randomised patients to prehabilitation (n = 18) or standard of care (n = 22). Nakajima et al. compared a cohort of patients undergoing prehabilitation to historical patients. Neither study determined a significant difference in outcomes except for reduced rates of delayed gastric emptying in one and a shorter length of stay in the other. Several studies report an improvement in lean muscle mass prior to surgery and one reported improvement in quality of life in those undergoing prehabilitation [109–114]. Although showing promising results, the collective interpretation of these studies is difficult owing to poor standardisation of exercise and nutritional interventions and paucity of participants. Table 4: Pre-operative areas for potential gain.

Table 3. Summary of prehabilitation studies for pancreatic resection.

	Year	Study Design	No.	Exercise Plan	Key Findings
Nakajima et al.	2019	Retrospective, cohort	76	30 days Unsupervised, self-reported exercise	Shorter length of stay in prehabilitation group (23 days vs. days, $p = 0.045$)
Ausania et al.	2019	Randomised controlled trial	18	2 weeks supervised and unsupervised, aerobic exercise	Reduction in DGE in prehabilitation group (5.6% vs. 40.9%, $p = 0.01$)
Florez Bedoya et al.	2019	Prospective, cohort	23	15 weeks unsupervised, self-reported, aerobic and resistance exercise	No comment on clinical outcomes Evidence of prehabilitation increasing tumour vascularity.
Marker et al.	2018	Case series	3	12–16 weeks, supervised, physiotherapist reported, hour long, 3× a week	Underpowered
Parker et al.	2018	Prospective, cohort	50	60 min per week unsupervised, self-reported aerobic and strengthening exercise	No comment on clinical outcomes Home based exercise programme feasible
Ngo-Huang et al.	2019	Prospective, cohort	50	2 weeks, unsupervised, self-reported, hour long aerobic exercise	Prehabilitation associated with improved physical function (6MWT, STS, GS improved from baseline, $p = 0.48, 0.03$ & 0.08, respectively) and HRQOL (Improved with increased LPA ($p = 0.01$)

6MWT = 6 min walk test, STS = Sit to stand, GS = Gait speed, HRQOL = Health Related Quality of Life, LPA = Light physical activity.

Table 4. Pre-operative areas for potential gain.

Areas for Gain Pre-Operatively	Problem	Intervention	Gain
Avoidance of pre-operative biliary drainage	- PBD related complications are common - Avoidable delay to surgery - Missed window of opportunity for curative surgery	- Upfront surgery	- Avoid PBD related complications - Reduce postoperative complications - Increase number of patients undergoing curative surgery - Improve overall survival
Correction of PEI related malnutrition	- PEI is highly prevalent and related to weight loss, reduced QoL, reduced survival - Under-prescribing of PERT - Inadequate dosing - Malnourished at baseline - Sarcopenia	- PERT prescribing for all - Education of wider team - Patient education - Dietetic monitoring - Consider PPI - Consider supplements	- Improve quality of life - Reduce weight loss - Reduce complications - Improve survival
Prehabilitation	- Older age group - Sarcopenia - Too 'frail' for treatment - Deconditioning	- Consider who is 'at risk' - Physiotherapy involvement - More research	- Potential to reduce some complications - Reduce length of stay - Potential to improve access to treatment
Old age/frailty	- Nihilistic attitudes towards older age - Elderly not receiving same standard of care despite proven benefit	- MDT decision making with geriatrician if able - Use of assessment tools. Such as CGA - Co-morbidities rather than chronological age as deciding factor.	- Improved access to curative treatment options for the elderly.

PEI = Pancreatic exocrine insufficiency, PBD = Pre-operative biliary drainage, QoL = Quality of life, PERT = Pancreatic enzyme replacement therapy, PPI = Proton pump inhibitor, CGA = Comprehensive geriatric assessment.

3. Peri-Operative Pathways

3.1. Enhanced Recovery after Surgery

Enhanced recovery after surgery (ERAS) is a multimodal approach to a patient's perioperative journey which aims to facilitate early return to the preoperative state [115]. Broadly, it facilitates sustained recovery and reduces complications. A secondary benefit is frequently a reduced length of stay.

The value of ERAS pathways in pancreatic surgery has been recommended on the basis of high level evidence in domains such as avoidance of hypothermia, use of wound catheters compared to epidural analgesia (EDA), use of somatostatin analogues to reduce CR-POPF [116]. protocols for thromboprophylaxis and antimicrobials and interventions for preoperative nutrition for patients with severe weight loss [36]. As patient reported outcomes (PROs) have become of particular importance in pancreatic cancer due to the elderly cohort of patients, a recent addition has been patient-centred PROs into the ERAS pathway [117,118].

The degree of compliance with ERAS pathways is strongly associated with clinical outcome [119]. With numerous components, intensive monitoring of the pathway with regular audit and a dedicated specialist nurse input improves compliance. An evaluation into the feasibility of an ERAS pathway after PD has demonstrated over 70% compliance achieved within a multicentre cohort study and was associated with a significant reduction of overall complications and length of stay [120].

ERAS after pancreatic surgery have been associated with a reduction in mild complications (Clavien Dindo grade I-II) significant improvements in overall morbidity and length of stay without any increase in readmission [121–125]. Effect on pancreatic specific complications is difficult to interpret as studies have variably included PD and distal pancreatectomy and ISGPS definitions have not been consistently reported for delayed gastric emptying (DGE) and postoperative pancreatic fistula (POPF) However, a lower incidence of DGE has been observed with no effect on POPF rate [122,123,125].

Implementation of ERAS pathways has been hindered due to the economic impact associated with the necessary resources required, namely a specialist nurse, audit and data collection and patient information booklets [126]. However, these costs, have been offset by the reduction in postoperative complications and subsequent hospital length of stay [127].

Though the short-term benefits are evident, long term benefits have also been suggested by one study where a relationship between increased compliance to the ERAS pathway and survival benefit has been found [128].

3.2. Reducing Complications from Surgery

Surgery alone, is a poor treatment for pancreatic cancer. Only with associated receipt of chemotherapy do patients gain a good chance for cure. One major barrier to patients receiving adjuvant therapy is the occurrence of post-operative complications. Thus, strategies to reduce these are attractive not only to improve perioperative outcomes but improve the delivery of adjuvant therapy. Post-operative pancreatic fistula (POPF) is the most frequent and severe complication after surgery [129]. Presently there is no widely accepted approach to reducing rates of clinically relevant POPF but a national study of early detection and minimally invasive treatment of POPF aims to determine whether the severity of POPF can be reduced [130].

An individual patient's risk of POPF varies hugely. It is somewhat remarkable that POPF rates are not routinely adjusted to take this into account. Individual surgeons risk adjustment and CUSUM analysis is a way for surgeons to objectively assess their outcomes [131]. Such strategies could help inform surgeons of optimal techniques.

Strategies to improve outcomes after complex procedures such as pancreatoduodenectomy, evolve from a critical understanding of events and outcomes. Without critical analysis background noise, variations in practice and organisational differences can make this task insensitive. Determining the root causes of mortality after pancreatectomy demonstrates this well [129]. Only by conducting in depth analyses of processes and outcomes can surgeons begin to understand fundamental reasons for failure. Solutions can then be developed which are designed to overcome problems which are prevalent at the local level. Solutions are likely to vary from centre to centre dependent upon variation in practice and outcome.

A further key improvement is to determine benchmarks of optimal outcomes. This strategy seeks to reduce the effect of variation in practice between centres by focussing on common factors between centres and avoiding outlier cases. In pancreatic cancer, this has allowed teams to compare outcomes to those of their peers after surgery for resectable cancer or with associated venous resection [132,133].

Taking the concept of assimilated gains, the Dutch are leading the way with a nationwide implementation of best practices based upon critical analysis of pathways and suboptimal outcomes with the PACAP-1 trial which seeks to improve outcomes and overall survival [134]. Table 5: Summary of Peri-operative areas for gain

Table 5. Summary of Peri-operative areas for gain.

Areas for Gain Peri-Operatively	Problem	Intervention	Gain
ERAS	- Protocol compliance - Standardisation of practice	- Standardised practices based upon best evidence - Routine audit	- Reduced complications - Reduced Hospital Costs - Reduced LoS
Reducing complications	- QI programs - Benchmarking - Root cause analysis	- Improved outcomes with POPF though systematic changes and better understanding of risk - Benchmarking and root cause analysis demonstrate where local outcomes fall below expected outcomes or those of peers	- Reduced complications and reduced harm from complications - Improved access to adjuvant chemotherapy - More rapid functional recovery after surgery
Correction of PEI related malnutrition	- See Table 2	- Junior Dr education - Patient education - PERT prescribing check - Dietetic review - See Table 4	- See Table 4

ERAS = Enhanced Recovery after Surgery, QI = Quality Improvement, POPF = Post-Operative Pancreatic Fistula, LoS = Length of Stay, PERT = Pancreatic Exocrine Replacement Therapy.

4. Post-Operative Pathways

Post-operative strategies should be designed to enhance functional recovery, maximise uptake of adjuvant chemotherapy and delivering appropriate surveillance. Care should be continuous and multidisciplinary, with continued nutritional consideration (as outlined in the pre-operative section). Functional decline and lack of chemotherapy uptake is more pronounced in elderly.

4.1. Adjuvant Therapy in Resectable Pancreatic Cancer

The benefit for adjuvant therapy is without question. Alone surgery achieves cure in less than 10% of patients [3,135]. Currently, a multimodal approach is the standard of care where 6 months of mFOLFIRINOX based on the results of PRODIGE-24 RCT for those with a sufficient performance status, or a combination of gemcitabine and capecitabine based on ESPAC-4 RCT [136,137]. Patients not sufficiently fit for combination therapy may still benefit from gemcitabine. The role of adjuvant therapy following neoadjuvant therapy and resection, however, is less clear. A recent multi-centre international study demonstrated that adjuvant chemotherapy following NAT, was only of benefit among patients with node positive disease [138].

Widespread variation in the use of adjuvant therapy is clear between and within countries. For example, studies demonstrate that 51% of patients receive adjuvant therapy in the USA, 54% in the Netherlands, 66% in Japan and 74% in Canada. Widespread variation within countries is also evident [139–142]. Within the Netherlands, rates of adjuvant therapy varied from 26 to 74% between health care providers. Sociodemographic variation explains some variation with deprived patients less likely to receive therapy [143]. Advanced age is a common factor associated with underuse of adjuvant therapy and will be considered separately below. However, such wide differences cannot be explained by demographic differences alone. Such data clearly points at systematic variation. Such variation is clearly undesirable and yet, despite the clear advantage of adjuvant therapy, there is little emphasis upon ensuring that patients chances of receiving therapy are optimized [144]. This low completion rate of the full therapeutic sequence may in part be explained by the reticence to initiate adjuvant chemotherapy following postoperative complications or poor performance status. However, ESPAC-3 has addressed this issue of time to initiate and optimal duration of chemotherapy [145]. Within this study, 68% of patients completed all six cycles of chemotherapy and for these patients, overall survival was significantly favoured. In those who did complete therapy, there was no difference in survival when comparing those who started earlier than eight weeks compared to those who started between 8 and 12 weeks, therefore time to initiation of chemotherapy was an important prognostic factor in favour of later treatment. Thus, this study concluded that completion of chemotherapy rather than early initiation was more important for survival.

Centralised cancer surgery is widely practiced. However, centralised chemotherapy is not standard practice. There is evidence that concentrating adjuvant therapy to a dedicated regional service increases the proportion of patients that receive therapy [146]. Overcoming nihilistic views and patients fear of therapy are important strategies as many patients choose not to pursue chemotherapy and clinicians not referring patients for chemotherapy is a mindset in great need of change [147].

A further variable that must be considered is not simply whether a patient receives adjuvant therapy but that efforts must focus upon an individualised approach where patients receive a regime that is as strong as can be tolerated for that individual. Incremental gains of multiagent therapy are seen over single agent gemcitabine [3,135,137]. Yet, there is very little data upon strategies to optimise not just the delivery of adjuvant therapy but also the regimen that is delivered. Some evidence supports centralised care to deliver more multiagent therapy [147].

Liquid biopsies are a novel way to diagnose cancer at an early stage, aid in prognostic evaluation [148], determine targets for therapy [149] and to evaluate cancer recurrence after treatment. The technique involves determining cancer DNA, vesicles and tumour cells in circulating blood [150,151]. Nomograms can be used to stratify patient risk for selection to treatment and may influence the choice of NAT, surgery or nature of adjuvant chemotherapy [152–156].

4.2. Benefits of and Access to Chemotherapy in the Elderly Population

After resection of pancreatic cancer, disease free survival (DFS) and disease specific survival (DSS) appear similar between elderly and younger patients, but overall survival (OS) is shorter, a possible reflection that elderly patients are less likely to receive adjuvant chemotherapy [86,157–159]. Elderly patients have just as much benefit from adjuvant therapy as younger patients and when chemotherapy use is stratified between young and older patients overall survival is the same [160]. The CONKO-001 trial had no upper age limit and specifically demonstrated that those over 65 show a similar improvement in OS and DFS as have numerous other studies evaluating adjuvant chemotherapy for pancreatic cancer [137,159,161–163]. This benefit is maintained when considering more aggressive regimens in the elderly such as FOLFIRINOX or neo-adjuvant chemotherapy [164–166].

Consequently, strategies to increase the use of chemotherapy in the elderly, such as centralisation of oncology services and measures to address frailty, yield major benefits [146,167]. The comprehensive geriatric assessment (CGA) is recommended by the Society for International Oncology in Geriatrics as a useful decision making tool for older people with malignancy [168]. There are several studies suggesting that the CGA can be useful in predicting functional decline, toxicity and overall survival [169,170] The CGA is lengthy and time consuming, a more practical approach, as recommended by the National Comprehensive Cancer Network, the European Organisation for Research and Treatment of Cancer and the International Society of Geriatric Oncology is to use a short frailty screening tool (such as the Fried score, the Clinical Frailty Scale or the Geriatric 8) to identify those who require a full screening [171–177].

Like surgery, the benefits of chemotherapy are not lessened by age and therefore older patients with appropriate performance status should not be denied access. Treatment decisions should be made in a multidisciplinary setting and include the use of a frailty screening tool and the input of a geriatrician to avoid discrepancies in treatment based on chronological age [95,96].

Since there are no published accepted standards for the proportion of patients that receive adjuvant therapy after pancreatic cancer surgery there is lack of clarity about what is acceptable practice. Thus, local audit and benchmarking one's practice against peers is an essential step in the standardisation of practices. Quality improvement programs could further enhance delivery of adjuvant chemotherapy if they were to target those patients most at risk of not receiving therapy, i.e., to overcome barriers presented by age, frailty and good functional recovery after surgery.

4.3. Surveillance after Resection of Pancreatic Cancer

Surveillance after resection of other cancer types is routine and evidence based. The notion is simple, that early detection of recurrence is more likely to identify disease at an earlier asymptomatic phase when patients are more likely to have preserved performance status and ultimately more likely to receive treatment. Most guidelines, including those from the European Society for Medical Oncology (ESMO) and International Association of Pancreatology/European Pancreatic Club (IAP/EPC), do not recommend routine surveillance after pancreatic cancer resection due to the poor prognosis and limited treatment options available for recurrence [178,179]. The nature of surveillance protocols typically involve CT scans at 3 or 6 month intervals supplemented by CA19-9 analysis. The optimal interval and impact of surveillance programs remain to be seen. It may be that artificial intelligence may help refine and improve surveillance programs; there is currently much interest in AI as a tool to facilitate the diagnosis of breast cancer within screening programs.

In the setting of recurrent pancreatic cancer there are an increasing number of treatment strategies. Despite this, many patients fail to receive palliative therapy. However, an individualised approach to treating recurrent pancreatic cancer is logical. Around half of all patients recur with local only disease [180]. Whilst systemic therapy seeks to control occult metastatic disease local therapies in the form of high intensity radiotherapy or ablation can be delivered [181]. Given that many patients are elderly, frail or may have had poor experience with systemic therapy local therapy can be delivered with more less disruption and more satisfaction for the patient. Targeted therapy of oligometastatic disease also offers alternative options for a limited number of patients. Furthermore, surveillance is desired by patients and clinicians alike [182,183]. Table 6: Areas for Post-operative gain.

Table 6. Areas for Post-operative gain.

Areas for Gain Post-Operatively	Problem	Intervention	Gain
Adjuvant chemotherapy	- Nihilism and under-utilisation of adjuvant chemotherapy	- Establish standards of practice and benchmarks for the proportion of patients that receive adjuvant therapy - QI programs to address frailty, advanced age and recovery after surgery	- Improved uptake of adjuvant therapy - Improved survival - Standardised practices
Surveillance	- Lack of standardised practice - Nihilism	- Implement surveillance programs	- Improved detection of early recurrence - Improved treatment rates - Improved duration of survival
Nutrition	- See Table 4	- Education of local physicians and those in palliative care - See Table 4	- See Table 4

QI = Quality improvement.

5. Novel Areas for Review

Though this body of work focusses upon areas where benefit can be clearly derived using existing evidence base there are areas with an emerging evidence base where benefit may be derived if practices are adopted.

Pancreatic surgery is associated with a high rate of cancer recurrence. Improving the staging pathways and novel approaches to treatment of the surgical margin are ways to improve outcomes.

Early cancer recurrence, even within ninety days of surgery, has to be considered a failure of staging [129]. The addition of routine Positron Emission Topography (PET) or Magnetic resonance imaging (MRI) scanning can help detect occult cancer. PET scanning, within a randomised trial, upstaged 20% of patients, preventing futile surgery [184]. However, it is important to note that the routine use of PET-CT is still debatable as it cause delays to resection and the potentially false positive results that may erroneously prevent surgery [185,186]. MRI can upstage 10–24% of patients with occult liver metastases where diffusion weight images can identify lesions under 5 mm, being more sensitive than computerised tomography (CT) or PET-CT [187–189]. These tests need to be considered carefully, however, as false positive results can be caused by common scenarios such as abscesses secondary to cholangitis and can delay treatment.

Failure of surgery to clear the margin is an Achilles heel of pancreatoduodenectomy. Local recurrence is very high after surgery, positive margins are associated with reduced survival and therefore it is necessary to consider how outcomes can be improved [190,191]. Neoadjuvant therapy (NAT) is associated with a higher rate of R0 resections, though it is important to consider results on an intention to treat basis [192,193]. There is much interest in NAT for resectable pancreatic cancer. Ongoing clinical trials will help determine the evidence base for this treatment. There are many retrospective cohort studies which are at risk of various bias including selection and survivor bias and until well conducted trial data is available it is not possible to make a clear statement [194]. Intraoperative frozen section has been used to identify positive pancreatic transection margins and the role of extending resections has been explored in numerous studies, but systematic review fails to observe a benefit to this practice [193]. Similarly, extending lymphadenectomy is not associated with greater survival but with morbidity [195,196]. The standard approach to pancreatoduodenectomy leaves perineural tissue around the superior mesenteric artery. It is this margin which is most frequently positive on histologic analysis. An artery first approach has a theoretical advantage that it can clear periadventitial tissues but clinical studies fail to demonstrate benefit in terms of improving R0 margin status [197,198]. Intraoperative radiotherapy has been long considered as an adjunct to improving margin status but no high-level evidence yet exists [199]. The addition of stereotactic ablative radiotherapy within a NAT program does not appear to improve R0 rates [200]. Irreversible electroporation has gained interest, predominantly surrounding control of locally advanced pancreatic cancer though the technology could be applied to improve margin control at resectable cancer. However, concerns over safety and a lack of high level evidence remain [201]. There is thus much work to be done in this area and focussing efforts on the problem of the surgical margin could reduce local recurrence.

Peritoneal metastases are less common than local recurrent or liver metastases but when they occur are associated with very poor outcomes. Positive intraoperative peritoneal cytology correlates with poor oncologic outcomes, in the absence of visible metastatic disease [202]. Among patients with cytology positive, or even macroscopic peritoneal disease, intraperitoneal chemotherapy can control ascites and some patients can go on to achieve surgical resection [203,204]. Such experience is limited to Japan. The remarkable outcomes indicate a potential role for intraperitoneal therapy, challenge current beliefs about pancreatic cancer biology and prognosis and merit a wider review.

Personalised medicine in pancreatic cancer care is most strongly associated with defining an individual's cancer genetics. Large multinational, multicentre organisations/trials are ongoing such as precisionpanc (https://precisionpanc.org, accessed on 10 January 2021). There have, however, been many negative trials of genetic targets among patients with metastatic pancreatic cancer which include MEK inhibitors, IGFR inhibitors, mTOR inhibitors, TRK inhibitors, NOTCH inhibitors, TGF-β inhibitors, immunotherapy or vaccine therapy [205]. Established genetic targets in resectable pancreatic cancer are thus largely unclear; the most actionable mutation is BRCA1-2 which is identified in approximately 5% of patients [206]. Patients with these tumours are sensitive to platinum agents and thus will be treated by inclusion of oxaliplatin in therapy regimens [207]. This target has also been exploited by the PARP inhibitor Olaparib [208].

6. Conclusions

This review sought to elucidate key areas of variation, undertreatment and pathway changes where improvements can be realised with little effort. Novel therapeutic options will present themselves in the future, but it would be remiss of any team caring for this cohort of patients to inadequately utilise current evidence and implement optimal treatment pathways. There is a disconnect between funding for research to establish novel treatments far outstripping funding to implement best care at the level of the health care provider/organisation. It is essential that surgeons understand that surgery is just one part of a complex pathway and that they are ideally placed to act as change agents to optimise broader pathway improvements. Some changes can be clearly applied to the majority, if not all patients, such as PERT among those undergoing pancreatoduodenectomy. Other interventions can never be applied to all patients. There will always be some jaundiced patients with resectable cancer that undergo PBD or some patients who never receive adjuvant therapy. Locally, nationally or internationally accepted benchmarks are required to understand what is achievable and to help teams identify areas of poor performance. Collaborative multicentre, multinational studies are an essential part of assessing and improving patient care in the 21st century and teams are encouraged to develop and take part in these ventures. Through the aggregation of marginal gains, our patients can realise better outcomes and experience in the near future.

Author Contributions: K.J.R.: Conception and design, Supervision, Writing—Review and editing; R.P. and S.P.-B.; Research and writing—original draft preparation, in equal parts. All authors have read and agreed to the published version of the manuscript.

Funding: This research received no external funding.

Institutional Review Board Statement: Not applicable.

Informed Consent Statement: Not applicable.

Data Availability Statement: Not applicable.

Conflicts of Interest: The authors declare no conflict of interest.

References

1. Rahib, L.; Smith, B.D.; Aizenberg, R.; Rosenzweig, A.B.; Fleshman, J.M.; Matrisian, L.M. Projecting Cancer Incidence and Deaths to 2030: The Unexpected Burden of Thyroid, Liver, and Pancreas Cancers in the United States. *Cancer Res.* **2014**, *74*, 2913–2921. [CrossRef]
2. Rawla, P.; Sunkara, T.; Gaduputi, V. Epidemiology of Pancreatic Cancer: Global Trends, Etiology and Risk Factors. *World J. Oncol.* **2019**, *10*, 10–27. [CrossRef] [PubMed]
3. Neoptolemos, J.; Dunn, J.; Stocken, D.; Almond, J.; Link, K.; Beger, H.; Bassi, C.; Falconi, M.; Pederzoli, P.; Dervenis, C.; et al. Adjuvant chemoradiotherapy and chemotherapy in resectable pancreatic cancer: A randomised controlled trial. *Lancet* **2001**, *358*, 1576–1585. [CrossRef]
4. Panagiotopoulou, I.G.; Bennett, J.; Tweedle, E.M.; Di Saverio, S.; Gourgiotis, S.; Hardwick, R.H.; Wheeler, J.; Davies, R.J. Enhancing the emergency general surgical service: An example of the aggregation of marginal gains. *Ann. R. Coll. Surg. Engl.* **2019**, *101*, 479–486. [CrossRef] [PubMed]
5. Thomson, K.J.; Peggs, K.S. Allogeneic transplantation in the UK: An aggregation of marginal gains? *Br. J. Haematol.* **2013**, *163*, 149–159. [CrossRef] [PubMed]
6. Durrand, J.W.; Batterham, A.M.; Danjoux, G.R. Pre-habilitation. I: Aggregation of marginal gains. *Anaesthesia* **2014**, *69*, 403–406. [CrossRef] [PubMed]
7. Haeno, H.; Gonen, M.; Davis, M.B.; Herman, J.M.; Iacobuzio-Donahue, C.A.; Michor, F. Computational Modeling of Pancreatic Cancer Reveals Kinetics of Metastasis Suggesting Optimum Treatment Strategies. *Cell* **2012**, *148*, 362–375. [CrossRef]
8. Lygidakis, N.J.; Van Der Heyde, M.N.; Lubbers, M.J. Evaluation of preoperative biliary drainage in the surgical management of pancreatic head carcinoma. *Acta Chir. Scand.* **1987**, *153*, 665–668.
9. Whipple, A.O.; Parsons, W.B.; Mullins, C.R. Treatment of Carcinoma of the Ampulla Of Vater. *Ann. Surg.* **1935**, *102*, 763–779. [CrossRef]
10. Glenn, F.; Evans, J.A.; Mujahed, Z.; Thorbjarnarson, B. Percutaneous transhepatic cholangiography. *Ann. Surg.* **1962**, *156*, 451–460. [CrossRef]
11. Phoa, S.S.K.S.; Reeders, J.W.A.J.; Rauws, E.A.J.; De Wit, L.; Gouma, D.J.; Laméris, J.S. Spiral computed tomography for preoperative staging of potentially resectable carcinoma of the pancreatic head. *Br. J. Surg.* **1999**, *86*, 789–794. [CrossRef]
12. Katz, M.H.G.; Marsh, R.; Herman, J.M.; Shi, Q.; Collison, E.; Venook, A.P.; Kindler, H.L.; Alberts, S.R.; Philip, P.; Lowy, A.M.; et al. Borderline Resectable Pancreatic Cancer: Need for Standardization and Methods for Optimal Clinical Trial Design. *Ann. Surg. Oncol.* **2013**, *20*, 2787–2795. [CrossRef]
13. Van der Gaag, N.A.; de Castro, S.M.; Rauws, E.A.; Bruno, M.J.; van Eijck, C.H.; Kuipers, E.J.; Gerritsen, J.G.M.; Rutten, J.-P.; Greve, J.W.; Hesselink, E.J.; et al. Preoperative biliary drainage for periampullary tumors causing obstructive jaundice; DR ainage vs. (direct) OP eration (DROP-trial). *BMC Surg.* **2007**, *7*, 3.
14. Sahora, K.; Morales-Oyarvide, V.; Ferrone, C.; Fong, Z.V.; Warshaw, A.L.; And, K.D.L.; Castillo, C.F.-D. Preoperative biliary drainage does not increase major complications in pancreaticoduodenectomy: A large single center experience from the Massachusetts General Hospital. *J. Hepatobiliary Pancreat. Sci.* **2016**, *23*, 181–187. [CrossRef]
15. Herzog, T.; Belyaev, O.; Akkuzu, R.; Hölling, J.; Uhl, W.; Chromik, A.M. The Impact of Bile Duct Cultures on Surgical Site Infections in Pancreatic Surgery. *Surg. Infect.* **2015**, *16*, 443–449. [CrossRef]
16. Mohammed, S.; Evans, C.; VanBuren, G.; Hodges, S.E.; Silberfein, E.; Artinyan, A.; Mo, Q.; Issazadeh, M.; McElhany, A.L.; Fisher, W.E. Treatment of bacteriobilia decreases wound infection rates after pancreaticoduodenectomy. *HPB* **2014**, *16*, 592–598. [CrossRef]
17. Cavell, L.K.; Allen, P.J.; Vinoya, C.; Eaton, A.A.; Gonen, M.; Gerdes, H.; Mendelsohn, R.B.; D'Angelica, M.I.; Kingham, P.T.; Fong, Y.; et al. Biliary Self-Expandable Metal Stents Do Not Adversely Affect Pancreaticoduodenectomy. *Am. J. Gastroenterol.* **2013**, *108*, 1168–1173. [CrossRef]
18. Coates, J.M.; Beal, S.H.; Russo, J.E.; Vanderveen, K.A.; Chen, S.L.; Bold, R.J.; Canter, R.J. Negligible Effect of Selective Preoperative Biliary Drainage on Perioperative Resuscitation, Morbidity, and Mortality in Patients Undergoing Pancreaticoduodenectomy. *Arch. Surg.* **2009**, *144*, 841–847. [CrossRef]
19. Tol, J.A.M.G.; Van Hooft, J.E.; Timmer, R.; Kubben, F.J.G.M.; Van Der Harst, E.; De Hingh, I.H.J.T.; Vleggaar, F.P.; Molenaar, I.Q.; Keulemans, Y.C.A.; Boerma, D.; et al. Metal or plastic stents for preoperative biliary drainage in resectable pancreatic cancer. *Gut* **2016**, *65*, 1981–1987. [CrossRef]

20. Liu, P.; Lin, H.; Chen, Y.; Wu, Y.-S.; Tang, M.; Liu, C. Comparison of Metal and Plastic Stents for Preoperative Biliary Drainage in Resectable and Borderline Resectable Periampullary Cancer: A Meta-Analysis and System Review. *J. Laparoendosc. Adv. Surg. Tech.* **2018**, *28*, 1074–1082. [CrossRef]
21. Lee, P.J.; Podugu, A.; Wu, D.; Lee, A.C.; Stevens, T.; Windsor, J.A. Preoperative biliary drainage in resectable pancreatic cancer: A systematic review and network meta-analysis. *HPB* **2018**, *20*, 477–486. [CrossRef] [PubMed]
22. Sanjeevi, S.; Ivanics, T.; Lundell, L.; Kartalis, N.; Andrén-Sandberg, Å.; Blomberg, J.; Del Chiaro, M.; Ansorge, C. Impact of delay between imaging and treatment in patients with potentially curable pancreatic cancer. *Br. J. Surg.* **2016**, *103*, 267–275. [CrossRef] [PubMed]
23. Glant, J.A.; Waters, J.A.; House, M.G.; Zyromski, N.J.; Nakeeb, A.; Pitt, H.A.; Lillemoe, K.D.; Schmidt, C.M. Does the interval from imaging to operation affect the rate of unanticipated metastasis encountered during operation for pancreatic adenocarcinoma? *Surgery* **2011**, *150*, 607–616. [CrossRef] [PubMed]
24. Raman, S.P.; Reddy, S.; Weiss, M.J.; Manos, L.L.; Cameron, J.L.; Zheng, L.; Herman, J.M.; Hruban, R.H.; Fishman, E.K.; Wolfgang, C.L. Impact of the time interval between MDCT imaging and surgery on the accuracy of identifying metastatic disease in patients with pancreatic cancer. *Am. J. Roentgenol.* **2015**, *204*, W37–W42. [CrossRef]
25. Müller, P.C.; Hodson, J.; Kuemmerli, C.; Kalisvaart, M.; Pande, R.; Roberts, K.J. Effect of time to surgery in resectable pancreatic cancer: A systematic review and meta-analysis. *Langenbeck's Arch. Surg.* **2020**, *405*, 293–302. [CrossRef]
26. Pande, R.; Hodson, J.; Marudanayagam, R.; Chatzizacharis, N.A.; Dasari, B.; Muiesan, P.; Sutcliffe, R.P.; Mirza, D.F.; Isaac, J.; Roberts, K.J. Survival Advantage of Upfront Surgery for Pancreatic Head Cancer Without Preoperative Biliary Drainage. *Front. Oncol.* **2020**, *10*, 526514. [CrossRef]
27. Sauvanet, A.; Boher, J.-M.; Paye, F.; Bachellier, P.; Cuhna, A.S.; Le Treut, Y.-P.; Adham, M.; Mabrut, J.-Y.; Chiche, L.; Delpero, J.-R. Severe Jaundice Increases Early Severe Morbidity and Decreases Long-Term Survival after Pancreaticoduodenectomy for Pancreatic Adenocarcinoma. *J. Am. Coll. Surg.* **2015**, *221*, 380–389. [CrossRef]
28. National Guideline A. *National Institute for Health and Care Excellence: Clinical Guidelines. Pancreatic Cancer in Adults: Diagnosis and Management*; National Institute for Health and Care Excellence: London, UK, 2018.
29. Pande, R.; Hodson, J.; Marudanayagam, R.; Mirza, D.; Isaac, J.; Roberts, K.J. Venous resection at pancreaticoduodenectomy can be safely performed in the presence of jaundice. *Hepatobiliary Pancreat. Dis. Int.* **2020**, *19*, 488–491. [CrossRef]
30. Dolejs, S.; Zarzaur, B.L.; Zyromski, N.J.; Pitt, H.A.; Riall, T.S.; Hall, B.L.; Behrman, S.W. Does Hyperbilirubinemia Contribute to Adverse Patient Outcomes Following Pancreatoduodenectomy? *J. Gastrointest. Surg.* **2017**, *21*, 647–656. [CrossRef]
31. El Nakeeb, A.; Salem, A.; Mahdy, Y.; El Dosoky, M.; Said, R.; Ellatif, M.A.; Ezzat, H.; Elsabbagh, A.M.; Hamed, H.; Abd Alah, T.; et al. Value of preoperative biliary drainage on postoperative outcome after pancreaticoduodenectomy: A case-control study. *Asian J. Surg.* **2018**, *41*, 155–162. [CrossRef]
32. Yoon, K.W.; Heo, J.S.; Choi, D.W.; Choi, S.H. Factors affecting long-term survival after surgical resection of pancreatic ductal adenocarcinoma. *J. Korean Surg. Soc.* **2011**, *81*, 394–401. [CrossRef]
33. Berberat, P.; Künzli, B.; Gulbinas, A.; Ramanauskas, T.; Kleeff, J.; Müller, M.; Wagner, M.; Friess, H.; Büchler, M. An audit of outcomes of a series of periampullary carcinomas. *Eur. J. Surg. Oncol.* **2009**, *35*, 187–191. [CrossRef]
34. Topal, B.; Aerts, R.; Hendrickx, T.; Fieuws, S.; Penninckx, F. Determinants of complications in pancreaticoduodenectomy. *Eur. J. Surg. Oncol.* **2007**, *33*, 488–492. [CrossRef]
35. Gilsdorf, R.B.; Spanos, P. Factors influencing morbidity and mortality in pancreaticoduodenectomy. *Ann Surg.* **1973**, *177*, 332–337.
36. MMelloul, E.; Lassen, K.; Roulin, D.; Grass, F.; Perinel, J.; Adham, M.; Wellge, E.B.; Kunzler, F.; Besselink, M.G.; Asbun, H.; et al. Guidelines for Perioperative Care for Pancreatoduodenectomy: Enhanced Recovery After Surgery (ERAS) Recommendations 2019. *World J. Surg.* **2020**, *44*, 2056–2084. [CrossRef]
37. Li, Z.; Zhang, Z.; Hu, W.; Zeng, Y.; Liu, X.; Mai, G.; Zhang, Y.; Lu, H.; Tian, B. Pancreaticoduodenectomy with preoperative obstructive jaundice: Drainage or not. *Pancreas* **2009**, *38*, 379–386. [CrossRef]
38. Pamecha, V.; Patil, N.S.; Kumar, S.; Rajendran, V.; Gupta, S.; Sasturkar, S.V.; Sinha, P.K.; Arora, A.; Agarwal, N.; Baghmar, S. Upfront pancreaticoduodenectomy in severely jaundiced patients: Is it safe? *J. Hepatobiliary Pancreat. Sci.* **2019**, *26*, 524–533. [CrossRef]
39. Van der Gaag, N.A.; Rauws, E.A.; van Eijck, C.H.; Bruno, M.J.; van der Harst, E.; Kubben, F.J.; Gerritsen, J.J.G.M.; Greve, J.W.; Gerhards, M.F.; de Hingh, I.H.J.T.; et al. Preoperative biliary drainage for cancer of the head of the pancreas. *N. Engl. J. Med.* **2010**, *362*, 129–137. [CrossRef]
40. Padillo, F.J.; Andicoberry, B.; Naranjo, A.; Miño, G.; Pera, C.; Sitges-Serra, A. Anorexia and the effect of internal biliary drainage on food intake in patients with obstructive jaundice. *J. Am. Coll. Surg.* **2001**, *192*, 584–590. [CrossRef]
41. Padillo, F.J.; Andicoberry, B.; Muntane, J.; Lozano, J.M.; Miño, G.; Sitges-Serra, A.; Pera-Madrazo, C. Factors Predicting Nutritional Derangements in Patients with Obstructive Jaundice: Multivariate Analysis. *World J. Surg.* **2001**, *25*, 413–418. [CrossRef]
42. Tomasulo, P.A.; Levin, J.; Murphy, P.A.; Winkelstein, J.A. Biological activities of tritiated endotoxins: Correlation of the Limulus lysate assay with rabbit pyrogen and complement-activation assays for endotoxin. *J. Lab. Clin. Med.* **1977**, *89*, 308–315. [PubMed]
43. Mullen, J.L.; Buzby, G.P.; Matthews, D.C.; Smale, B.F.; Rosato, E.F. Reduction of operative morbidity and mortality by combined preoperative and postoperative nutritional support. *Ann. Surg.* **1980**, *192*, 604–613. [CrossRef] [PubMed]

44. Buzby, G.P.; Williford, W.O.; Peterson, O.L.; Crosby, L.O.; Page, C.P.; Reinhardt, G.F.; Mullen, J.L. A randomized clinical trial of total parenteral nutrition in malnourished surgical patients: The rationale and impact of previous clinical trials and pilot study on protocol design. *Am. J. Clin. Nutr.* **1988**, *47* (Suppl. S2), 357–365. [CrossRef]
45. Von Meyenfeldt, M.F.; Meijerink, W.J.; Rouflart, M.M.; Builmaassen, M.T.; Soeters, P.B. Perioperative nutritional support: A randomised clinical trial. *Clin. Nutr.* **1992**, *11*, 180–186. [CrossRef]
46. Roberts, K.; Bannister, C.; Schrem, H. Enzyme replacement improves survival among patients with pancreatic cancer: Results of a population based study. *Pancreatology* **2019**, *19*, 114–121. [CrossRef] [PubMed]
47. Benini, L.; Amodio, A.; Campagnola, P.; Agugiaro, F.; Cristofori, C.; Micciolo, R.; Magro, A.; Gabbrielli, A.; Cabrini, G.; Moser, L.; et al. Fecal elastase-1 is useful in the detection of steatorrhea in patients with pancreatic diseases but not after pancreatic resection. *Pancreatology* **2013**, *13*, 38–42. [CrossRef] [PubMed]
48. Tseng, D.S.; Molenaar, I.Q.; Besselink, M.G.; van Eijck, C.H.; Borel Rinkes, I.H.; van Santvoort, H.C. Pancreatic Exocrine Insufficiency in Patients With Pancreatic or Periampullary Cancer: A Systematic Review. *Pancreas* **2016**, *45*, 325–330. [CrossRef] [PubMed]
49. Sikkens, E.C.M.; Cahen, D.L.; de Wit, J.; Looman, C.W.; van Eijck, C.; Bruno, M.J. A prospective assessment of the natural course of the exocrine pancreatic function in patients with a pancreatic head tumor. *J. Clin. Gastroenterol.* **2014**, *48*, e43–e46. [CrossRef]
50. Lemaire, E.; O'Toole, D.; Sauvanet, A.; Hammel, P.; Belghiti, J.; Ruszniewski, P. Functional and morphological changes in the pancreatic remnant following pancreaticoduodenectomy with pancreaticogastric anastomosis. *Br. J. Surg.* **2000**, *87*, 434–438. [CrossRef]
51. Singh, V.K.; Haupt, M.E.; Geller, D.E.; Hall, J.A.; Diez, P.M.Q. Less common etiologies of exocrine pancreatic insufficiency. *World J. Gastroenterol.* **2017**, *23*, 7059–7076. [CrossRef]
52. Sikkens, E.C.M.; Cahen, D.L.; de Wit, J.; Looman, C.W.; van Eijck, C.; Bruno, M.J. Prospective assessment of the influence of pancreatic cancer resection on exocrine pancreatic function. *Br. J. Surg.* **2014**, *101*, 109–113. [CrossRef]
53. Dominguez-Muñoz, J.E. Diagnosis and treatment of pancreatic exocrine insufficiency. *Curr. Opin. Gastroenterol.* **2018**, *34*, 349–354. [CrossRef]
54. Johnson, C.D.; Williamson, N.; Solingen, G.J.-V.; Arbuckle, R.; Johnson, C.; Simpson, S.; Staab, D.; Dominguez-Munoz, E.; Levy, P.; Connett, G.; et al. Psychometric evaluation of a patient-reported outcome measure in pancreatic exocrine insufficiency (PEI). *Pancreatology* **2019**, *19*, 182–190. [CrossRef]
55. Johnson, C.D.; Arbuckle, R.; Bonner, N.; Connett, G.; Dominguez-Munoz, E.; Levy, P.; Staab, D.; Williamson, N.; Lerch, M.M. Qualitative Assessment of the Symptoms and Impact of Pancreatic Exocrine Insufficiency (PEI) to Inform the Development of a Patient-Reported Outcome (PRO) Instrument. *Patient Patient Centered Outcomes Res.* **2017**, *10*, 615–628. [CrossRef]
56. Sikkens, E.C.M.; Cahen, D.L.; de Wit, J.; Looman, C.W.; van Eijck, C.; Bruno, M.J. The daily practice of pancreatic enzyme replacement therapy after pancreatic surgery: A northern European survey: Enzyme replacement after surgery. *J Gastrointest Surg.* **2012**, *16*, 1487–1492. [CrossRef]
57. RICOCHET Study Group; West Midlands Research Collaborative. Receipt of Curative Resection or Palliative Care for Hepatopancreaticobiliary Tumours (RICOCHET): Protocol for a Nationwide Collaborative Observational Study. *JMIR Res. Protoc.* **2019**, *8*, e13566. [CrossRef]
58. Landers, A.; Muircroft, W.; Brown, H. Pancreatic enzyme replacement therapy (PERT) for malabsorption in patients with metastatic pancreatic cancer. *BMJ Support. Palliat. Care* **2014**, *6*, 75–79. [CrossRef]
59. Barkin, J.A.; Westermann, A.; Hoos, W.; Moravek, C.; Matrisian, L.; Wang, H.; Shemanski, L.; Barkin, J.S.; Rahib, L. Frequency of Appropriate Use of Pancreatic Enzyme Replacement Therapy and Symptomatic Response in Pancreatic Cancer Patients. *Pancreas* **2019**, *48*, 780–786. [CrossRef]
60. Lindkvist, B. Diagnosis and treatment of pancreatic exocrine insufficiency. *World J. Gastroenterol.* **2013**, *19*, 7258–7566. [CrossRef]
61. Laterza, L.; Scaldaferri, F.; Bruno, G.; Agnes, A.; Boškoski, I.; Ianiro, G.; Gerardi, V.; Ojetti, V.; Alfieri, S.; Gasbarrini, A. Pancreatic function assessment. *Eur. Rev. Med. Pharmacol. Sci.* **2013**, *17* (Suppl. S2), 65–71.
62. Dominguez-Munoz, J.E.; Nieto, L.; Vilarino, M.; Lourido, M.V.; Iglesias-Garcia, J. Development and Diagnostic Accuracy of a Breath Test for Pancreatic Exocrine Insufficiency in Chronic Pancreatitis. *Pancreas* **2016**, *45*, 241–247. [CrossRef]
63. Lindkvist, B.; Phillips, M.E.; Domínguez-Muñoz, J.E. Clinical, anthropometric and laboratory nutritional markers of pancreatic exocrine insufficiency: Prevalence and diagnostic use. *Pancreatology* **2015**, *15*, 589–597. [CrossRef]
64. Partelli, S.; Frulloni, L.; Minniti, C.; Bassi, C.; Barugola, G.; D'Onofrio, M.; Crippa, S.; Falconi, M. Faecal elastase-1 is an independent predictor of survival in advanced pancreatic cancer. *Dig. Liver Dis.* **2012**, *44*, 945–951. [CrossRef] [PubMed]
65. Gooden, H.M.; White, K.J. Pancreatic cancer and supportive care—Pancreatic exocrine insufficiency negatively impacts on quality of life. *Support. Care Cancer* **2013**, *21*, 1835–1841. [CrossRef]
66. Van Dijk, S.M.; Heerkens, H.D.; Tseng, D.S.J.; Intven, M.; Molenaar, I.Q.; van Santvoort, H.C. Systematic review on the impact of pancreatoduodenectomy on quality of life in patients with pancreatic cancer. *HPB* **2018**, *20*, 204–215. [CrossRef]
67. Heerkens, H.D.; Van Berkel, L.; Tseng, D.S.; Monninkhof, E.M.; Van Santvoort, H.C.; Hagendoorn, J.; Rinkes, I.H.B.; Lips, I.M.; Intven, M.; Molenaar, I.Q. Long-term health-related quality of life after pancreatic resection for malignancy in patients with and without severe postoperative complications. *HPB* **2018**, *20*, 188–195. [CrossRef]

68. Roberts, K.J.; Schrem, H.; Hodson, J.; Angelico, R.; Dasari, B.V.M.; Coldham, C.A.; Marudanayagam, R.; Sutcliffe, R.P.; Muiesan, P.; Isaac, J.; et al. Pancreas exocrine replacement therapy is associated with increased survival following pancreatoduodenectomy for periampullary malignancy. *HPB* **2017**, *19*, 859–867. [CrossRef]
69. Seiler, C.M.; Izbicki, J.; Varga-Szabó, L.; Czako, L.; Fiók, J.; Sperti, C.; Lerch, M.M.; Pezzilli, R.; Vasileva, G.; Pap, A.; et al. Randomised clinical trial: A 1-week, double-blind, placebo-controlled study of pancreatin 25 000 Ph. Eur. minimicrospheres (Creon 25000 MMS) for pancreatic exocrine insufficiency after pancreatic surgery, with a 1-year open-label extension. *Aliment. Pharmacol. Ther.* **2013**, *37*, 691–702. [CrossRef]
70. Braga, M.; Cristallo, M.; De Franchis, R.; Mangiagalli, A.; Zerbi, A.; Agape, D.; Primignani, M.; Di Carlo, V. Pancreatic enzyme replacement therapy in post-pancreatectomy patients. *Int. J. Pancreatol.* **1989**, *5*, 37–44.
71. Landers, A.; Brown, H.; Strother, M. The effectiveness of pancreatic enzyme replacement therapy for malabsorption in advanced pancreatic cancer, a pilot study. *Palliat. Care Res. Treat.* **2019**, *12*, 1178224218825270. [CrossRef] [PubMed]
72. Domínguez-Muñoz, J.E.; Iglesias-García, J.; Iglesias-Rey, M.; Figueiras, A.; Vilariño-Insua, M. Effect of the administration schedule on the therapeutic efficacy of oral pancreatic enzyme supplements in patients with exocrine pancreatic insufficiency: A randomized, three-way crossover study. *Aliment. Pharmacol. Ther.* **2005**, *21*, 993–1000. [CrossRef] [PubMed]
73. Dominguez-Munoz, J.E.; Iglesias-Garcia, J.; Iglesias-Rey, M.; Vilarino-Insua, M. Optimising the therapy of exocrine pancreatic insufficiency by the association of a proton pump inhibitor to enteric coated pancreatic extracts. *Gut* **2006**, *55*, 1056–1057. [CrossRef] [PubMed]
74. Kim, E.; Kang, J.S.; Han, Y.; Kim, H.; Kwon, W.; Kim, J.R.; Kim, S.-W.; Jang, J.-Y. Influence of preoperative nutritional status on clinical outcomes after pancreatoduodenectomy. *HPB* **2018**, *20*, 1051–1061. [CrossRef]
75. Kim, E.; Lee, D.-H.; Jang, J.-Y. Effects of Preoperative Malnutrition on Postoperative Surgical Outcomes and Quality of Life of Elderly Patients with Periampullary Neoplasms: A Single-Center Prospective Cohort Study. *Gut Liver* **2019**, *13*, 690–697. [CrossRef] [PubMed]
76. Gianotti, L.; Besselink, M.G.; Sandini, M.; Hackert, T.; Conlon, K.; Gerritsen, A.; Griffin, O.; Fingerhut, A.; Probst, P.; Abu Hilal, M.; et al. Nutritional support and therapy in pancreatic surgery: A position paper of the International Study Group on Pancreatic Surgery (ISGPS). *Surgery* **2018**, *164*, 1035–1048. [CrossRef]
77. Powell-Brett, S.; Carino, N.D.L.; Roberts, K. Understanding pancreatic exocrine insufficiency and replacement therapy in pancreatic cancer. *Eur. J. Surg. Oncol.* **2021**, *47*, 539–544. [CrossRef] [PubMed]
78. Aida, T.; Furukawa, K.; Suzuki, D.; Shimizu, H.; Yoshidome, H.; Ohtsuka, M.; Kato, A.; Yoshitomi, H.; Miyazaki, M. Preoperative immunonutrition decreases postoperative complications by modulating prostaglandin E2 production and T-cell differentiation in patients undergoing pancreatoduodenectomy. *Surgery* **2014**, *155*, 124–133. [CrossRef]
79. Gade, J.; Levring, T.; Hillingsø, J.; Hansen, C.P.; Andersen, J.R. The Effect of Preoperative Oral Immunonutrition on Complications and Length of Hospital Stay After Elective Surgery for Pancreatic Cancer—A Randomized Controlled Trial. *Nutr. Cancer* **2016**, *68*, 225–233. [CrossRef]
80. Hamza, N.; Darwish, A.; O'Reilly, D.A.; Denton, J.; Sheen, A.J.; Chang, D.; Sherlock, D.J.; Ammori, B.J. Perioperative Enteral Immunonutrition Modulates Systemic and Mucosal Immunity and the Inflammatory Response in Patients With Periampullary Cancer Scheduled for Pancreaticoduodenectomy: A Randomized Clinical Trial. *Pancreas* **2015**, *44*, 41–52. [CrossRef]
81. Silvestri, S.; Franchello, A.; Deiro, G.; Galletti, R.; Cassine, D.; Campra, D.; Bonfanti, D.; De Carli, L.; Fop, F.; Fronda, G. Preoperative oral immunonutrition versus standard preoperative oral diet in well nourished patients undergoing pancreaticoduodenectomy. *Int. J. Surg.* **2016**, *31*, 93–99. [CrossRef]
82. Yang, F.-A.; Chen, Y.-C.; Tiong, C. Immunonutrition in Patients with Pancreatic Cancer Undergoing Surgical Intervention: A Systematic Review and Meta-Analysis of Randomized Controlled Trials. *Nutrition* **2020**, *12*, 2798. [CrossRef] [PubMed]
83. Riall, T.S.; Sheffield, K.M.; Kuo, Y.-F.; Townsend, C.M., Jr.; Goodwin, J.S. Resection Benefits Older Adults with Locoregional Pancreatic Cancer Despite Greater Short-Term Morbidity and Mortality. *J. Am. Geriatr. Soc.* **2011**, *59*, 647–654. [CrossRef] [PubMed]
84. Kanda, M.; Fujii, T.; Suenaga, M.; Takami, H.; Inokawa, Y.; Yamada, S.; Kobayashi, D.; Tanaka, C.; Sugimoto, H.; Nomoto, S.; et al. Pancreatoduodenectomy With Portal Vein Resection Is Feasible and Potentially Beneficial for Elderly Patients With Pancreatic Cancer. *Pancreas* **2014**, *43*, 951–958. [CrossRef] [PubMed]
85. National Cancer Equality Inititative; Pharmaceutical Oncology Initiative. *The Impact of Patient Age on Clinical Decision-Making in Oncology*; Department of Health Cancer Policy Team: London, UK, 2012.
86. Tan, E.; Song, J.; Lam, S.; D'Souza, M.; Crawford, M.; Sandroussi, C. Postoperative outcomes in elderly patients undergoing pancreatic resection for pancreatic adenocarcinoma: A systematic review and meta-analysis. *Int. J. Surg.* **2019**, *72*, 59–68. [CrossRef]
87. Amin, S.; Lucas, A.L.; Frucht, H. Evidence for treatment and survival disparities by age in pancreatic adenocarcinoma: A population-based analysis. *Pancreas* **2013**, *42*, 249–253. [CrossRef]
88. Nipp, R.; Tramontano, A.C.; Kong, C.Y.; Pandharipande, P.; Dowling, E.C.; Schrag, D.; Hur, C. Disparities in cancer outcomes across age, sex, and race/ethnicity among patients with pancreatic cancer. *Cancer Med.* **2018**, *7*, 525–535. [CrossRef]
89. Chandrabalan, V.V.; McMillan, D.C.; Carter, R.; Kinsella, J.; McKay, C.J.; Carter, C.R.; Dickson, E.J. Pre-operative cardiopulmonary exercise testing predicts adverse post-operative events and non-progression to adjuvant therapy after major pancreatic surgery. *HPB* **2013**, *15*, 899–907. [CrossRef]
90. Thomas, G.; Tahir, M.R.; Bongers, B.C.; Kallen, V.L.; Slooter, G.D.; van Meeteren, N.L. Prehabilitation before major intra-abdominal cancer surgery: A systematic review of randomised controlled trials. *Eur. J. Anaesthesiol.* **2019**, *36*, 933–945. [CrossRef]

91. West, M.A.; Parry, M.G.; Lythgoe, D.; Barben, C.P.; Kemp, G.J.; Grocott, M.P.W.; Jack, S. Cardiopulmonary exercise testing for the prediction of morbidity risk after rectal cancer surgery. *Br. J. Surg.* **2014**, *101*, 1166–1172. [CrossRef]
92. Minnella, E.M.; Awasthi, R.; Loiselle, S.E.; Agnihotram, R.V.; Ferri, L.E.; Carli, F. Effect of Exercise and Nutrition Prehabilitation on Functional Capacity in Esophagogastric Cancer Surgery: A Randomized Clinical Trial. *JAMA Surg.* **2018**, *153*, 1081–1089. [CrossRef]
93. Dunne, D.F.J.; Jack, S.; Jones, R.P.; Jones, L.; Lythgoe, D.T.; Malik, H.Z.; Poston, G.J.; Palmer, D.H.; Fenwick, S.W. Randomized clinical trial of prehabilitation before planned liver resection. *Br. J. Surg.* **2016**, *103*, 504–512. [CrossRef]
94. Bhatia, C.; Kayser, B. Preoperative high-intensity interval training is effective and safe in deconditioned patients with lung cancer: A randomized clinical trial. *J. Rehabil. Med.* **2019**, *51*, 712–718. [CrossRef]
95. Kerr, J.; Anderson, C.; Lippman, S.M. Physical activity, sedentary behaviour, diet, and cancer: An update and emerging new evidence. *Lancet Oncol.* **2017**, *18*, e457–e471. [CrossRef]
96. Wilson, R.J.T.; Davies, S.; Yates, D.; Redman, J.; Stone, M. Impaired functional capacity is associated with all-cause mortality after major elective intra-abdominal surgery. *Br. J. Anaesth.* **2010**, *105*, 297–303. [CrossRef]
97. McGuigan, A.; Kelly, P.; Turkington, R.C.; Jones, C.; Coleman, H.G.; McCain, R.S. Pancreatic cancer: A review of clinical diagnosis, epidemiology, treatment and outcomes. *World J. Gastroenterol.* **2018**, *24*, 4846–4861. [CrossRef]
98. Akahori, T.; Sho, M.; Kinoshita, S.; Nagai, M.; Nishiwada, S.; Tanaka, T.; Tamamoto, T.; Ohbayashi, C.; Hasegawa, M.; Kichikawa, K.; et al. Prognostic Significance of Muscle Attenuation in Pancreatic Cancer Patients Treated with Neoadjuvant Chemoradiotherapy. *World J. Surg.* **2015**, *39*, 2975–2982. [CrossRef]
99. Sandini, M.; Patino, M.; Ferrone, C.R.; Alvarez-Pérez, C.A.; Honselmann, K.C.; Paiella, S.; Catania, M.; Riva, L.; Tedesco, G.; Casolino, R.; et al. Association Between Changes in Body Composition and Neoadjuvant Treatment for Pancreatic Cancer. *JAMA Surg.* **2018**, *153*, 809–815. [CrossRef]
100. Mackay, T.M.; Smits, F.J.; Roos, D.; Bonsing, B.A.; Bosscha, K.; Busch, O.R.; Creemers, G.J.; van Dam, R.M.; van Eijck, C.H.J.; Gerhardet, M.F.; et al. The risk of not receiving adjuvant chemotherapy after resection of pancreatic ductal adenocarcinoma: A nationwide analysis. *HPB* **2020**, *22*, 233–240. [CrossRef]
101. Bundred, J.; Kamarajah, S.K.; Roberts, K.J. Body composition assessment and sarcopenia in patients with pancreatic cancer: A systematic review and meta-analysis. *HPB* **2019**, *21*, 1603–1612. [CrossRef]
102. Giles, C.; Cummins, S. Prehabilitation before cancer treatment. *BMJ* **2019**, *366*, l5120. [CrossRef]
103. Kamarajah, S.K.; Bundred, J.; Weblin, J.; Tan, B.H. Critical appraisal on the impact of preoperative rehabilitation and outcomes after major abdominal and cardiothoracic surgery: A systematic review and meta-analysis. *Surgery* **2020**, *167*, 540–549. [CrossRef] [PubMed]
104. Barberan-Garcia, A.; Ubre, M.; Pascual-Argente, N.; Risco, R.; Faner, J.; Balust, J.; Lacy, A.; Puig-Junoy, J.; Roca, J.; Martinez-Palli, G. Post-discharge impact and cost-consequence analysis of prehabilitation in high-risk patients undergoing major abdominal surgery: Secondary results from a randomised controlled trial. *Br. J. Anaesth.* **2019**, *123*, 450–456. [CrossRef] [PubMed]
105. Levett, D.Z.; Edwards, M.; Grocott, M.; Mythen, M. Preparing the patient for surgery to improve outcomes. *Best Pr. Res. Clin. Anaesthesiol.* **2016**, *30*, 145–157. [CrossRef] [PubMed]
106. Carli, F.; Scheede-Bergdahl, C. Prehabilitation to Enhance Perioperative Care. *Anesthesiol. Clin.* **2015**, *33*, 17–33. [CrossRef] [PubMed]
107. Gillis, C.; Buhler, K.; Bresee, L.; Carli, F.; Gramlich, L.; Culos-Reed, N.; Sajobi, T.T.; Fenton, T.R. Effects of Nutritional Prehabilitation, With and Without Exercise, on Outcomes of Patients Who Undergo Colorectal Surgery: A Systematic Review and Meta-analysis. *Gastroenterology* **2018**, *155*, 391–410.e4. [CrossRef] [PubMed]
108. Heger, P.; Probst, P.; Wiskemann, J.; Steindorf, K.; Diener, M.K.; Mihaljevic, A.L. A Systematic Review and Meta-analysis of Physical Exercise Prehabilitation in Major Abdominal Surgery (PROSPERO 2017 CRD42017080366). *J. Gastrointest. Surg.* **2020**, *24*, 1375–1385. [CrossRef] [PubMed]
109. Ausania, F.; Senra, P.; Meléndez, R.; Caballeiro, R.; Ouviña, R.; Casal-Núñez, E. Prehabilitation in patients undergoing pancreaticoduodenectomy: A randomized controlled trial. *Rev. Esp. Enferm. Dig.* **2019**, *111*, 603–608. [CrossRef] [PubMed]
110. Nakajima, H.; Yokoyama, Y.; Inoue, T.; Nagaya, M.; Mizuno, Y.; Kadono, I.; Nishiwaki, K.; Nishida, Y.; Nagino, M. Clinical Benefit of Preoperative Exercise and Nutritional Therapy for Patients Undergoing Hepato-Pancreato-Biliary Surgeries for Malignancy. *Ann. Surg. Oncol.* **2018**, *26*, 264–272. [CrossRef]
111. Florez Bedoya, C.A.; Cardoso, A.C.F.; Parker, N.; Ngo-Huang, A.; Petzel, M.Q.; Kim, M.P.; Fogelman, D.; Romero, S.G.; Wang, H.; Park, M.; et al. Exercise during preoperative therapy increases tumor vascurity in pancreatic tumor patients. *Sci. Rep.* **2019**, *9*, 13966. [CrossRef]
112. Marker, R.J.; Peters, J.C.; Purcell, W.T.; Jankowski, C.A. Effects of Preoperative Exercise on Physical Fitness and Body Composition in Pancreatic Cancer Survivors Receiving Neoadjuvant Therapy: A Case Series. *Rehabil. Oncol.* **2018**, *36*, E1–E9. [CrossRef]
113. Parker, N.H.; Ngo-Huang, A.; Lee, R.E.; O'Connor, D.P.; Basen-Engquist, K.M.; Petzel, M.Q.; Wang, X.; Xiao, L.; Fogelman, D.R.; Schadler, K.L.; et al. Physical activity and exercise during preoperative pancreatic cancer treatment. *Support. Care Cancer* **2018**, *27*, 2275–2284. [CrossRef]
114. Ngo-Huang, A.; Parker, N.H.; Bruera, E.; Lee, R.E.; Simpson, R.; O'Connor, D.P.; Petzel, M.Q.B.; Fontillas, R.C.; Schadler, K.; Xiao, L.; et al. Home-Based Exercise Prehabilitation During Preoperative Treatment for Pancreatic Cancer Is Associated With Improvement in Physical Function and Quality of Life. *Integr. Cancer Ther.* **2019**, *18*, 1534735419894061. [CrossRef]

115. Ljungqvist, O.; Scott, M.; Fearon, K.C. Enhanced Recovery After Surgery: A Review. *JAMA Surg.* **2017**, *152*, 292–298. [CrossRef]
116. Li, T.; D'Cruz, R.T.; Lim, S.Y.; Shelat, V.G.; Tianpei, L.; Yang, L.S. Somatostatin analogues and the risk of post-operative pancreatic fistulas after pancreatic resection—A systematic review & meta-analysis. *Pancreatology* **2020**, *20*, 158–168.
117. De Rosa, P.; Jewell, A. The potential use for patient reported outcome measures in people with pancreatic cancer, with a specific focus on older patients. *Eur. J. Surg. Oncol.* **2021**, *47*, 495–502. [CrossRef]
118. Van Rijssen, L.B.; Gerritsen, A.; Henselmans, I.; Sprangers, M.A.; Jacobs, M.; Bassi, C.; Busch, O.R.; Fernandez-Del Castillo, C.; Fong, Z.V.; He, F.; et al. Core Set of Patient-reported Outcomes in Pancreatic Cancer (COPRAC): An International Delphi Study Among Patients and Health Care Providers. *Ann. Surg.* **2019**, *270*, 158–164. [CrossRef]
119. ERAS Compliance Group. The Impact of Enhanced Recovery Protocol Compliance on Elective Colorectal Cancer Resection: Results From an International Registry. *Ann. Surg.* **2015**, *261*, 1153–1159. [CrossRef]
120. Roulin, D.; Melloul, E.; Wellg, B.E.; Izbicki, J.; Vrochides, D.; Adham, M.; Hübner, M.; Demartines, N. Feasibility of an Enhanced Recovery Protocol for Elective Pancreatoduodenectomy: A Multicenter International Cohort Study. *World J. Surg.* **2020**, *44*, 2761–2769. [CrossRef]
121. Coolsen, M.M.E.; Van Dam, R.M.; Van Der Wilt, A.A.; Slim, K.; Lassen, K.; DeJong, C.H.C. Systematic Review and Meta-analysis of Enhanced Recovery After Pancreatic Surgery with Particular Emphasis on Pancreaticoduodenectomies. *World J. Surg.* **2013**, *37*, 1909–1918. [CrossRef]
122. Xiong, J.; Szatmary, P.; Huang, W.; de la Iglesia-Garcia, D.; Nunes, Q.M.; Xia, Q.; Hu, W.; Sutton, R.; Liu, X.; Raraty, M.G. Enhanced Recovery After Surgery Program in Patients Undergoing Pancreaticoduodenectomy: A PRISMA-Compliant Systematic Review and Meta-Analysis. *Medicine* **2016**, *95*, e3497. [CrossRef]
123. Ji, H.-B.; Zhu, W.-T.; Wei, Q.; Wang, X.-X.; Wang, H.-B.; Chen, Q.-P. Impact of enhanced recovery after surgery programs on pancreatic surgery: A meta-analysis. *World J. Gastroenterol.* **2018**, *24*, 1666–1678. [CrossRef] [PubMed]
124. Cao, Y.; Gu, H.-Y.; Huang, Z.-D.; Wu, Y.-P.; Zhang, Q.; Luo, J.; Zhang, C.; Fu, Y. Impact of Enhanced Recovery After Surgery on Postoperative Recovery for Pancreaticoduodenectomy: Pooled Analysis of Observational Study. *Front. Oncol.* **2019**, *9*, 687. [CrossRef]
125. Sun, Y.-M.; Wang, Y.; Mao, Y.-X.; Wang, W. The Safety and Feasibility of Enhanced Recovery after Surgery in Patients Undergoing Pancreaticoduodenectomy: An Updated Meta-Analysis. *BioMed Res. Int.* **2020**, *2020*, 7401276. [CrossRef] [PubMed]
126. Roulin, D.; Najjar, P.; Demartines, N. Enhanced Recovery After Surgery Implementation: From Planning to Success. *J. Laparoendosc. Adv. Surg. Tech.* **2017**, *27*, 876–879. [CrossRef] [PubMed]
127. Kagedan, D.J.; Devitt, K.S.; St-Germain, A.T.; Ramjaun, A.; Cleary, S.P.; Wei, A.C. The economics of recovery after pancreatic surgery: Detailed cost minimization analysis of an enhanced recovery program. *HPB* **2017**, *19*, 1026–1033. [CrossRef] [PubMed]
128. Passeri, M.; Lyman, W.B.; Murphy, K.; Iannitti, D.; Martinie, J.; Baker, E.; Vrochides, D. Implementing an ERAS Protocol for Pancreaticoduodenectomy Does Not Affect Oncologic Outcomes when Compared with Traditional Recovery. *Am. Surg.* **2020**, *86*, e81–e83. [CrossRef] [PubMed]
129. Vollmer, C.M.; The Pancreatic Surgery Mortality Study Group; Sanchez, N.; Gondek, S.; McAuliffe, J.C.; Kent, T.S.; Christein, J.D.; Callery, M.P. A Root-Cause Analysis of Mortality Following Major Pancreatectomy. *J. Gastrointest. Surg.* **2011**, *16*, 89–103. [CrossRef]
130. Smits, F.J.; Henry, A.C.; Van Eijck, C.H.; Besselink, M.G.; Busch, O.R.; Arntz, M.; Bollen, T.L.; Van Delden, O.M.; Heuvel, D.V.D.; Van Der Leij, C.; et al. Care after pancreatic resection according to an algorithm for early detection and minimally invasive management of pancreatic fistula versus current practice (PORSCH-trial): Design and rationale of a nationwide stepped-wedge cluster-randomized trial. *Trials* **2020**, *21*, 389. [CrossRef]
131. Roberts, K.J.; Boteon, A.; Marcon, F.; Abradelo, M.; Dasari, B.; Muiesan, P.; Marudanayagam, R.; Sutcliffe, R.P.; Isaac, J.; Mirza, D.F. Risk adjusted assessment of individual surgeon's pancreatic fistula outcomes. *HPB* **2020**, *22*, 452–460. [CrossRef]
132. Sánchez-Velázquez, P.; Muller, X.; Malleo, G.; Park, J.; Hwang, H.; Napoli, N.; Javed, A.; Inoue, Y.; Beghdadi, N.; Kalisvaart, M.; et al. Benchmarks in pancreatic surgery. A novel tool for unbiased outcome comparisons. *HPB* **2020**, *22*, S383. [CrossRef]
133. Raptis, D.A.; Sánchez-Velázquez, P.; Machairas, N.; Sauvanet, A.; De Leon, A.R.; Oba, A.; Koerkamp, B.G.; Lovasik, B.; Chan, C.; Yeo, C.J.; et al. Defining Benchmark Outcomes for Pancreatoduodenectomy With Portomesenteric Venous Resection. *Ann. Surg.* **2020**, *272*, 731–737. [CrossRef]
134. Mackay, T.M.; Dutch Pancreatic Cancer Group; Smits, F.J.; Latenstein, A.E.J.; Bogte, A.; Bonsing, B.A.; Bos, H.; Bosscha, K.; Brosens, L.A.A.; Hol, L.; et al. Impact of nationwide enhanced implementation of best practices in pancreatic cancer care (PACAP-1): A multicenter stepped-wedge cluster randomized controlled trial. *Trials* **2020**, *21*, 334. [CrossRef]
135. Conroy, T.; Hammel, P.; Hebbar, M.; Ben Abdelghani, M.; Wei, A.C.; Raoul, J.-L.; Choné, L.; Francois, E.; Artru, P.; Biagi, J.J.; et al. FOLFIRINOX or Gemcitabine as Adjuvant Therapy for Pancreatic Cancer. *N. Engl. J. Med.* **2018**, *379*, 2395–2406. [CrossRef]
136. Conroy, T.; Hammel, P.; Hebbar, M.; Ben Abdelghani, M.; Wei, A.C.-C.; Raoul, J.-L.; Chone, L.; Francois, E.; Artru, P.; Biagi, J.J.; et al. Unicancer GI PRODIGE 24/CCTG PA.6 trial: A multicenter international randomized phase III trial of adjuvant mFOLFIRINOX versus gemcitabine (gem) in patients with resected pancreatic ductal adenocarcinomas. *J. Clin. Oncol.* **2018**, *36*, LBA4001. [CrossRef]
137. Neoptolemos, J.P.; Palmer, D.H.; Ghaneh, P.; Psarelli, E.E.; Valle, J.W.; Halloran, C.M.; Faluyi, O.; O'Reilly, D.A.; Cunningham, D.; Wadsley, J.; et al. Comparison of adjuvant gemcitabine and capecitabine with gemcitabine monotherapy in patients with resected pancreatic cancer (ESPAC-4): A multicentre, open-label, randomised, phase 3 trial. *Lancet* **2017**, *389*, 1011–1024. [CrossRef]

138. Van Roessel, S.; van Veldhuisen, E.; Klompmaker, S.; Janssen, Q.P.; Abu Hilal, M.; Alseidi, A.; Balduzzi, A.; Balzano, G.; Bassi, C.; Berrevoet, F.; et al. Evaluation of Adjuvant Chemotherapy in Patients With Resected Pancreatic Cancer After Neoadjuvant FOLFIRINOX Treatment. *JAMA Oncol.* **2020**, *6*, 1–8. [CrossRef] [PubMed]
139. Sata, N.; Kurashina, K.; Nagai, H.; Nagakawa, T.; Ishikawa, O.; Ohta, T.; Oka, M.; Kinoshita, H.; Kimura, W.; Shimada, H.; et al. The effect of adjuvant and neoadjuvant chemo(radio)therapy on survival in 1679 resected pancreatic carcinoma cases in Japan: Report of the national survey in the 34th annual meeting of Japanese Society of Pancreatic Surgery. *J. Hepatobiliary Pancreat. Surg.* **2009**, *16*, 485–492. [CrossRef]
140. Bakens, M.J.; van der Geest, L.G.; van Putten, M.; van Laarhoven, H.W.; Creemers, G.-J.; Besselink, M.G.; Lemmens, V.E.; de Hingh, I.H.; Dutch Pancreatic Cancer Group. The use of adjuvant chemotherapy for pancreatic cancer varies widely between hospitals: A nationwide population-based analysis. *Cancer Med.* **2016**, *5*, 2825–2831. [CrossRef]
141. Kagedan, D.; Dixon, M.; Raju, R.; Li, Q.; Elmi, M.; Shin, E.; Liu, N.; El-Sedfy, A.; Paszat, L.; Kiss, A.; et al. Predictors of Adjuvant Treatment for Pancreatic Adenocarcinoma at the Population Level. *Curr. Oncol.* **2016**, *23*, 334–342. [CrossRef]
142. Mayo, S.C.; Gilson, M.M.; Herman, J.M.; Cameron, J.L.; Nathan, H.; Edil, B.H.; Choti, M.A.; Schulick, R.D.; Wolfgang, C.L.; Pawlik, T.M. Management of Patients with Pancreatic Adenocarcinoma: National Trends in Patient Selection, Operative Management, and Use of Adjuvant Therapy. *J. Am. Coll. Surg.* **2012**, *214*, 33–45. [CrossRef]
143. Kagedan, D.J.; Abraham, L.; Goyert, N.; Li, Q.; Paszat, L.F.; Kiss, A.; Earle, C.C.; Mittmann, N.; Coburn, N.G. Beyond the dollar: Influence of sociodemographic marginalization on surgical resection, adjuvant therapy, and survival in patients with pancreatic cancer. *Cancer* **2016**, *122*, 3175–3182. [CrossRef] [PubMed]
144. Van der Geest, L.G.M.; van Eijck, C.H.J.; Groot Koerkamp, B.; Lemmens, V.; Busch, O.R.; Vissers, P.A.J.; Wilmink, J.W.; Besselink, M.G.; Dutch Pancreatic Cancer Group. Trends in treatment and survival of patients with nonresected, nonmetastatic pancreatic cancer: A population-based study. *Cancer Med.* **2018**, *7*, 4943–4951. [CrossRef] [PubMed]
145. Neoptolemos, J.P.; Stocken, D.D.; Friess, H.; Bassi, C.; Dunn, J.A.; Hickey, H.; Beger, H.; Fernandez-Cruz, L.; Dervenis, C.; Lacaine, F.; et al. A Randomized Trial of Chemoradiotherapy and Chemotherapy after Resection of Pancreatic Cancer. *N. Engl. J. Med.* **2004**, *350*, 1200–1210. [CrossRef] [PubMed]
146. Faluyi, O.O.; Connor, J.L.; Chatterjee, M.; Ikin, C.; Wong, H.; Palmer, D.H. Advanced pancreatic adenocarcinoma outcomes with transition from devolved to centralised care in a regional Cancer Centre. *Br. J. Cancer* **2017**, *116*, 424–431. [CrossRef] [PubMed]
147. Fisher, A.V.; Ma, Y.; Wang, X.; Campbell-Flohr, S.A.; Rathouz, P.J.; Ronnekleiv-Kelly, S.M.; Abbott, D.E.; Weber, S.M. National Trends in Centralization of Surgical Care and Multimodality Therapy for Pancreatic Adenocarcinoma. *J. Gastrointest. Surg.* **2019**, *24*, 2021–2029. [CrossRef]
148. Sorenson, G.D.; Pribish, D.M.; Valone, F.H.; Memoli, V.A.; Bzik, D.J.; Yao, S.L. Soluble normal and mutated DNA sequences from single-copy genes in human blood. *Cancer Epidemiol. Biomark. Prev.* **1994**, *3*, 67–71.
149. Glantz, M.J.; Cole, B.F.; Glantz, L.K.; Cobb, J.; Mills, P.; Lekos, A.; Walters, B.C.; Recht, L.D. Cerebrospinal fluid cytology in patients with cancer: Minimizing false-negative results. *Cancer* **1998**, *82*, 733–739. [CrossRef]
150. Anker, P.; Stroun, M.; Maurice, P.A. Spontaneous release of DNA by human blood lymphocytes as shown in an in vitro system. *Cancer Res.* **1975**, *35*, 2375–2382.
151. Stroun, M.; Lyautey, J.; Lederrey, C.; Olson-Sand, A.; Anker, P. About the possible origin and mechanism of circulating DNA apoptosis and active DNA release. *Clin. Chim. Acta* **2001**, *313*, 139–142. [CrossRef]
152. Kim, N.; Han, I.W.; Ryu, Y.; Hwang, D.W.; Heo, J.S.; Choi, D.W.; Shin, S.H. Predictive Nomogram for Early Recurrence after Pancreatectomy in Resectable Pancreatic Cancer: Risk Classification Using Preoperative Clinicopathologic Factors. *Cancers* **2020**, *12*, 137. [CrossRef]
153. Brennan, M.F.; Kattan, M.W.; Klimstra, D.; Conlon, K. Prognostic Nomogram for Patients Undergoing Resection for Adenocarcinoma of the Pancreas. *Ann. Surg.* **2004**, *240*, 293–298. [CrossRef]
154. Ferrone, C.R.; Kattan, M.W.; Tomlinson, J.S.; Thayer, S.P.; Brennan, M.F.; Warshaw, A.L. Validation of a Postresection Pancreatic Adenocarcinoma Nomogram for Disease-Specific Survival. *J. Clin. Oncol.* **2005**, *23*, 7529–7535. [CrossRef]
155. He, C.; Mao, Y.; Wang, J.; Duan, F.; Lin, X.; Li, S. Nomograms predict long-term survival for patients with periampullary adenocarcinoma after pancreatoduodenectomy. *BMC Cancer* **2018**, *18*, 327. [CrossRef]
156. Li, H.-B.; Zhou, J.; Zhao, F.-Q. A Prognostic Nomogram for Disease-Specific Survival in Patients with Pancreatic Ductal Adenocarcinoma of the Head of the Pancreas Following Pancreaticoduodenectomy. *Med. Sci. Monit.* **2018**, *24*, 6313–6321. [CrossRef]
157. Parmar, A.D.; Vargas, G.M.; Tamirisa, N.P.; Sheffield, K.M.; Riall, T.S. Trajectory of care and use of multimodality therapy in older patients with pancreatic adenocarcinoma. *Surgery* **2014**, *156*, 280–289. [CrossRef]
158. Frakes, J.M.; Strom, T.; Springett, G.M.; Hoffe, S.E.; Balducci, L.; Hodul, P.; Malafa, M.P.; Shridhar, R. Resected pancreatic cancer outcomes in the elderly. *J. Geriatr. Oncol.* **2015**, *6*, 127–132. [CrossRef]
159. Nagrial, A.M.; Chang, D.K.; Nguyen, N.Q.; Johns, A.L.; Chantrill, L.A.; Humphris, J.L.; Chin, V.T.; Samra, J.S.; Gill, A.J.; Pajic, M.; et al. Adjuvant chemotherapy in elderly patients with pancreatic cancer. *Br. J. Cancer* **2013**, *110*, 313–319. [CrossRef]
160. Shin, S.H.; Park, Y.; Hwang, D.W.; Song, K.B.; Lee, J.H.; Kwon, J.; Yoo, C.; Alshammary, S.; Kim, S.C. Prognostic Value of Adjuvant Chemotherapy Following Pancreaticoduodenectomy in Elderly Patients With Pancreatic Cancer. *Anticancer. Res.* **2019**, *39*, 1005–1012. [CrossRef]

161. Oettle, H.; Neuhaus, P.; Hochhaus, A.; Hartmann, J.T.; Gellert, K.; Ridwelski, K.; Niedergethmann, M.; Zülke, C.; Fahlke, J.; Arning, M.B.; et al. Adjuvant chemotherapy with gemcitabine and long-term outcomes among patients with resected pancreatic cancer: The CONKO-001 randomized trial. *JAMA* **2013**, *310*, 1473–1481. [CrossRef]
162. Neoptolemos, J.P.; Stocken, D.D.; Bassi, C.; Ghaneh, P.; Cunningham, D.; Goldstein, D.; Padbury, R.; Moore, M.J.; Gallinger, S.; Mariette, C.; et al. Adjuvant chemotherapy with fluorouracil plus folinic acid vs gemcitabine following pancreatic cancer resection: A randomized controlled trial. *JAMA* **2010**, *304*, 1073–1081. [CrossRef]
163. Miyamoto, D.T.; Mamon, H.J.; Ryan, D.P.; Willett, C.G.; Ancukiewicz, M.; Kobayashi, W.K.; Blaszkowsky, L.; Castillo, C.F.-D.; Hong, T.S. Outcomes and Tolerability of Chemoradiation Therapy for Pancreatic Cancer Patients Aged 75 Years or Older. *Int. J. Radiat. Oncol.* **2010**, *77*, 1171–1177. [CrossRef]
164. Miura, J.T.; Krepline, A.N.; George, B.; Ritch, P.S.; Erickson, B.A.; Johnston, F.M.; Oshima, K.; Christians, K.K.; Evans, D.B.; Tsai, S. Use of neoadjuvant therapy in patients 75 years of age and older with pancreatic cancer. *Surgery* **2015**, *158*, 1545–1555. [CrossRef] [PubMed]
165. Li, X.; Huang, D.-B.; Zhang, Q.; Guo, C.-X.; Fu, Q.-H.; Zhang, X.-C.; Tang, T.-Y.; Su, W.; Chen, Y.-W.; Chen, W.; et al. The efficacy and toxicity of chemotherapy in the elderly with advanced pancreatic cancer. *Pancreatology* **2020**, *20*, 95–100. [CrossRef] [PubMed]
166. Mizrahi, J.D.; Rogers, J.E.; Hess, K.R.; Wolff, R.A.; Varadhachary, G.R.; Javle, M.M.; Shroff, R.T.; Ho, L.; Fogelman, D.R.; Raghav, K.P.; et al. Modified FOLFIRINOX in pancreatic cancer patients Age 75 or older. *Pancreatology* **2020**, *20*, 501–504. [CrossRef] [PubMed]
167. Kalsi, T.; Babic-Illman, G.; Ross, P.; Maisey, N.; Hughes, S.; Fields, P.E.; Martin, F.C.; Wang, Y.; Harari, D. The impact of comprehensive geriatric assessment interventions on tolerance to chemotherapy in older people. *Br. J. Cancer* **2015**, *112*, 1435–1444. [CrossRef] [PubMed]
168. Overcash, J.; Ford, N.; Kress, E.; Ubbing, C.; Williams, N. Comprehensive Geriatric Assessment as a Versatile Tool to Enhance the Care of the Older Person Diagnosed with Cancer. *Geriatrics* **2019**, *4*, 39. [CrossRef] [PubMed]
169. Hurria, A.; Togawa, K.; Mohile, S.G.; Owusu, C.; Klepin, H.D.; Gross, C.P.; Lichtmnan, S.M.; Gajra, A.; Bhatia, S.; Katheria, V.; et al. Predicting chemotherapy toxicity in older adults with cancer: A prospective multicenter study. *J. Clin. Oncol.* **2011**, *29*, 3457–3465. [CrossRef]
170. Puts, M.T.E.; Santos, B.; Hardt, J.; Monette, J.; Girre, V.; Atenafu, E.G.; Springall, E.; Alibhai, S.M.H. An update on a systematic review of the use of geriatric assessment for older adults in oncology. *Ann. Oncol.* **2014**, *25*, 307–315. [CrossRef]
171. Hurria, A.; Wildes, T.; Blair, S.L.; Browner, I.S.; Cohen, H.J.; DeShazo, M.; Dotan, E.; Edil, B.H.; Extermann, M.; Ganti, A.K.P.; et al. Senior Adult Oncology, Version 2.2014. *J. Natl. Compr. Cancer Netw.* **2014**, *12*, 82–126. [CrossRef]
172. Wildiers, H.; Heeren, P.; Puts, M.; Topinkova, E.; Janssen-Heijnen, M.L.G.; Extermann, M.; Falandry, C.; Artz, A.; Brain, E.; Colloca, G.; et al. International Society of Geriatric Oncology Consensus on Geriatric Assessment in Older Patients With Cancer. *J. Clin. Oncol.* **2014**, *32*, 2595–2603. [CrossRef]
173. Extermann, M.; Aapro, M.; Bernabei, R.; Cohen, H.J.; Droz, J.-P.; Lichtman, S.; Mor, V.; Monfardini, S.; Repetto, L.; Sørbye, L.; et al. Use of comprehensive geriatric assessment in older cancer patients: Recommendations from the task force on CGA of the International Society of Geriatric Oncology (SIOG). *Crit. Rev. Oncol. Hematol.* **2005**, *55*, 241–252. [CrossRef]
174. Pallis, A.; Fortpied, C.; Wedding, U.; Van Nes, M.; Penninckx, B.; Ring, A.; Lacombe, D.; Monfardini, S.; Scalliet, P.; Wildiers, H. EORTC elderly task force position paper: Approach to the older cancer patient. *Eur. J. Cancer* **2010**, *46*, 1502–1513. [CrossRef] [PubMed]
175. Fried, L.P.; Tangen, C.M.; Walston, J.D.; Newman, A.B.; Hirsch, C.; Gottdiener, J.S.; Seeman, T.E.; Tracy, R.P.; Kop, W.J.; Burke, G.L.; et al. Frailty in Older Adults: Evidence for a Phenotype. *J. Gerontol. Ser. A Boil. Sci. Med. Sci.* **2001**, *56*, M146–M156. [CrossRef]
176. Rockwood, K.; Song, X.; Macknight, C.; Bergman, H.; Hogan, D.B.; McDowell, I.; Mitnitski, A. A global clinical measure of fitness and frailty in elderly people. *Can. Med. Assoc. J.* **2005**, *173*, 489–495. [CrossRef]
177. Bellera, C.A.; Rainfray, M.; Mathoulin-Pélissier, S.; Mertens, C.; Delva, F.; Fonck, M.; Soubeyran, P.L. Screening older cancer patients: First evaluation of the G-8 geriatric screening tool. *Ann. Oncol.* **2012**, *23*, 2166–2172. [CrossRef]
178. Ducreux, M.; Cuhna, A.S.; Caramella, C.; Hollebecque, A.; Burtin, P.; Goéré, D.; Seufferlein, T.; Haustermans, K.; Van Laethem, J.L.; Conroy, T.; et al. Cancer of the pancreas: ESMO Clinical Practice Guidelines for diagnosis, treatment and follow-up. *Ann. Oncol.* **2015**, *26*, v56–v68. [CrossRef]
179. Takaori, K.; Bassi, C.; Biankin, A.; Brunner, T.B.; Cataldo, I.; Campbell, F.; Cunningham, D.; Falconi, M.; Frampton, A.E.; Furuse, J.; et al. International Association of Pancreatology (IAP)/European Pancreatic Club (EPC) consensus review of guidelines for the treatment of pancreatic cancer. *Pancreatology* **2016**, *16*, 14–27. [CrossRef]
180. Jones, R.P.; Psarelli, E.E.; Jackson, R.; Ghaneh, P.; Halloran, C.M.; Palmer, D.H.; Campbell, F.; Valle, J.W.; Faluyi, O.; O'Reilly, D.; et al. Patterns of Recurrence After Resection of Pancreatic Ductal Adenocarcinoma: A Secondary Analysis of the ESPAC-4 Randomized Adjuvant Chemotherapy Trial. *JAMA Surg.* **2019**, *154*, 1038–1048. [CrossRef]
181. Goldsmith, C.; Plowman, P.N.; Green, M.M.; Dale, R.G.; Price, P.M. Stereotactic ablative radiotherapy (SABR) as primary, adjuvant, consolidation and re-treatment option in pancreatic cancer: Scope for dose escalation and lessons for toxicity. *Radiat. Oncol.* **2018**, *13*, 204. [CrossRef]
182. Elberg Dengsø, K.; Tjørnhøj-Thomsen, T.; Oksbjerg Dalton, S.; Marcel Christensen, B.; Hillingsø, J.; Thomsen, T. It's all about the CA-19-9. A longitudinal qualitative study of patients' experiences and perspectives on follow-up after curative surgery for cancer in the pancreas, duodenum or bile-duct. *Acta Oncol.* **2019**, *58*, 642–649. [CrossRef]

183. Deobald, R.G.; Cheng, E.S.W.; Ko, Y.-J.; Wright, F.C.; Karanicolas, P.J. A qualitative study of patient and clinician attitudes regarding surveillance after a resection of pancreatic and peri-ampullary cancer. *HPB* **2015**, *17*, 409–415. [CrossRef] [PubMed]
184. Ghaneh, P.; Hanson, R.; Titman, A.; Lancaster, G.; Plumpton, C.; Lloyd-Williams, H.; Yeo, S.T.; Edwards, R.T.; Johnson, C.; Abu Hilal, M.; et al. PET-PANC: Multicentre prospective diagnostic accuracy and health economic analysis study of the impact of combined modality 18fluorine-2-fluoro-2-deoxy-d-glucose positron emission tomography with computed tomography scanning in the diagnosis and management of pancreatic cancer. *Health Technol. Assess.* **2018**, *22*, 1–114. [PubMed]
185. Palmieri, L.-J.; Coriat, R. 18F-FDG PET/CT in pancreatic adenocarcinoma: On the edge of a paradigm shift? *Diagn. Interv. Imaging* **2019**, *100*, 731–733. [CrossRef]
186. Wang, L.; Dong, P.; Wang, W.; Tian, B. Positron emission tomography modalities prevent futile radical resection of pancreatic cancer: A meta-analysis. *Int. J. Surg.* **2017**, *46*, 119–125. [CrossRef]
187. Riviere, D.M.; Van Geenen, E.J.M.; Van Der Kolk, B.M.; Nagtegaal, I.D.; Radema, S.A.; Van Laarhoven, C.J.H.M.; Hermans, J.J. Improving preoperative detection of synchronous liver metastases in pancreatic cancer with combined contrast-enhanced and diffusion-weighted MRI. *Abdom. Radiol.* **2019**, *44*, 1756–1765. [CrossRef]
188. Marion-Audibert, A.-M.; Vullierme, M.-P.; Ronot, M.; Mabrut, J.-Y.; Sauvanet, A.; Zins, M.; Cuilleron, M.; Sa-Cunha, A.; Lévy, P.; Rode, A. Routine MRI With DWI Sequences to Detect Liver Metastases in Patients With Potentially Resectable Pancreatic Ductal Carcinoma and Normal Liver CT: A Prospective Multicenter Study. *Am. J. Roentgenol.* **2018**, *211*, W217–W225. [CrossRef]
189. Jeon, S.K.; Lee, J.M.; Joo, I.; Lee, N.H.; Ahn, S.J.; Woo, H.; Lee, M.S.; Jang, J.-Y.; Han, J.K. Correction to: Magnetic resonance with diffusion-weighted imaging improves assessment of focal liver lesions in patients with potentially resectable pancreatic cancer on CT. *Eur. Radiol.* **2018**, *28*, 4315. [CrossRef]
190. Kalisvaart, M.; Broadhurst, D.; Marcon, F.; Pande, R.; Schlegel, A.; Sutcliffe, R.; Marudanayagam, R.; Mirza, D.; Chatzizacharias, N.; Abradelo, M.; et al. Recurrence patterns of pancreatic cancer after pancreatoduodenectomy: Systematic review and a single-centre retrospective study. *HPB* **2020**, *22*, 1240–1249. [CrossRef]
191. Butler, J.R.; Ahmad, S.A.; Katz, M.H.; Cioffi, J.L.; Zyromski, N.J. A systematic review of the role of periadventitial dissection of the superior mesenteric artery in affecting margin status after pancreatoduodenectomy for pancreatic adenocarcinoma. *HPB* **2016**, *18*, 305–311. [CrossRef]
192. Versteijne, E.; Vogel, J.A.; Besselink, M.G.; Busch, O.R.C.; Wilmink, J.W.; Daams, J.G.; van Eijck, C.H.J.; Koerkamp, B.G.; Rasch, C.R.N.; van Tienhoven, G. Meta-analysis comparing upfront surgery with neoadjuvant treatment in patients with resectable or borderline resectable pancreatic cancer. *Br. J. Surg.* **2018**, *105*, 946–958. [CrossRef]
193. Petrucciani, N.; Nigri, G.; Debs, T.; Giannini, G.; Sborlini, E.; Antolino, L.; Aurello, P.; D'Angelo, F.; Gugenheim, J.; Ramacciato, G. Frozen section analysis of the pancreatic margin during pancreaticoduodenectomy for cancer: Does extending the resection to obtain a secondary R0 provide a survival benefit? Results of a systematic review. *Pancreatology* **2016**, *16*, 1037–1043. [CrossRef]
194. Schwarz, L.; Vernerey, D.; Bachet, J.B.; Tuech, J.J.; Portales, F.; Michel, P.; Cunha, A.S. Resectable pancreatic adenocarcinoma neo-adjuvant FOLF(IRIN)OX-based chemotherapy—A multicenter, non-comparative, randomized, phase II trial (PANACHE01-PRODIGE48 study). *BMC Cancer* **2018**, *18*, 762. [CrossRef]
195. Wang, W.; He, Y.; Wu, L.; Ye, L.; Yao, L.; Tang, Z. Efficacy of extended versus standard lymphadenectomy in pancreatoduodenectomy for pancreatic head adenocarcinoma. An update meta-analysis. *Pancreatology* **2019**, *19*, 1074–1080. [CrossRef]
196. Dasari, B.V.M.; Pasquali, S.; Vohra, R.S.; Smith, A.M.; Taylor, M.A.; Sutcliffe, R.P.; Muiesan, P.; Roberts, K.J.; Isaac, J.; Mirza, D.F. Extended Versus Standard Lymphadenectomy for Pancreatic Head Cancer: Meta-Analysis of Randomized Controlled Trials. *J. Gastrointest. Surg.* **2015**, *19*, 1725–1732. [CrossRef]
197. Sabater, L.; Cugat, E.; Serrablo, A.; Suarez-Artacho, G.; Diez-Valladares, L.; Santoyo-Santoyo, J.; Martín-Pérez, E.; Ausania, F.; Lopez-Ben, S.; Jover-Navalon, J.M.; et al. Does the Artery-first Approach Improve the Rate of R0 Resection in Pancreatoduodenectomy?: A Multicenter, Randomized, Controlled Trial. *Ann. Surg.* **2019**, *270*, 738–746. [CrossRef]
198. Negoi, I.; Hostiuc, S.; Runcanu, A.; Negoi, R.I.; Beuran, M. Superior mesenteric artery first approach versus standard pancreaticoduodenectomy: A systematic review and meta-analysis. *Hepatobiliary Pancreat. Dis. Int.* **2017**, *16*, 127–138. [CrossRef]
199. Hiraoka, T.; Uchino, R.; Kanemitsu, K.; Toyonaga, M.; Saitoh, N.; Nakamura, I.; Tashiro, S.; Miyauchi, Y. Combination of intraoperative radiation with resection of cancer of the pancreas. *Int. J. Pancreatol.* **1990**, *7*, 201–207.
200. Katz, M.H.G.; Ou, F.S.; Herman, J.M.; Ahmad, S.A.; Wolpin, B.; Marsh, R.; Behr, S.; Shi, Q.; Chuong, M.; Schwartz, L.H.; et al. Alliance for clinical trials in oncology (ALLIANCE) trial A021501: Preoperative extended chemotherapy vs. chemotherapy plus hypofractionated radiation therapy for borderline resectable adenocarcinoma of the head of the pancreas. *BMC Cancer* **2017**, *17*, 505. [CrossRef]
201. Lafranceschina, S.; Brunetti, O.; DelVecchio, A.; Conticchio, M.; Ammendola, M.; Currò, G.; Piardi, T.; De'Angelis, N.; Silvestris, N.; Memeo, R. Systematic Review of Irreversible Electroporation Role in Management of Locally Advanced Pancreatic Cancer. *Cancers* **2019**, *11*, 1718. [CrossRef]
202. Tsuchida, H.; Fujii, T.; Mizuma, M.; Satoi, S.; Igarashi, H.; Eguchi, H.; Kuroki, T.; Shimizu, Y.; Tani, M.; Tanno, S.; et al. Prognostic importance of peritoneal washing cytology in patients with otherwise resectable pancreatic ductal adenocarcinoma who underwent pancreatectomy: A nationwide, cancer registry–based study from the Japan Pancreas Society. *Surgery* **2019**, *166*, 997–1003. [CrossRef] [PubMed]

203. Yamada, S.; Fujii, T.; Yamamoto, T.; Takami, H.; Yoshioka, I.; Yamaki, S.; Sonohara, F.; Shibuya, K.; Motoi, F.; Hirano, S.; et al. Phase I/II study of adding intraperitoneal paclitaxel in patients with pancreatic cancer and peritoneal metastasis. *BJS* **2020**, *107*, 1811–1817. [CrossRef]
204. Satoi, S.; Fujii, T.; Yanagimoto, H.; Motoi, F.; Kurata, M.; Takahara, N.; Yamada, S.; Yamamoto, T.; Mizuma, M.; Honda, G.; et al. Multicenter Phase II Study of Intravenous and Intraperitoneal Paclitaxel With S-1 for Pancreatic Ductal Adenocarcinoma Patients With Peritoneal Metastasis. *Ann. Surg.* **2017**, *265*, 397–401. [CrossRef]
205. Lai, E.; Puzzoni, M.; Ziranu, P.; Pretta, A.; Impera, V.; Mariani, S.; Liscia, N.; Soro, P.; Musio, F.; Persano, M.; et al. New therapeutic targets in pancreatic cancer. *Cancer Treat. Rev.* **2019**, *81*, 101926. [CrossRef] [PubMed]
206. Holter, S.; Borgida, A.; Dodd, A.; Grant, R.; Semotiuk, K.; Hedley, D.; Dhani, N.; Narod, S.; Akbari, M.; Moore, M.; et al. Germline BRCA Mutations in a Large Clinic-Based Cohort of Patients With Pancreatic Adenocarcinoma. *J. Clin. Oncol.* **2015**, *33*, 3124–3129. [CrossRef] [PubMed]
207. Waddell, N.; Initiative, A.P.C.G.; Pajic, M.; Patch, A.-M.; Chang, D.K.; Kassahn, K.S.; Bailey, P.; Johns, A.L.; Miller, D.; Nones, K.; et al. Whole genomes redefine the mutational landscape of pancreatic cancer. *Nat. Cell Biol.* **2015**, *518*, 495–501. [CrossRef] [PubMed]
208. Golan, T.; Hammel, P.; Reni, M.; Van Cutsem, E.; Macarulla, T.; Hall, M.J.; Park, J.-O.; Hochhauser, D.; Arnold, D.; Oh, D.-Y.; et al. Maintenance Olaparib for Germline BRCA-Mutated Metastatic Pancreatic Cancer. *N. Engl. J. Med.* **2019**, *381*, 317–327. [CrossRef] [PubMed]

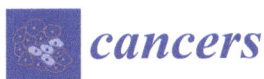 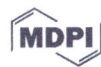

Article

Predictive Features of Malignancy in Branch Duct Type Intraductal Papillary Mucinous Neoplasm of the Pancreas: A Meta-Analysis

Wooil Kwon [†], Youngmin Han [†], Yoonhyeong Byun, Jae Seung Kang, Yoo Jin Choi, Hongbeom Kim and Jin-Young Jang *

Department of Surgery and Cancer Research Institute, Seoul National University College of Medicine, Seoul 03080, Korea; willdoc@snu.ac.kr (W.K.); views@snu.ac.kr (Y.H.); yoonhyeong@snu.ac.kr (Y.B.); 74398@snuh.org (J.S.K.); 74401@snuh.org (Y.J.C.); surgeonkhb@snu.ac.kr (H.K.)
* Correspondence: jangjy4@snu.ac.kr; Tel.: +82-2-2072-2914; Fax: +82-2-766-3975
† These authors contributed equally to this paper as first authors.

Received: 31 July 2020; Accepted: 11 September 2020; Published: 14 September 2020

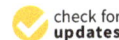

Simple Summary: Currently, there are several guidelines that are widely used to establish the treatment strategy for branch duct type intraductal papillary mucinous neoplasms. Although there are some common grounds, there are discrepancies on which features they adopt, how much each feature is weighted, and how the features are combined. Furthermore, some of the features are based on lower level evidences or expert opinions. The aim of this meta-analysis was to investigate important clinical, radiological, and biochemical risk factors for malignancy and their impact as predictors. This study found symptom, size, cyst wall thickening, presence of mural nodule, change in main pancreatic duct caliber, lymphadenopathy, CA 19-9, and CEA as risk factors. Lymphadenopathy (odd ratio [OR]: 8.55), abrupt caliber change (OR: 7.41), and mural nodule (OR: 4.10) had the highest odd ratios. We expect the higher level evidences of this study to help shape better guidelines and reduce discrepancies among future guidelines.

Abstract: The current guidelines on branch duct type intraductal papillary mucinous neoplasm (BD-IPMN) recommend various predictive features of malignancy as well as different treatment strategies. This study aimed to identify the risk factors for malignancy with higher level of evidence. A meta-analysis was performed on 40 literatures published between 2000 and 2019. These literatures included 6301 patients with pathologically proven IPMN. Malignancy was defined as high-grade dysplasia and invasive carcinoma. It was significantly associated with symptoms (odds ratio [OR] 1.35, confidence interval [CI] 1.01–1.79), size ≥ 3 cm (OR 1.90, CI 1.51–2.40), cystic wall thickening (OR 2.53, CI 1.50–4.27), mural nodule (OR 4.10, CI 3.38–4.97), main pancreatic duct dilatation (OR 2.98, CI 2.11–4.21), abrupt caliber change of the pancreatic duct (OR 7.41, CI 2.49–22.06), lymphadenopathy (OR 8.55, CI 3.25–22.51), elevated carbohydrate antigen 19-9 (OR 4.01, CI 2.55–6.28), and elevated carcinoembryonic antigen (OR 2.04, CI 1.60–2.61). Multilocular cysts and multiple cysts did not show a significant association with malignancy. This study examined the clinical, radiological, and biochemical features of BD-IPMN, often used as malignancy predictors according to the widely used guidelines. The results confirmed that all the features currently being used are valid.

Keywords: branch duct intraductal papillary mucinous neoplasm; risk factor; malignancy; meta-analysis

1. Introduction

Branch duct type intraductal papillary mucinous neoplasm (BD-IPMN) is a well-known premalignant lesion of the pancreas. The prevalence of BD-IPMN-associated malignancy is reportedly over 24% [1]. Nearly four decades have passed since the first report of IPMN by Ohashi et al. [2], but our understanding of IPMN is still limited. Particularly, the ability to predict malignancy and set an appropriate treatment plan is far from satisfactory. Given that pancreatic cancer is the fourth leading cause of cancer mortality [3], the clinical implications of this shortcoming are grave. To make matters worse, the incidence of IPMN is on a steady rise, as incidental detections are increasing due to better access to heath check-ups and increased use of cross-sectional imaging studies [4,5]. The current situation poses a great challenge for pancreatic surgeons and physicians.

Many investigations have been conducted, results have been produced, and the endeavor continues. Currently, there are several management guidelines for IPMN. Among them, the most frequently referenced are those by the American Gastroenterological Association (AGA) [6], European Study Group on Cystic Tumours of the Pancreas [7,8], and International Association of Pancreatology (IAP) [1,9,10]. Although all these guidelines have some commonalities, they do differ with respect to certain surgical treatment indications and surveillance strategies. Another issue is that few of these guidelines cite studies with lower levels of evidences, while others cite experts' opinions.

The first step in producing high-quality treatment guidelines for BD-IPMN is to clarify the risk factors for malignancy. Therefore, a meta-analysis was performed to identify the clinically important risk factors for malignancy and their impact. This study investigated the comprehensive factors including clinical, radiological, and biochemical factors that could be acquired preoperatively.

2. Results

2.1. Search Results

The search process is described in Figure 1. A thorough literature search on MEDLINE identified 472 publications that were potentially relevant to this study. A total of, 412 studies were excluded after screening. Of the remaining 60 publications, 17 were excluded after detailed review due to insufficient data regarding worrisome features/high-risk stigmata, absence of pathological data, insufficient sample size, or overlap with another study. When an overlapping study cohort was found, the larger sample study was chosen. If there were results regarding worrisome features/high-risk stigmata in a smaller overlapping study that was not addressed in the larger one, it was still included. Finally, 40 publications were included in the analysis [11–50]. The publication bias was assessed visually by inspecting the funnel plot for asymmetry.

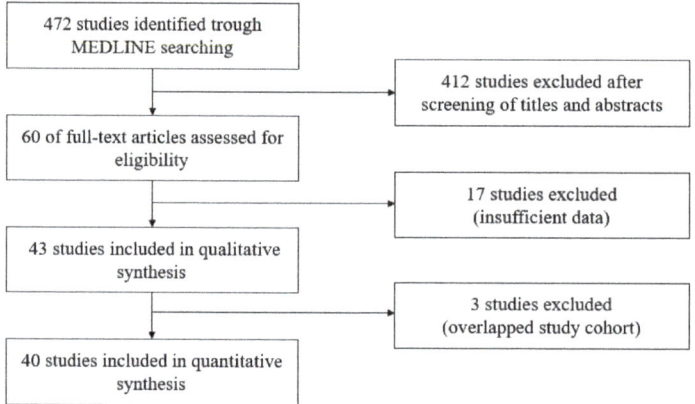

Figure 1. A flow diagram of the inclusion criteria of studies eligible for meta-analysis.

2.2. Characteristics of Included Studies

The characteristics of the included publications are described in Table 1. This study included 40 publications with 6301 patients diagnosed with IPMN, of which histological data of 4241 patients diagnosed with benign IPMN and 2060 with malignant IPMN were identified. In all studies, malignant IPMN was defined as invasive carcinoma and high-grade dysplasia. Terms such as invasive cancer, intraductal papillary mucinous carcinoma (IPMC), and invasive IPMN were considered equivalent to invasive carcinoma. Non-invasive carcinoma, carcinoma in situ, and IPMC in situ were considered equivalent to high-grade dysplasia.

2.3. Clinical Symptoms

Data regarding symptoms were extractable in 15 studies [12,15,19,20,23,25,27,31,33,35,36,38,40–42]. In these studies, 840 patients (54.8%) presented symptoms, and malignancy was reported in 28.6% of patients with symptoms and 27.4% without symptoms. The odds ratio (OR) of having symptoms was 1.35 (95% confidence interval [CI] 1.01–1.79, $p = 0.040$) (Table 2, Figure 2a).

2.4. Characteristics of Cyst

Data regarding cyst size were obtained from 22 studies with 4446 patients [12,15–17,20–22,24–26,30–33,36–38,40,41,43,48,49], and the risk of malignancy was examined for a reference size of 3 cm. The malignancy rate in cysts ≥ 3 cm and < 3 cm in size was 38.7% and 25.7%, respectively. Cysts of size ≥ 3 cm significantly increased the risk of malignancy with an OR of 1.90 (95% CI 1.51–2.40, $p < 0.001$) (Table 2, Figure 2b).

Data regarding cystic wall thickening was extracted from nine studies with 689 patients [13,14,17,18,34,37,38,40,43], and wall thickening was found in 15.2% of the cases. Moreover, 51.4% of the patients with wall thickening reported malignancy as compared to 23.6% of those without wall thickening. Wall thickening was significantly associated with malignancy with OR of 2.53 (95% CI 1.50–4.27, $p < 0.001$) (Table 2, Figure 2c).

Multilocularity and multiplicity was analyzed in seven [17,20,21,34,37,40,47] and eight studies [12,15,17,21,35,37,40,47], respectively. Malignancy rate of multilocular and unilocular cysts was 27.0% and 22.2%, respectively. Furthermore, the malignancy rate of single and multiple cysts was 26.6% and 24.0%, respectively. Notably, neither of the features was associated with an increased risk of malignancy (multilocularity: OR 0.92, 95% CI 0.63–1.35, $p = 0.680$; multiplicity: OR 0.76, 95% CI 0.55–1.04, $p = 0.090$) (Table 2, Figure 2d,e).

Table 1. Characteristics of included studies.

Study	Year	Study Period	No. of Patients	Mean Age (Years)	Male/Female	Type of IPMN	Benign	Malignant	Malignancy Proportion (%)	Diagnostic Modality
Akahoshi et al. [11]	2018	2006–2017	50	68	33/17	BD	33	17	34.0%	CT, MRI
Akita et al. [12]	2011	1992–2007	32	62.6	19/13	BD	20	12	37.5%	CT, MRI, MRCP
Arikawa et al. [13]	2011	2003–2008	25	65.2	20/5	BD	17	8	32.0%	CT, MRCP, EUS
Aso et al. [14]	2014	2006–2013	70	N/A	N/A	BD	42	28	40.0%	CT, MRCP, EUS
Attiyeh et al. [15]	2018	2005–2015	381	67	160/221	BD	276	105	27.6%	Not stated
Bournet et al. [16]	2009	1988–2005	53	63.9	52/47	BD, mixed	29	24	24.2%	CT, MRCP, EUS, ERCP
Carbognin et al. [17]	2006	1995–2005	29	Benign 64.7 Malignant 62.2	17/12	BD, mixed	11	18	62.1%	CT, MRI, MRCP
Chiu et al. [18]	2006	1995–2005	40	N/A	N/A	BD, MD, mixed	30	10	25.0%	CT
Correa-Gallego et al. [19]	2013	1994–2010	123	68	50/73	BD	87	36	29.3%	Not stated
Dortch et al. [20]	2015	2002–2013	66	68	26/42	BD	54	12	18.2%	CT, MRCP, EUS, FNA
Fritz et al. [21]	2014	2004–2012	233	N/A	95/138	BD	177	56	24.0%	CT, MRI
Harima et al. [22]	2015	2009–2014	15	N/A	N/A	BD	1	14	93.3%	CT, EUS
Hirono et al. [23]	2017	1999–2015	109	N/A	46/63	BD	52	57	52.3%	CT, EUS
Jang et al. [24]	2017	1992–2012	2258	65.0	1408/850	BD	1429	829	36.7%	CT, EUS
Kato et al. [25]	2015	1994–2012	47	66.2	30/17	BD	25	22	46.8%	Not stated
Kim YI et al. [26]	2015	1997–2013	324	62	179/145	BD	282	42	13.0%	CT, MRCP, EUS, ERCP
Kim TH et al. [27]	2015	2004–2012	177	63	108/69	BD	138	39	22.0%	CT, EUS
Koshita et al. [28]	2017	2005–2014	28	62.2	17/11	BD	14	14	50.0%	CT, MRCP, EUS, ERCP
Lee et al. [29]	2014	2002–2011	84	64.7	55/29	BD	68	16	19.0%	EUS
Maguchi et al. [30]	2011	N/A	29	N/A	N/A	BD	20	9	31.0%	CT, EUS
Mimura et al. [31]	2010	1998–2009	43	Benign 66.0 Malignant 66.7	29/14	BD, mixed	23	20	46.5%	CT, EUS
Nagai et al. [32]	2009	1984–2007	84	63	48/36	BD	47	37	44.0%	CT, ERCP, MRI, EUS
Nguyen et al. [33]	2015	1996–2012	66	69	26/42	BD	51	15	22.7%	CT, MRI, EUS
Ogawa et al. [34]	2008	2000–2006	49	64.9	39/20	BD	22	27	55.1%	CT
Ohno et al. [35]	2012	2001–2009	30	65.1	15/15	BD	19	11	63.3%	CT, ERCP, CE-EUS
Ohtsuka et al. [36]	2012	1990–2009	99	N/A	60/39	BD	77	22	22.2%	CT, MRCP, US, EUS
Ridtitid et al. [37]	2016	2001–2013	135	65.2	71/64	BD	117	18	13.3%	CT, MRI, EUS
Robles et al. [38]	2014	2006–2014	120	57.9	65/55	BD	84	36	30.0%	CT, MRI, EUS
Rodriguez et al. [39]	2007	1990–2005	145	67*	62/83	BD	113	32	22.1%	CEUS, CT, MRI
Sahora et al. [40]	2013	1995–2012	217	N/A	82/135	BD, mixed	169	48	22.1%	CT, MRI, MRCP, EUS
Salvia et al. [41]	2007	2000–2003	20	58	10/10	BD	18	2	10.0%	US, MRI, MRCP, CEUS, EUS, ERCP
Schmidt et al. [42]	2007	1991–2006	103	63	50/53	BD	83	20	19.4%	CT, MRI, ERCP, EUS
Seo et al. [43]	2016	2011–2013	60	64.3	35/25	BD	52	8	13.3%	CT, MRI
Serikawa et al. [44]	2006	1992–2005	56	65.8	42/14	BD	49	7	10.3%	US, EUS, CT, ERCP, MRCP
Shimizu et al. [45]	2020	1996–2014	466	67.9	274/192	BD	208	258	55.4%	CT, EUS, MRCP
Strauss et al. [46]	2016	2004–2012	168	N/A	N/A	BD	126	42	25.0%	CT, MRI, MRCP
Takeshita et al. [47]	2008	2002–2006	46	65	28/25	BD	38	8	17.4%	CT
Tang et al. [48]	2008	1995–2006	31	66.5	10/21	BD	26	5	16.1%	CT, MRI, MRCP, ERCP, EUS
Wong et al. [49]	2013	2000–2010	105	68	47/58	BD	43	62	59.0%	CT, MRI, EUS
Woo et al. [50]	2009	1998–2005	85	63	50/35	BD	71	14	16.5%	CT, EUS, ERCP, MR

N/A, not available; IPMN, intraductal papillary mucinous neoplasm; BD, branch duct; MD, main duct; CT, computed tomography; MRI, magnetic resonance image; MRCP, magnetic resonance cholangiopancreatography; ERCP, endoscopic retrograde cholangiopancreatography; US, ultrasonography; CEUS, contrast-enhanced ultrasonography; EUS, endoscopic ultrasonography; CE-EUS, contrast-enhanced endoscopic ultrasonography; FNA, fine needle aspiration. * in median.

Table 2. Summary of clinical, radiographic, and biochemical parameters.

Parameters	No. Studies	No. of Patient	No. of Positive Feature (%)	No. of Malignancy (%)	No. of Malignancy among Positive Features (%)	No. of Malignancy among Negative Features (%)	OR	95% CI	p-Value
Symptoms (+)	16	2844	1089 (38.3)	966 (34.0)	369 (33.9)	597 (34.0)	1.35	1.01, 1.79	0.040
Cyst size (≥3 cm)	22	4446	2091 (47.0)	1414 (31.8)	814 (38.9)	605 (25.7)	1.90	1.51, 2.40	<0.001
Wall thickening	9	689	105 (15.2)	192 (27.9)	54 (51.4)	138 (23.6)	2.53	1.50, 4.27	<0.001
Multilocular	7	741	389 (52.5)	183 (24.7)	105 (27.0)	78 (22.2)	0.92	0.63, 1.35	0.68
Multiplicity	8	1058	350 (33.1)	272 (25.7)	84 (24.0)	188 (26.6)	0.76	0.55, 1.04	0.09
Mural nodule	25	4495	1610 (35.8)	1434 (31.9)	845 (52.5)	589 (20.4)	4.10	3.38, 4.97	<0.001
MPD dilatation	15	3499	1482 (42.4)	1190 (34.0)	698 (47.1)	492 (24.4)	2.98	2.11, 4.21	<0.001
>5 mm	8	3098	1305 (42.1)	1031 (33.3)	607 (46.5)	424 (23.6)	2.85	1.90, 4.26	<0.001
>6 mm	5	270	107 (39.6)	125 (46.3)	70 (65.4)	55 (33.7)	3.86	1.63, 9.11	0.002
>7 mm	2	131	70 (53.4)	72 (55.0)	21 (30.0)	13 (21.3)	2.69	0.42, 17.16	0.29
Abrupt caliber change	4	467	34 (7.3)	74 (15.8)	18 (52.9)	56 (12.9)	7.41	2.49, 22.06	<0.001
Lymphadenopathy	4	390	70 (17.9)	70 (17.9)	14 (20.0)	56 (15.3)	8.55	3.25, 22.51	<0.001
CA 19-9 (>37 U/mL)	8	3279	477 (14.5)	1073 (32.7)	295 (61.8)	778 (27.8)	4.01	2.55, 6.28	<0.001
CEA (>5 ng/mL)	4	2405	301 (12.5)	912 (37.9)	161 (53.5)	751 (35.7)	2.04	1.60, 2.61	<0.001

OR, odd ratio; CI, confidence interval; MPD, main pancreatic duct; CA, carbohydrate antigen; CEA, carcinoembryonic antigen.

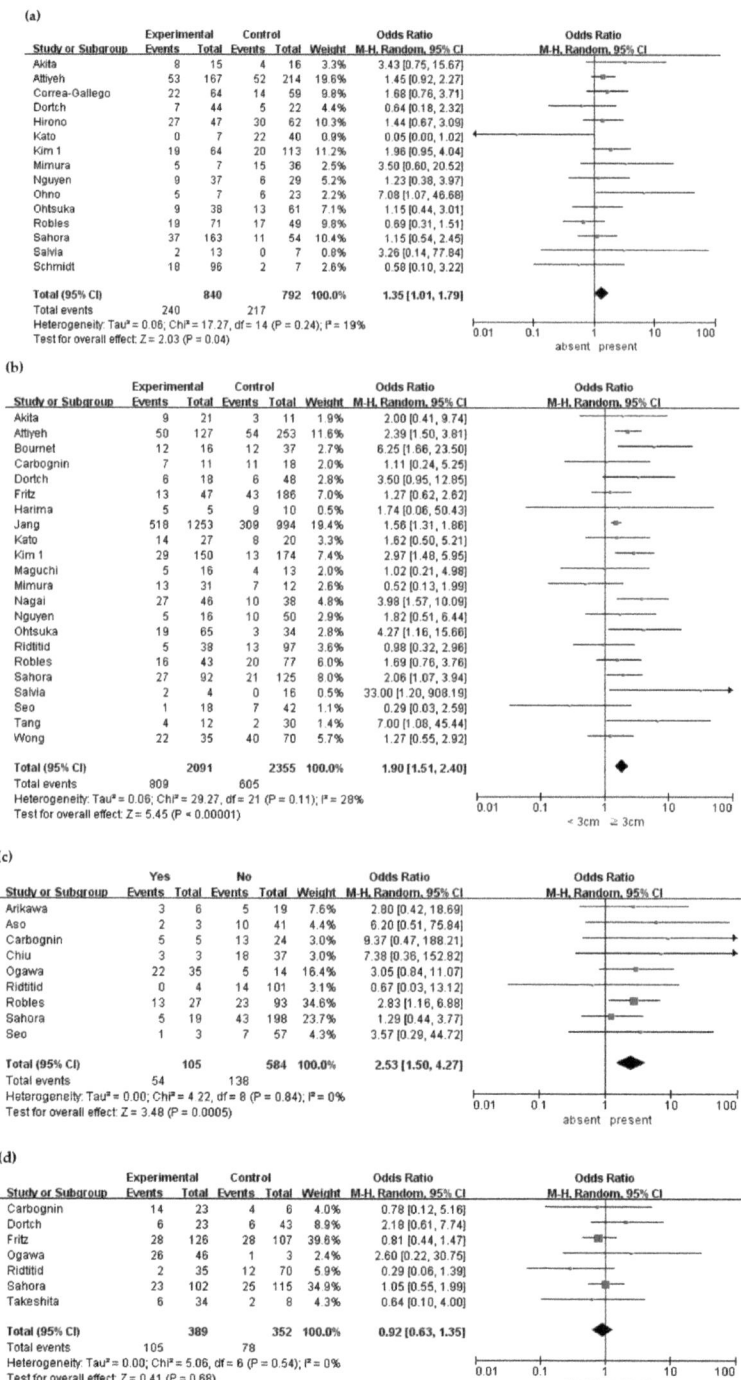

Figure 2. Cont.

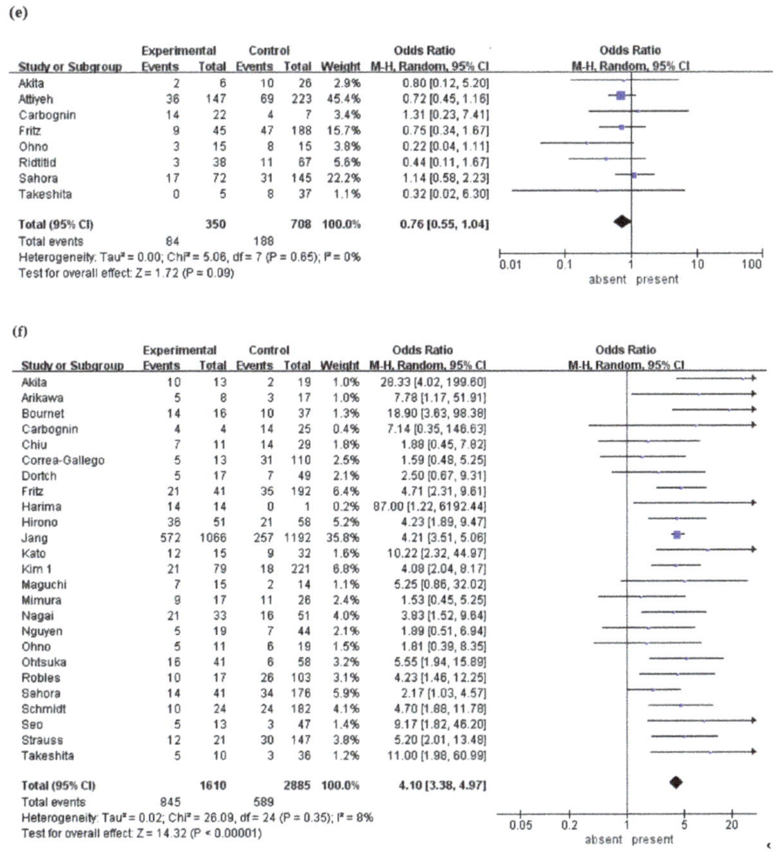

Figure 2. Forest plot showing the incidence of malignancy in BD-IPMN stratified by symptoms, characteristics of the cyst, and presence of mural nodule. (**a**) symptom. (**b**) cyst size. (**c**) cyst wall thickening. (**d**) multilocular cyst. (**e**) multiple cyst. and (**f**) mural nodule.

2.5. Mural Nodule

Mural nodule was the most frequently investigated parameter observed in 25 studies and cohort of 4495 patients [12,13,16–26,30–33,35,36,38,40,42,43,46,47]. The prevalence of mural nodule in BD-IPMN was 35.8%, and the pooled malignancy rate was 31.9%. The malignancy rate was 52.5% in the presence of mural nodule and 20.4% in its absence. The presence of mural nodule resulted in a four-fold increase in the malignancy risk. The pooled OR was 4.10 (95% CI 3.38–4.97, $p < 0.001$) (Table 2, Figure 2f).

2.6. Changes in Main Pancreatic Duct

Several studies examined the size of the main pancreatic duct, but they all had different cut-off values. The reference size was 5 mm in eight studies [22,24–26,37,38,40,43], 6 mm in five studies [16,30–32,34], and 7 mm in two studies [12,36]. For pancreatic ducts of size 5 mm, the OR was 2.85 (95% CI 1.90–4.26, $p < 0.001$), and a malignancy rate of 46.5% for ducts > 5 mm. The ORs for main pancreatic ducts >6 and 7 mm were 3.86 (95% CI 1.63–9.11, $p = 0.002$) and 2.69 (95% CI 0.42–17.16, $p = 0.29$), respectively. Overall, the OR for dilatation of the main pancreatic duct was 2.98 (95% CI 2.11–4.21, $p < 0.001$) (Table 2, Figure 3a).

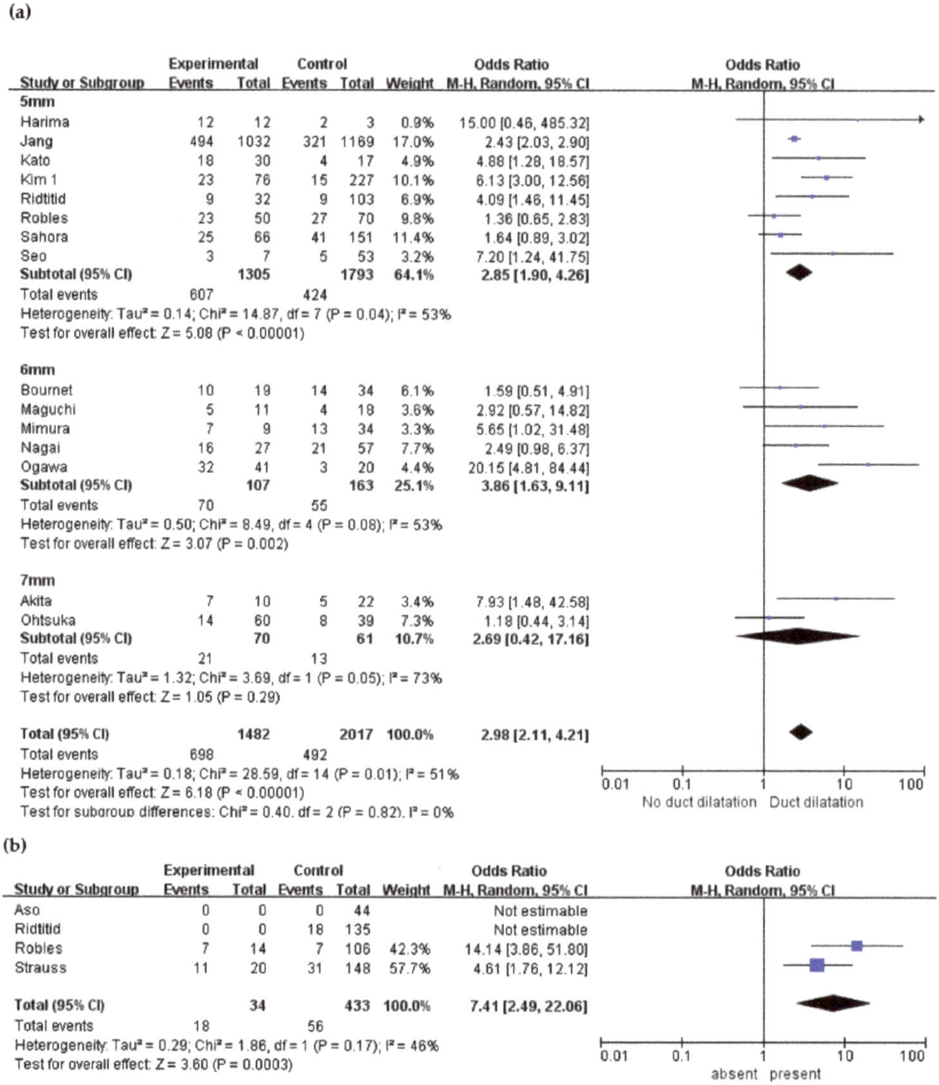

(a)

Study or Subgroup	Experimental Events	Total	Control Events	Total	Weight	Odds Ratio M-H, Random, 95% CI
5mm						
Harima	12	12	2	3	0.9%	15.00 [0.46, 485.32]
Jang	494	1032	321	1169	17.0%	2.43 [2.03, 2.90]
Kato	18	30	4	17	4.9%	4.88 [1.28, 18.57]
Kim 1	23	76	15	227	10.1%	6.13 [3.00, 12.56]
Ridtitid	9	32	9	103	6.9%	4.09 [1.46, 11.45]
Robles	23	50	27	70	9.8%	1.36 [0.65, 2.83]
Sahora	25	66	41	151	11.4%	1.64 [0.89, 3.02]
Seo	3	7	5	53	3.2%	7.20 [1.24, 41.75]
Subtotal (95% CI)		1305		1793	64.1%	2.85 [1.90, 4.26]
Total events	607		424			
Heterogeneity: Tau² = 0.14; Chi² = 14.87, df = 7 (P = 0.04); I² = 53%						
Test for overall effect: Z = 5.08 (P < 0.00001)						
6mm						
Bournet	10	19	14	34	6.1%	1.59 [0.51, 4.91]
Maguchi	5	11	4	18	3.6%	2.92 [0.57, 14.82]
Mimura	7	9	13	34	3.3%	5.65 [1.02, 31.48]
Nagai	16	27	21	57	7.7%	2.49 [0.98, 6.37]
Ogawa	32	41	3	20	4.4%	20.15 [4.81, 84.44]
Subtotal (95% CI)		107		163	25.1%	3.86 [1.63, 9.11]
Total events	70		55			
Heterogeneity: Tau² = 0.50; Chi² = 8.49, df = 4 (P = 0.08); I² = 53%						
Test for overall effect: Z = 3.07 (P = 0.002)						
7mm						
Akita	7	10	5	22	3.4%	7.93 [1.48, 42.58]
Ohtsuka	14	60	8	39	7.3%	1.18 [0.44, 3.14]
Subtotal (95% CI)		70		61	10.7%	2.69 [0.42, 17.16]
Total events	21		13			
Heterogeneity: Tau² = 1.32; Chi² = 3.69, df = 1 (P = 0.05); I² = 73%						
Test for overall effect: Z = 1.05 (P = 0.29)						
Total (95% CI)		1482		2017	100.0%	2.98 [2.11, 4.21]
Total events	698		492			
Heterogeneity: Tau² = 0.18; Chi² = 28.59, df = 14 (P = 0.01); I² = 51%						
Test for overall effect: Z = 6.18 (P < 0.00001)						
Test for subgroup differences: Chi² = 0.40, df = 2 (P = 0.82), I² = 0%						

No duct dilatation / Duct dilatation

(b)

Study or Subgroup	Experimental Events	Total	Control Events	Total	Weight	Odds Ratio M-H, Random, 95% CI
Aso	0	0	0	44		Not estimable
Ridtitid	0	0	18	135		Not estimable
Robles	7	14	7	106	42.3%	14.14 [3.86, 51.80]
Strauss	11	20	31	148	57.7%	4.61 [1.76, 12.12]
Total (95% CI)		34		433	100.0%	7.41 [2.49, 22.06]
Total events	18		56			
Heterogeneity: Tau² = 0.29; Chi² = 1.86, df = 1 (P = 0.17); I² = 46%						
Test for overall effect: Z = 3.60 (P = 0.0003)						

absent / present

Figure 3. Forest plot demonstrates the incidence of malignancy in BD-IPMN in relation to change in main pancreatic duct. Forest plot stratified (**a**) by the diameter of pancreatic duct and (**b**) by abrupt caliber change.

Four studies examined the caliber change in the pancreatic duct in 467 patients [14,37,38,46]. Among 34 patients with an abrupt change in caliber, 18 patients (52.9%) had malignant BD-IPMN with OR of 7.41 (95% CI 2.49–22.06, $p < 0.001$) (Table 2, Figure 3b).

2.7. Lymphadenopathy

Four studies examining lymphadenopathy had a pooled cohort of 390 patients [14,17,21,43]. The prevalence of lymphadenopathy was 6.2%. The malignancy rate in these patients was 58.3% as compared to 15.3% in those without lymphadenopathy. The OR for lymphadenopathy was the highest among all parameters at 8.55 (95% CI 3.25–22.51, $p < 0.001$) (Table 2, Figure 4).

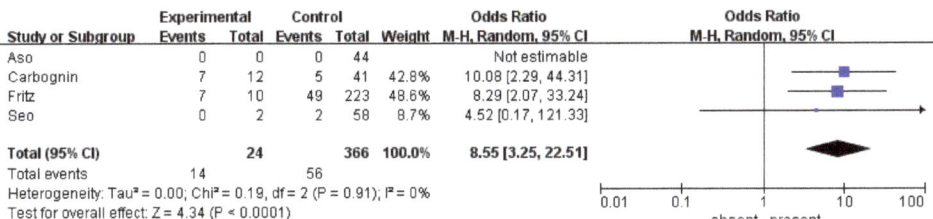

Figure 4. Forest plot demonstrates the incidence of malignancy in BD-IPMN stratified by the presence of lymphadenopathy.

2.8. Biochemical Markers

Carbohydrate antigen (CA) 19-9 with a cut-off level of 37 U/mL was examined in eight studies [15,21,23–26,36,40]. Among 3279 pooled patients, 477 patients (14.5%) had elevated CA 19-9 levels, of which 61.8% had malignant BD-IPMN, whereas only 27.8% of the normal CA 19-9 patients showed malignancy. The OR was 4.01 (95% CI 2.55–6.28, $p < 0.001$) (Table 2 and Figure 5a).

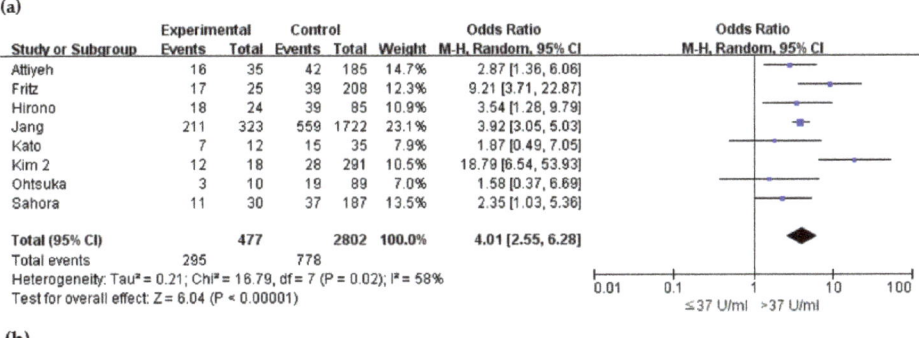

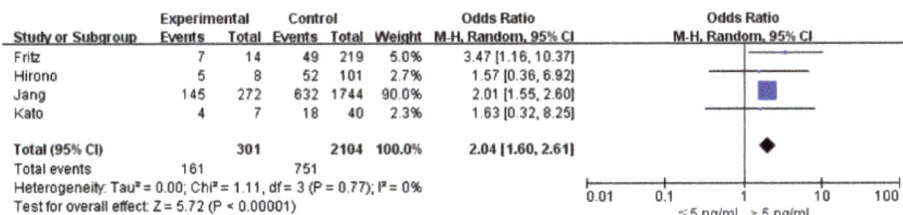

Figure 5. Forest plot demonstrates the incidence of malignancy in BD-IPMN in relation to biochemical markers. (**a**) carbohydrate antigen 19-9 and (**b**) carcinoembryonic antigen.

There were four studies [21,23–25] with pooled cohort of 2405 patients that reported the presence of carcinoembryonic antigen (CEA) with a cut-off level of 5 ng/mL. The malignancy rate among patients with elevated CEA and normal CEA was 53.5% and 35.7%, respectively. The OR for elevated CEA was 2.04 (95% CI 1.60–2.61, $p < 0.001$) (Table 2, Figure 5b).

3. Discussion

This study revealed that the parameters of symptoms, size, cystic wall thickening, presence of mural nodule, change in main pancreatic duct caliber, lymphadenopathy, CA 19-9, and CEA were the predictive features of malignancy in BD-IPMN. On the other hand, multilocularity of cyst and multiple cysts were not malignancy predictors.

The findings are in accordance with most of the widely used guidelines. The AGA guideline utilizes size, dilated main pancreatic duct, solid component, and positive cytology to determine the treatment strategy [6]. Reference size ≥ 3 cm, dilated main pancreatic duct, and associated solid component were considered risk factors, and presence of at least two of these would warrant endoscopic ultrasound-fine needle aspiration (EUS-FNA). In the case of positive cytology or presence of a solid component and a dilated pancreatic duct, surgery is indicated. Since this guideline is for asymptomatic neoplastic pancreatic cysts, the symptoms were not considered.

Unlike the conservative AGA guidelines, the European study group proposes a more aggressive approach in BD-IPMN patients [7,8]. Presence of jaundice, positive cytology, enhancing mural nodule (≥5 mm), solid mass, and main pancreatic duct ≥10 mm are absolute indicators for surgery. Growth rate ≥5 mm/year, elevated serum CA 19-9 level, main pancreatic duct dilatation between 5–9.9 mm, cyst diameter ≥40 mm, new onset diabetes mellitus, acute pancreatitis, and enhancing mural nodule (<5 mm) are relative indicators wherein healthy patients may opt for surgery.

The IAP guidelines stratify the features into high-risk stigmata and worrisome features. The high-risk stigmata and worrisome features warrant surgery and EUS, respectively. High-risk stigmata include obstructive jaundice in a patient with cystic lesion of the head of the pancreas, enhancing mural nodule ≥5 mm, and main pancreatic duct ≥10 mm. Worrisome features include cyst ≥3 cm, enhancing mural nodule <5 mm, thickened/enhancing cyst walls, main duct size 5–9 mm, abrupt change in caliber of pancreatic duct with distal pancreatic atrophy, lymphadenopathy, increased CA 19-9 serum level, and cystic growth rate ≥5 mm/2 years. The features used by the IAP and European study group are similar. However, the IAP guidelines are slightly more conservative, wherein surgery is decided based on the EUS findings in patients with worrisome features.

In this study, all the features were included to validate those featuring in various guidelines. In addition, other features such as locularity, multiplicity, and CEA serum level were explored. The parameter of symptoms showed a significant association with malignancy. However, the symptoms could be heterogenous and often vague. They consisted of one or combinations of clinical findings such as abdominal pain, weight loss, pancreatitis, and jaundice. Therefore, it is difficult to define what symptom to look for and determine the appropriate treatment strategy. Notably, jaundice was found to be a significant predictor of malignancy by several studies [15,27,38,42]. In particular, a nomogram developed by Attiyeh et al. [15] automatically assigned a predicted probability of high-risk disease of "1" to patients with jaundice. Another symptom that showed high association with malignancy was weight loss. Among five studies that examined weight loss separately [15,19,20,33,42], all studies except one [33] found weight loss to be significantly associated with malignancy. While many symptoms depend on the patient's report and tend to be subjective, jaundice and weight loss are symptoms that can be objectively quantified. Therefore, instead of considering symptoms as a whole, utilizing jaundice and weight loss to predict malignancy seemed reasonable, and studies defining the cut-off values for these symptoms should be warranted. Nevertheless, jaundice and weight loss are symptoms often associated with overt cancer and may have limited value in predicting earlier malignant transformation such as high-grade dysplasia. Our results showed that 27.4% of asymptomatic patients reported malignancy, demonstrating that absence of symptoms does not assure the absence of malignancy. Therefore, radiologic and biochemical changes may be more important in early detection of malignant transformations.

Previously, a cyst size of 3 cm was considered an absolute indication of BD-IPMN [10,51,52]. However, subsequent studies found that size alone was insufficient to predict malignancy, and although size correlated with malignancy risk, the safe cut-off limit was unclear [53–56]. The European study group does not consider a cyst size of 3 cm as an absolute indication, but rather considers the presence of other risk factors as determining factors, unless the diameter reaches 4 cm [7]. The IAP also stepped down the 3-cm size criteria from an absolute indication to a worrisome feature since the 2012 consensus guidelines [1,9]. Likewise, although the AGA states that size ≥3 cm increases the risk of malignancy by three times [57], size is not the sole determinant of the strategy [6]. In the present study, size ≥3 cm

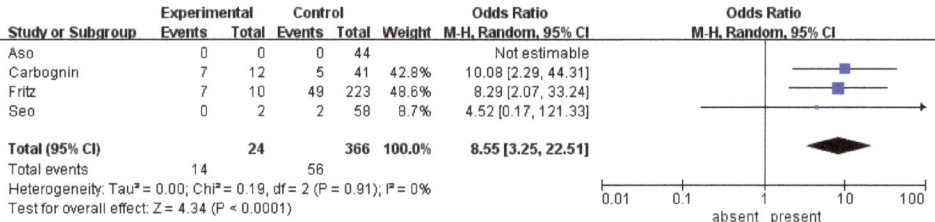

Figure 4. Forest plot demonstrates the incidence of malignancy in BD-IPMN stratified by the presence of lymphadenopathy.

2.8. Biochemical Markers

Carbohydrate antigen (CA) 19-9 with a cut-off level of 37 U/mL was examined in eight studies [15,21,23–26,36,40]. Among 3279 pooled patients, 477 patients (14.5%) had elevated CA 19-9 levels, of which 61.8% had malignant BD-IPMN, whereas only 27.8% of the normal CA 19-9 patients showed malignancy. The OR was 4.01 (95% CI 2.55–6.28, $p < 0.001$) (Table 2 and Figure 5a).

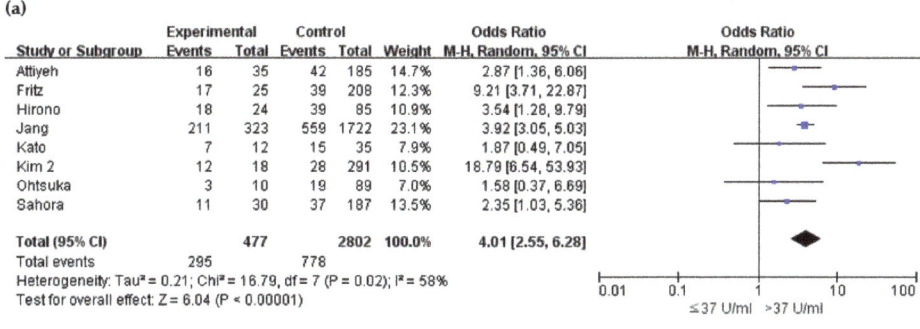

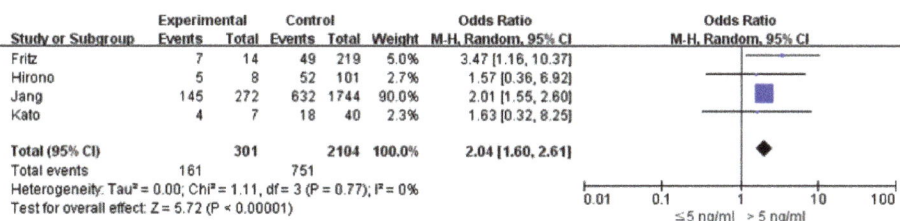

Figure 5. Forest plot demonstrates the incidence of malignancy in BD-IPMN in relation to biochemical markers. (**a**) carbohydrate antigen 19-9 and (**b**) carcinoembryonic antigen.

There were four studies [21,23–25] with pooled cohort of 2405 patients that reported the presence of carcinoembryonic antigen (CEA) with a cut-off level of 5 ng/mL. The malignancy rate among patients with elevated CEA and normal CEA was 53.5% and 35.7%, respectively. The OR for elevated CEA was 2.04 (95% CI 1.60–2.61, $p < 0.001$) (Table 2, Figure 5b).

3. Discussion

This study revealed that the parameters of symptoms, size, cystic wall thickening, presence of mural nodule, change in main pancreatic duct caliber, lymphadenopathy, CA 19-9, and CEA were the predictive features of malignancy in BD-IPMN. On the other hand, multilocularity of cyst and multiple cysts were not malignancy predictors.

The findings are in accordance with most of the widely used guidelines. The AGA guideline utilizes size, dilated main pancreatic duct, solid component, and positive cytology to determine the treatment strategy [6]. Reference size ≥ 3 cm, dilated main pancreatic duct, and associated solid component were considered risk factors, and presence of at least two of these would warrant endoscopic ultrasound-fine needle aspiration (EUS-FNA). In the case of positive cytology or presence of a solid component and a dilated pancreatic duct, surgery is indicated. Since this guideline is for asymptomatic neoplastic pancreatic cysts, the symptoms were not considered.

Unlike the conservative AGA guidelines, the European study group proposes a more aggressive approach in BD-IPMN patients [7,8]. Presence of jaundice, positive cytology, enhancing mural nodule (≥5 mm), solid mass, and main pancreatic duct ≥10 mm are absolute indicators for surgery. Growth rate ≥5 mm/year, elevated serum CA 19-9 level, main pancreatic duct dilatation between 5–9.9 mm, cyst diameter ≥40 mm, new onset diabetes mellitus, acute pancreatitis, and enhancing mural nodule (<5 mm) are relative indicators wherein healthy patients may opt for surgery.

The IAP guidelines stratify the features into high-risk stigmata and worrisome features. The high-risk stigmata and worrisome features warrant surgery and EUS, respectively. High-risk stigmata include obstructive jaundice in a patient with cystic lesion of the head of the pancreas, enhancing mural nodule ≥5 mm, and main pancreatic duct ≥10 mm. Worrisome features include cyst ≥3 cm, enhancing mural nodule <5 mm, thickened/enhancing cyst walls, main duct size 5–9 mm, abrupt change in caliber of pancreatic duct with distal pancreatic atrophy, lymphadenopathy, increased CA 19-9 serum level, and cystic growth rate ≥5 mm/2 years. The features used by the IAP and European study group are similar. However, the IAP guidelines are slightly more conservative, wherein surgery is decided based on the EUS findings in patients with worrisome features.

In this study, all the features were included to validate those featuring in various guidelines. In addition, other features such as locularity, multiplicity, and CEA serum level were explored. The parameter of symptoms showed a significant association with malignancy. However, the symptoms could be heterogenous and often vague. They consisted of one or combinations of clinical findings such as abdominal pain, weight loss, pancreatitis, and jaundice. Therefore, it is difficult to define what symptom to look for and determine the appropriate treatment strategy. Notably, jaundice was found to be a significant predictor of malignancy by several studies [15,27,38,42]. In particular, a nomogram developed by Attiyeh et al. [15] automatically assigned a predicted probability of high-risk disease of "1" to patients with jaundice. Another symptom that showed high association with malignancy was weight loss. Among five studies that examined weight loss separately [15,19,20,33,42], all studies except one [33] found weight loss to be significantly associated with malignancy. While many symptoms depend on the patient's report and tend to be subjective, jaundice and weight loss are symptoms that can be objectively quantified. Therefore, instead of considering symptoms as a whole, utilizing jaundice and weight loss to predict malignancy seemed reasonable, and studies defining the cut-off values for these symptoms should be warranted. Nevertheless, jaundice and weight loss are symptoms often associated with overt cancer and may have limited value in predicting earlier malignant transformation such as high-grade dysplasia. Our results showed that 27.4% of asymptomatic patients reported malignancy, demonstrating that absence of symptoms does not assure the absence of malignancy. Therefore, radiologic and biochemical changes may be more important in early detection of malignant transformations.

Previously, a cyst size of 3 cm was considered an absolute indication of BD-IPMN [10,51,52]. However, subsequent studies found that size alone was insufficient to predict malignancy, and although size correlated with malignancy risk, the safe cut-off limit was unclear [53–56]. The European study group does not consider a cyst size of 3 cm as an absolute indication, but rather considers the presence of other risk factors as determining factors, unless the diameter reaches 4 cm [7]. The IAP also stepped down the 3-cm size criteria from an absolute indication to a worrisome feature since the 2012 consensus guidelines [1,9]. Likewise, although the AGA states that size ≥3 cm increases the risk of malignancy by three times [57], size is not the sole determinant of the strategy [6]. In the present study, size ≥3 cm increased the malignancy risk by two times. Although size is a significant factor, its impact is not as great as that of other features. Hence, size alone has a limited potential in predicting malignancy.

Wall thickening is a feature considered exclusively in the guidelines by IAP. It was introduced in the 2012 consensus guideline [1]. In this study, wall thickening increased the malignancy risk by 2.5 times. However, it is uncertain whether the wall thickening was accompanied by enhancement in the studies. Other cystic characteristics such as multilocularity or multiplicity of cysts did not increase the risk of malignancy.

Mural nodule is one of the strongest and most consistent risk factors in all the guidelines. Mural nodule is an absolute indication according to the European study group, and it could be an indication if it is accompanied by main pancreatic duct dilatation >5 mm according to the AGA guidelines. The AGA found that solid component increased the risk by almost eight times after reviewing 816 patients in seven studies [57]. They found that the incidence of malignancy was 73% in patients with a mural nodule as compared to 23% in those without a mural nodule. In 25 studies with 4495 patients, the malignancy rate was 52.5% in those with a mural nodule and 20.4% in those without. Furthermore, this study found that the malignancy risk was four times higher in patients with mural nodule. Nevertheless, mural nodule is one of the highly predictive factors of malignancy. Recently, enhancement and size of mural nodule have received attention, and these factors were applied to the IAP and European study group guidelines [1,8,58–61]. However, the diagnostic performances vary according to the imaging modality used, and meta-analysis cannot be conducted with the limited number of studies. Therefore, this study did not sub-analyze the mural nodule feature by size or enhancement, and future studies are needed to clarify the effect of these factors.

The main pancreatic duct change is another consistent risk factor of malignancy. The European study group, AGA, and IAP guidelines include main pancreatic duct dilatation. The AGA did not provide a definition of main duct dilation, whereas the European study group and IAP defined duct dilatation as dilatation >5 mm [1,6–9,57]. The IAP and European study group further stratified the risk level according to the extent of dilatation. Main duct dilation between 5–9 mm and >1 cm is considered as worrisome feature and high-risk stigmata by the IAP, or as a relative and absolute indication by the European study group. In contrast, the AGA requires that the solid component be accompanied by main duct dilatation for it to qualify as an indication. Interestingly, the AGA did not find a significant association between dilated pancreatic duct and malignancy (OR, 2.38, 95% CI 0.71–8.00), but included it in their guidelines because the review was performed with resected IPMNs [6,57]. Nevertheless, the main duct dilatation is a well-recognized risk factor that was also confirmed in this meta-analysis. However, the reference cut-off values vary according to studies, and each guideline weighs the same criteria differently. Future efforts are required to reach a consensus. Another change often studied and considered in the IAP guidelines is the abrupt change in caliber. Although this may overlap with main duct dilatation and may be considered an extreme form of dilatation, its OR was the second highest in this study at 7.41. However, this was based only on four studies, and the true predictive value needs further validation.

Lymphadenopathy was recently added to the IAP guidelines during the 2017 revision [9]. There are no references to lymphadenopathy in the European study group or AGA guidelines. Although least attention was given to lymphadenopathy, it demonstrated the highest OR, showing 8.5 times increased risk of malignancy. There were only four studies with a pooled cohort of 390 patients, of which 6.2% had lymphadenopathy. More studies are needed to accurately evaluate the impact of lymphadenopathy in predicting the malignancy in BD-IPMN cases.

Finally, a biochemical marker, CA 19-9, was indicated as a relative risk factor in the European guidelines and as a worrisome feature in the revised 2017 IAP guidelines [7,9]. This study showed that elevated CA 19-9 above 37 U/mL had four times higher risk of malignancy, which is similar to the risk associated with mural nodule. In addition to CA 19-9, the role of CEA was examined, which posed twice the risk of malignancy when elevated above 5 ng/mL. However, only four studies were examined and its actual role needs to be further studied for a definitive conclusion.

There are several limitations in this study. First, all the studies included in this meta-analysis were observational studies, and potential biases are likely to be greater in such studies. Thus, the results should always be interpreted with caution. Second, the studies were conducted on resected IPMNs, thus limiting the knowledge regarding the natural course of the disease. Conversely, this ensures the most accurate pathologic diagnosis. Third, some features had slightly different or more specified definitions in the guidelines, e.g., for "enhanced" wall thickening, and different values for duct dilatations. However, for analysis with an adequate population, the features could not be too narrowly defined. Finally, as the risk of malignancy is likely to increase, an analysis of risk by combination of features or creating a predictive model would have been informative.

4. Materials and Methods

4.1. Literature Search Strategy

A literature search was conducted using the MEDLINE to identify a relevant study about the outcomes in patients with worrisome features or high-risk stigmata of IPMN and malignancy proven by surgery or biopsy. A combination of search terms, including IPMN, computed tomography (CT), magnetic resonance image (MRI), EUS, malignancy, worrisome features, or predictive features, were used.

4.2. Inclusion/Exclusion Criteria

Studies were included if they met the following criteria: written in English, full-article, publication year between January 2000 and May 2019, patient with BD-IPMN diagnosed by CT, MRI or EUS and final pathological diagnosis by surgical resection or biopsy, and >10 patients in the study. We excluded case reports, case series with small sample size (<10 patients), review articles, editorials, consensus proceedings, studies without pathological diagnosis, not within field of interest, and insufficient or overlapping data.

4.3. Data Extraction and Quality Assessment

Two reviewers (W.K. and Y.H.) independently extracted the data from each study and resolved their disagreements by discussion or by consulting a third reviewer (J-Y.J.). The following data were collected from the studies that met the criteria. (1) Study—publication year, study design, and study location. (2) Cases—total number of BD-IPMN patients, frequency of pathologic malignancy in BD-IPMN, age, and sex. (3) Cystic morphology—maximum cyst size, presence of mural nodules, and maximum diameter of main pancreatic duct. (4) Clinical data—symptoms (jaundice, diabetes, pain, and weight loss), imaging methods, CA 19-9 level (normal value 0–37 U/mL), and CEA level (normal value 0–5 ng/mL). (5) Outcomes—cytology result and pathology result.

Malignant BD-IPMN was identified when there was histological evidence of BD-IPMN with invasive carcinoma or high-grade dysplasia after surgical resection, and cytological/histological evidence of high-grade dysplasia/malignant cells was found after FNA/biopsy of BD-IPMN with or without associated radiological signs of malignancy.

The choice of the articles included in this review were in accordance with the Preferred Reporting Items for Systematic Reviews and Meta-Analyses statement (PRISMA) [62], and a PRISMA flowchart was formulated (Figure 1) for transparency of the conclusions reached by the authors. The quality of included studies was assessed using the Newcastle Ottawa Scale [63] by two reviewers (W.K. and Y.H.).

4.4. Data Analysis

Interpretative analysis of the OR between positive and negative worrisome features in IPMN patients was performed. The OR of BD-IPMN with or without worrisome features/high-risk stigmata was calculated by dividing the total number of events by the total number of patients. If these specific data were not provided in a study, it was calculated by adding or subtracting the number of patients who had confirmed pathology and imaging data. The corresponding 95% CIs were calculated using exact methods. A meta-analysis of all eligible studies identified was then planned with the Review Manager software (RevMan) (version 5.3; The Cochrane Collaboration, The Nordic Cochrane Center, Copenhagen, Denmark) using a random-effects model. This model was used because we believe that the relevant variation in the risk is most likely a consequence of inter-study differences. Statistical analysis was performed for all stages of this meta-analysis in accordance with the MOOSE guidelines [64]. The quantity of heterogeneity and publication bias was assessed. A p-value < 0.050 was accepted as statistically significant.

5. Conclusions

This study examined the parameters used to predict malignancy as specified by the most commonly used guidelines. This not only included clinical and radiographic features, but also biochemical features. The results confirmed that all the currently used features are valid. However, each guideline utilizes certain features and weighs the impact of each feature differently, resulting in different treatment strategies in BD-IPMN patients presenting similar features. This study hopes to contribute in making future guidelines more compatible and standardized.

Author Contributions: Conceptualization, W.K. and J.-Y.J.; methodology, Y.H., Y.B., J.S.K., Y.J.C.; software, Y.H.; validation, Y.H., W.K. and J.-Y.J.; formal analysis, Y.H. and W.K.; investigation, W.K. and J.-Y.J.; resources, H.K. and J.-Y.J.; data curation, Y.B., J.S.K., Y.J.C., Y.H., and H.K.; writing—original draft preparation, W.K. and Y.H.; writing—review and editing, W.K., Y.H., H.K., and J.-Y.J.; visualization, W.K. and Y.H.; supervision, J.-Y.J.; project administration, Y.H.; funding acquisition, J.-Y.J. All authors have read and agreed to the published version of the manuscript.

Funding: This study was supported by grant no. 23-2017-0090 from the SNUH Research Fund.

Conflicts of Interest: The authors declare no conflict of interest.

References

1. Tanaka, M.; Fernandez-del Castillo, C.; Adsay, V.; Chari, S.; Falconi, M.; Jang, J.Y.; Kimura, W.; Levy, P.; Pitman, M.B.; Schmidt, C.M.; et al. International consensus guidelines 2012 for the management of IPMN and MCN of the pancreas. *Pancreatology* **2012**, *12*, 183–197. [CrossRef]
2. Ohashi, K.; Murakami, Y.; Maruyama, M. Four cases of "mucin-producing" cancer of the pancreas on specific findings of the papilla of Vater. *Prog. Dig. Endosc.* **1982**, *20*, 348–352.
3. Siegel, R.L.; Miller, K.D.; Jemal, A. Cancer statistics, 2019. *CA Cancer J. Clin.* **2019**, *69*, 7–34. [CrossRef] [PubMed]
4. Chang, Y.R.; Park, J.K.; Jang, J.Y.; Kwon, W.; Yoon, J.H.; Kim, S.W. Incidental pancreatic cystic neoplasms in an asymptomatic healthy population of 21,745 individuals: Large-scale, single-center cohort study. *Medicine (Baltimore)* **2016**, *95*, e5535. [CrossRef] [PubMed]
5. Fernandez-del Castillo, C.; Targarona, J.; Thayer, S.P.; Rattner, D.W.; Brugge, W.R.; Warshaw, A.L. Incidental pancreatic cysts: Clinicopathologic characteristics and comparison with symptomatic patients. *Arch. Surg.* **2003**, *138*, 423–427. [CrossRef]
6. Vege, S.S.; Ziring, B.; Jain, R.; Moayyedi, P.; Clinical Guidelines, C.; American Gastroenterology, A. American gastroenterological association institute guideline on the diagnosis and management of asymptomatic neoplastic pancreatic cysts. *Gastroenterology* **2015**, *148*, 819–822, quize 812–813. [CrossRef]
7. Del Chiaro, M.; Verbeke, C.; Salvia, R.; Kloppel, G.; Werner, J.; McKay, C.; Friess, H.; Manfredi, R.; Van Cutsem, E.; Lohr, M.; et al. European experts consensus statement on cystic tumours of the pancreas. *Dig. Liver Dis.* **2013**, *45*, 703–711. [CrossRef] [PubMed]
8. European Study Group on Cystic Tumours of the Pancreas. European evidence-based guidelines on pancreatic cystic neoplasms. *Gut* **2018**, *67*, 789–804. [CrossRef] [PubMed]
9. Tanaka, M.; Fernandez-Del Castillo, C.; Kamisawa, T.; Jang, J.Y.; Levy, P.; Ohtsuka, T.; Salvia, R.; Shimizu, Y.; Tada, M.; Wolfgang, C.L. Revisions of international consensus Fukuoka guidelines for the management of IPMN of the pancreas. *Pancreatology* **2017**, *17*, 738–753. [CrossRef] [PubMed]

10. Tanaka, M.; Chari, S.; Adsay, V.; Fernandez-del Castillo, C.; Falconi, M.; Shimizu, M.; Yamaguchi, K.; Yamao, K.; Matsuno, S. International consensus guidelines for management of intraductal papillary mucinous neoplasms and mucinous cystic neoplasms of the pancreas. *Pancreatology* **2006**, *6*, 17–32. [CrossRef] [PubMed]
11. Akahoshi, K.; Ono, H.; Akasu, M.; Ban, D.; Kudo, A.; Konta, A.; Tanaka, S.; Tanabe, M. Rapid growth speed of cysts can predict malignant intraductal mucinous papillary neoplasms. *J. Surg. Res.* **2018**, *231*, 195–200. [CrossRef] [PubMed]
12. Akita, H.; Takeda, Y.; Hoshino, H.; Wada, H.; Kobayashi, S.; Marubashi, S.; Eguchi, H.; Tanemura, M.; Mori, M.; Doki, Y.; et al. Mural nodule in branch duct-type intraductal papillary mucinous neoplasms of the pancreas is a marker of malignant transformation and indication for surgery. *Am. J. Surg.* **2011**, *202*, 214–219. [CrossRef] [PubMed]
13. Arikawa, S.; Uchida, M.; Uozumi, J.; Sakoda, J.; Kaida, H.; Kunou, Y.; Hirose, Y.; Abe, T.; Hayabuchi, N.; Naito, Y.; et al. Utility of multidetector row CT in diagnosing branch duct IPMNs of the pancreas compared with MR cholangiopancreatography and endoscopic ultrasonography. *Kurume Med. J.* **2011**, *57*, 91–100. [CrossRef] [PubMed]
14. Aso, T.; Ohtsuka, T.; Matsunaga, T.; Kimura, H.; Watanabe, Y.; Tamura, K.; Ideno, N.; Osoegawa, T.; Takahata, S.; Shindo, K.; et al. "High-risk stigmata" of the 2012 international consensus guidelines correlate with the malignant grade of branch duct intraductal papillary mucinous neoplasms of the pancreas. *Pancreas* **2014**, *43*, 1239–1243. [CrossRef] [PubMed]
15. Attiyeh, M.A.; Fernandez-Del Castillo, C.; Al Efishat, M.; Eaton, A.A.; Gonen, M.; Batts, R.; Pergolini, I.; Rezaee, N.; Lillemoe, K.D.; Ferrone, C.R.; et al. Development and Validation of a Multi-institutional Preoperative Nomogram for Predicting Grade of Dysplasia in Intraductal Papillary Mucinous Neoplasms (IPMNs) of the Pancreas: A Report from The Pancreatic Surgery Consortium. *Ann. Surg.* **2018**, *267*, 157–163. [CrossRef]
16. Bournet, B.; Kirzin, S.; Carrere, N.; Portier, G.; Otal, P.; Selves, J.; Musso, C.; Suc, B.; Moreau, J.; Fourtanier, G.; et al. Clinical fate of branch duct and mixed forms of intraductal papillary mucinous neoplasia of the pancreas. *J. Gastroenterol. Hepatol.* **2009**, *24*, 1211–1217. [CrossRef]
17. Carbognin, G.; Zamboni, G.; Pinali, L.; Chiara, E.D.; Girardi, V.; Salvia, R.; Mucelli, R.P. Branch duct IPMTs: Value of cross-sectional imaging in the assessment of biological behavior and follow-up. *Abdom. Imaging* **2006**, *31*, 320–325. [CrossRef]
18. Chiu, S.S.; Lim, J.H.; Lee, W.J.; Chang, K.T.; Oh, D.K.; Lee, K.T.; Lee, J.K.; Choi, S.H. Intraductal papillary mucinous tumour of the pancreas: Differentiation of malignancy and benignancy by CT. *Clin. Radiol.* **2006**, *61*, 776–783. [CrossRef]
19. Correa-Gallego, C.; Do, R.; Lafemina, J.; Gonen, M.; D'Angelica, M.I.; DeMatteo, R.P.; Fong, Y.; Kingham, T.P.; Brennan, M.F.; Jarnagin, W.R.; et al. Predicting dysplasia and invasive carcinoma in intraductal papillary mucinous neoplasms of the pancreas: Development of a preoperative nomogram. *Ann. Surg. Oncol.* **2013**, *20*, 4348–4355. [CrossRef]
20. Dortch, J.D.; Stauffer, J.A.; Asbun, H.J. Pancreatic Resection for Side-Branch Intraductal Papillary Mucinous Neoplasm (SB-IPMN): A Contemporary Single-Institution Experience. *J. Gastrointest. Surg.* **2015**, *19*, 1603–1609. [CrossRef]
21. Fritz, S.; Klauss, M.; Bergmann, F.; Strobel, O.; Schneider, L.; Werner, J.; Hackert, T.; Buchler, M.W. Pancreatic main-duct involvement in branch-duct IPMNs: An underestimated risk. *Ann. Surg.* **2014**, *260*, 848–855. [CrossRef]
22. Harima, H.; Kaino, S.; Shinoda, S.; Kawano, M.; Suenaga, S.; Sakaida, I. Differential diagnosis of benign and malignant branch duct intraductal papillary mucinous neoplasm using contrast-enhanced endoscopic ultrasonography. *World J. Gastroenterol.* **2015**, *21*, 6252–6260. [CrossRef]
23. Hirono, S.; Kawai, M.; Okada, K.I.; Miyazawa, M.; Shimizu, A.; Kitahata, Y.; Ueno, M.; Yanagisawa, A.; Yamaue, H. Factors Associated With Invasive Intraductal Papillary Mucinous Carcinoma of the Pancreas. *JAMA Surg.* **2017**, *152*, e165054. [CrossRef] [PubMed]
24. Jang, J.Y.; Park, T.; Lee, S.; Kim, Y.; Lee, S.Y.; Kim, S.W.; Kim, S.C.; Song, K.B.; Yamamoto, M.; Hatori, T.; et al. Proposed Nomogram Predicting the Individual Risk of Malignancy in the Patients with Branch Duct Type Intraductal Papillary Mucinous Neoplasms of the Pancreas. *Ann. Surg.* **2017**, *266*, 1062–1068. [CrossRef] [PubMed]

25. Kato, Y.; Takahashi, S.; Gotohda, N.; Konishi, M. Risk factors for malignancy in branched-type intraductal papillary mucinous neoplasms of the pancreas during the follow-up period. *World J. Surg.* **2015**, *39*, 244–250. [CrossRef] [PubMed]
26. Kim, Y.I.; Shin, S.H.; Song, K.B.; Hwang, D.W.; Lee, J.H.; Park, K.M.; Lee, Y.J.; Kim, S.C. Branch duct intraductal papillary mucinous neoplasm of the pancreas: Single-center experience with 324 patients who underwent surgical resection. *Korean J. Hepatobiliary Pancreat. Surg.* **2015**, *19*, 113–120. [CrossRef]
27. Kim, T.H.; Song, T.J.; Hwang, J.H.; Yoo, K.S.; Lee, W.J.; Lee, K.H.; Dong, S.H.; Park, C.H.; Park, E.T.; Moon, J.H.; et al. Predictors of malignancy in pure branch duct type intraductal papillary mucinous neoplasm of the pancreas: A nationwide multicenter study. *Pancreatology* **2015**, *15*, 405–410. [CrossRef]
28. Koshita, S.; Noda, Y.; Ito, K.; Kanno, Y.; Ogawa, T.; Masu, K.; Masaki, Y.; Horaguchi, J.; Oikawa, M.; Tsuchiya, T.; et al. Pancreatic juice cytology with immunohistochemistry to detect malignancy and histologic subtypes in patients with branch duct type intraductal papillary mucinous neoplasms of the pancreas. *Gastrointest. Endosc.* **2017**, *85*, 1036–1046. [CrossRef]
29. Lee, K.H.; Lee, S.J.; Lee, J.K.; Ryu, J.K.; Kim, E.Y.; Kim, T.H.; Moon, J.H.; Lee, W.J.; Cho, Y.K.; Kim, J.J. Prediction of malignancy with endoscopic ultrasonography in patients with branch duct-type intraductal papillary mucinous neoplasm. *Pancreas* **2014**, *43*, 1306–1311. [CrossRef]
30. Maguchi, H.; Tanno, S.; Mizuno, N.; Hanada, K.; Kobayashi, G.; Hatori, T.; Sadakari, Y.; Yamaguchi, T.; Tobita, K.; Doi, R.; et al. Natural history of branch duct intraductal papillary mucinous neoplasms of the pancreas: A multicenter study in Japan. *Pancreas* **2011**, *40*, 364–370. [CrossRef]
31. Mimura, T.; Masuda, A.; Matsumoto, I.; Shiomi, H.; Yoshida, S.; Sugimoto, M.; Sanuki, T.; Yoshida, M.; Fujita, T.; Kutsumi, H.; et al. Predictors of malignant intraductal papillary mucinous neoplasm of the pancreas. *J. Clin. Gastroenterol.* **2010**, *44*, e224–e229. [CrossRef] [PubMed]
32. Nagai, K.; Doi, R.; Ito, T.; Kida, A.; Koizumi, M.; Masui, T.; Kawaguchi, Y.; Ogawa, K.; Uemoto, S. Single-institution validation of the international consensus guidelines for treatment of branch duct intraductal papillary mucinous neoplasms of the pancreas. *J. Hepatobiliary Pancreat. Surg.* **2009**, *16*, 353–358. [CrossRef] [PubMed]
33. Nguyen, A.H.; Toste, P.A.; Farrell, J.J.; Clerkin, B.M.; Williams, J.; Muthusamy, V.R.; Watson, R.R.; Tomlinson, J.S.; Hines, O.J.; Reber, H.A.; et al. Current recommendations for surveillance and surgery of intraductal papillary mucinous neoplasms may overlook some patients with cancer. *J. Gastrointest. Surg.* **2015**, *19*, 258–265. [CrossRef] [PubMed]
34. Ogawa, H.; Itoh, S.; Ikeda, M.; Suzuki, K.; Naganawa, S. Intraductal papillary mucinous neoplasm of the pancreas: Assessment of the likelihood of invasiveness with multisection CT. *Radiology* **2008**, *248*, 876–886. [CrossRef]
35. Ohno, E.; Itoh, A.; Kawashima, H.; Ishikawa, T.; Matsubara, H.; Itoh, Y.; Nakamura, Y.; Hiramatsu, T.; Nakamura, M.; Miyahara, R.; et al. Malignant transformation of branch duct-type intraductal papillary mucinous neoplasms of the pancreas based on contrast-enhanced endoscopic ultrasonography morphological changes: Focus on malignant transformation of intraductal papillary mucinous neoplasm itself. *Pancreas* **2012**, *41*, 855–862. [PubMed]
36. Ohtsuka, T.; Kono, H.; Nagayoshi, Y.; Mori, Y.; Tsutsumi, K.; Sadakari, Y.; Takahata, S.; Morimatsu, K.; Aishima, S.; Igarashi, H.; et al. An increase in the number of predictive factors augments the likelihood of malignancy in branch duct intraductal papillary mucinous neoplasm of the pancreas. *Surgery* **2012**, *151*, 76–83. [CrossRef]
37. Ridtitid, W.; DeWitt, J.M.; Schmidt, C.M.; Roch, A.; Stuart, J.S.; Sherman, S.; Al-Haddad, M.A. Management of branch-duct intraductal papillary mucinous neoplasms: A large single-center study to assess predictors of malignancy and long-term outcomes. *Gastrointest. Endosc.* **2016**, *84*, 436–445. [CrossRef]
38. Robles, E.P.; Maire, F.; Cros, J.; Vullierme, M.P.; Rebours, V.; Sauvanet, A.; Aubert, A.; Dokmak, S.; Levy, P.; Ruszniewski, P. Accuracy of 2012 International Consensus Guidelines for the prediction of malignancy of branch-duct intraductal papillary mucinous neoplasms of the pancreas. *United Eur. Gastroenterol. J.* **2016**, *4*, 580–586. [CrossRef]
39. Rodriguez, J.R.; Salvia, R.; Crippa, S.; Warshaw, A.L.; Bassi, C.; Falconi, M.; Thayer, S.P.; Lauwers, G.Y.; Capelli, P.; Mino-Kenudson, M.; et al. Branch-duct intraductal papillary mucinous neoplasms: Observations in 145 patients who underwent resection. *Gastroenterology* **2007**, *133*, 72–79, quize 309–310. [CrossRef]

40. Sahora, K.; Mino-Kenudson, M.; Brugge, W.; Thayer, S.P.; Ferrone, C.R.; Sahani, D.; Pitman, M.B.; Warshaw, A.L.; Lillemoe, K.D.; Fernandez-del Castillo, C.F. Branch duct intraductal papillary mucinous neoplasms: Does cyst size change the tip of the scale? A critical analysis of the revised international consensus guidelines in a large single-institutional series. *Ann. Surg.* **2013**, *258*, 466–475. [CrossRef]
41. Salvia, R.; Crippa, S.; Falconi, M.; Bassi, C.; Guarise, A.; Scarpa, A.; Pederzoli, P. Branch-duct intraductal papillary mucinous neoplasms of the pancreas: To operate or not to operate? *Gut* **2007**, *56*, 1086–1090. [CrossRef] [PubMed]
42. Schmidt, C.M.; White, P.B.; Waters, J.A.; Yiannoutsos, C.T.; Cummings, O.W.; Baker, M.; Howard, T.J.; Zyromski, N.J.; Nakeeb, A.; DeWitt, J.M.; et al. Intraductal papillary mucinous neoplasms: Predictors of malignant and invasive pathology. *Ann. Surg.* **2007**, *246*, 644–651. [CrossRef] [PubMed]
43. Seo, N.; Byun, J.H.; Kim, J.H.; Kim, H.J.; Lee, S.S.; Song, K.B.; Kim, S.C.; Han, D.J.; Hong, S.M.; Lee, M.G. Validation of the 2012 International Consensus Guidelines Using Computed Tomography and Magnetic Resonance Imaging: Branch Duct and Main Duct Intraductal Papillary Mucinous Neoplasms of the Pancreas. *Ann. Surg.* **2016**, *263*, 557–564. [CrossRef] [PubMed]
44. Serikawa, M.; Sasaki, T.; Fujimoto, Y.; Kuwahara, K.; Chayama, K. Management of intraductal papillary-mucinous neoplasm of the pancreas: Treatment strategy based on morphologic classification. *J. Clin. Gastroenterol.* **2006**, *40*, 856–862. [CrossRef]
45. Shimizu, Y.; Hijioka, S.; Hirono, S.; Kin, T.; Ohtsuka, T.; Kanno, A.; Koshita, S.; Hanada, K.; Kitano, M.; Inoue, H.; et al. New Model for Predicting Malignancy in Patients with Intraductal Papillary Mucinous Neoplasm. *Ann. Surg.* **2020**, *272*, 155–162. [CrossRef]
46. Strauss, A.; Birdsey, M.; Fritz, S.; Schwarz-Bundy, B.D.; Bergmann, F.; Hackert, T.; Kauczor, H.U.; Grenacher, L.; Klauss, M. Intraductal papillary mucinous neoplasms of the pancreas: Radiological predictors of malignant transformation and the introduction of bile duct dilation to current guidelines. *Br. J. Radiol.* **2016**, *89*, 20150853. [CrossRef]
47. Takeshita, K.; Kutomi, K.; Takada, K.; Haruyama, T.; Fukushima, J.; Aida, R.; Takada, T.; Furui, S. Differential diagnosis of benign or malignant intraductal papillary mucinous neoplasm of the pancreas by multidetector row helical computed tomography: Evaluation of predictive factors by logistic regression analysis. *J. Comput. Assist. Tomogr.* **2008**, *32*, 191–197. [CrossRef]
48. Tang, R.S.; Weinberg, B.; Dawson, D.W.; Reber, H.; Hines, O.J.; Tomlinson, J.S.; Chaudhari, V.; Raman, S.; Farrell, J.J. Evaluation of the guidelines for management of pancreatic branch-duct intraductal papillary mucinous neoplasm. *Clin. Gastroenterol. Hepatol.* **2008**, *6*, 815–819, quiz 719. [CrossRef]
49. Wong, J.; Weber, J.; Centeno, B.A.; Vignesh, S.; Harris, C.L.; Klapman, J.B.; Hodul, P. High-grade dysplasia and adenocarcinoma are frequent in side-branch intraductal papillary mucinous neoplasm measuring less than 3 cm on endoscopic ultrasound. *J. Gastrointest. Surg.* **2013**, *17*, 78–84. [CrossRef]
50. Woo, S.M.; Ryu, J.K.; Lee, S.H.; Yoon, W.J.; Kim, Y.T.; Yoon, Y.B. Branch duct intraductal papillary mucinous neoplasms in a retrospective series of 190 patients. *Br. J. Surg.* **2009**, *96*, 405–411. [CrossRef]
51. Matsumoto, T.; Aramaki, M.; Yada, K.; Hirano, S.; Himeno, Y.; Shibata, K.; Kawano, K.; Kitano, S. Optimal management of the branch duct type intraductal papillary mucinous neoplasms of the pancreas. *J. Clin. Gastroenterol.* **2003**, *36*, 261–265. [CrossRef] [PubMed]
52. Sugiyama, M.; Izumisato, Y.; Abe, N.; Masaki, T.; Mori, T.; Atomi, Y. Predictive factors for malignancy in intraductal papillary-mucinous tumours of the pancreas. *Br. J. Surg.* **2003**, *90*, 1244–1249. [CrossRef]
53. Walsh, R.M.; Vogt, D.P.; Henderson, J.M.; Hirose, K.; Mason, T.; Bencsath, K.; Hammel, J.; Brown, N. Management of suspected pancreatic cystic neoplasms based on cyst size. *Surgery* **2008**, *144*, 677–684. [CrossRef] [PubMed]
54. Weinberg, B.M.; Spiegel, B.M.; Tomlinson, J.S.; Farrell, J.J. Asymptomatic pancreatic cystic neoplasms: Maximizing survival and quality of life using Markov-based clinical nomograms. *Gastroenterology* **2010**, *138*, 531–540. [CrossRef] [PubMed]
55. Jang, J.Y.; Kim, S.W.; Lee, S.E.; Yang, S.H.; Lee, K.U.; Lee, Y.J.; Kim, S.C.; Han, D.J.; Choi, D.W.; Choi, S.H.; et al. Treatment guidelines for branch duct type intraductal papillary mucinous neoplasms of the pancreas: When can we operate or observe? *Ann. Surg. Oncol.* **2008**, *15*, 199–205. [CrossRef]
56. Tanaka, M. Controversies in the management of pancreatic IPMN. *Nat. Rev. Gastroenterol. Hepatol.* **2011**, *8*, 56–60. [CrossRef] [PubMed]

57. Scheiman, J.M.; Hwang, J.H.; Moayyedi, P. American gastroenterological association technical review on the diagnosis and management of asymptomatic neoplastic pancreatic cysts. *Gastroenterology* **2015**, *148*, 824–848, e822. [CrossRef]
58. Uehara, H.; Ishikawa, O.; Katayama, K.; Kawada, N.; Ikezawa, K.; Fukutake, N.; Takakura, R.; Takano, Y.; Tanaka, S.; Takenaka, A. Size of mural nodule as an indicator of surgery for branch duct intraductal papillary mucinous neoplasm of the pancreas during follow-up. *J. Gastroenterol.* **2011**, *46*, 657–663. [CrossRef]
59. Marchegiani, G.; Andrianello, S.; Borin, A.; Dal Borgo, C.; Perri, G.; Pollini, T.; Romano, G.; D'Onofrio, M.; Gabbrielli, A.; Scarpa, A.; et al. Systematic review, meta-analysis, and a high-volume center experience supporting the new role of mural nodules proposed by the updated 2017 international guidelines on IPMN of the pancreas. *Surgery* **2018**, *163*, 1272–1279. [CrossRef]
60. Ohno, E.; Hirooka, Y.; Itoh, A.; Ishigami, M.; Katano, Y.; Ohmiya, N.; Niwa, Y.; Goto, H. Intraductal papillary mucinous neoplasms of the pancreas: Differentiation of malignant and benign tumors by endoscopic ultrasound findings of mural nodules. *Ann. Surg.* **2009**, *249*, 628–634. [CrossRef]
61. Kawada, N.; Uehara, H.; Nagata, S.; Tsuchishima, M.; Tsutsumi, M.; Tomita, Y. Mural nodule of 10 mm or larger as predictor of malignancy for intraductal papillary mucinous neoplasm of the pancreas: Pathological and radiological evaluations. *Pancreatology* **2016**, *16*, 441–448. [CrossRef]
62. Moher, D.; Liberati, A.; Tetzlaff, J.; Altman, D.G.; Group, P. Preferred reporting items for systematic reviews and meta-analyses: The PRISMA statement. *BMJ* **2009**, *339*, b2535. [CrossRef]
63. Higgins, J.P.T.; Thomas, J.; Chandler, J.; Cumpston, M.; Li, T.; Page, M.J.; Welch, V.A. *Cochrane Handbook for Systematic Reviews of Interventions*, version 6.0 (updated July 2019); Cochrane: London, UK, 2019; Available online: www.training.cochrane.org/handbook (accessed on 20 July 2020).
64. Stroup, D.F.; Berlin, J.A.; Morton, S.C.; Olkin, I.; Williamson, G.D.; Rennie, D.; Moher, D.; Becker, B.J.; Sipe, T.A.; Thacker, S.B. Meta-analysis of observational studies in epidemiology: A proposal for reporting. Meta-analysis Of Observational Studies in Epidemiology (MOOSE) group. *JAMA* **2000**, *283*, 2008–2012. [CrossRef]

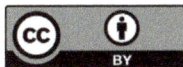

© 2020 by the authors. Licensee MDPI, Basel, Switzerland. This article is an open access article distributed under the terms and conditions of the Creative Commons Attribution (CC BY) license (http://creativecommons.org/licenses/by/4.0/).

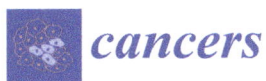

Systematic Review

Ductal Dilatation of ≥5 mm in Intraductal Papillary Mucinous Neoplasm Should Trigger the Consideration for Pancreatectomy: A Meta-Analysis and Systematic Review of Resected Cases

Y.H. Andrew Wu [1,†], Atsushi Oba [1,2,†], Laurel Beaty [1,3], Kathryn L. Colborn [1,3,4], Salvador Rodriguez Franco [1,5], Ben Harnke [6], Cheryl Meguid [1], Daniel Negrini [1,7], Roberto Valente [1,8], Steven Ahrendt [1,9], Richard D. Schulick [1,9] and Marco Del Chiaro [1,9,*]

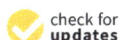

Citation: Wu, Y.H.A.; Oba, A.; Beaty, L.; Colborn, K.L.; Rodriguez Franco, S.; Harnke, B.; Meguid, C.; Negrini, D.; Valente, R.; Ahrendt, S.; et al. Ductal Dilatation of ≥5 mm in Intraductal Papillary Mucinous Neoplasm Should Trigger the Consideration for Pancreatectomy: A Meta-Analysis and Systematic Review of Resected Cases. *Cancers* **2021**, *13*, 2031. https://doi.org/10.3390/cancers13092031

Academic Editors: Niccola Funel and Sohei Satoi

Received: 2 March 2021
Accepted: 19 April 2021
Published: 22 April 2021

Publisher's Note: MDPI stays neutral with regard to jurisdictional claims in published maps and institutional affiliations.

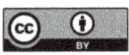

Copyright: © 2021 by the authors. Licensee MDPI, Basel, Switzerland. This article is an open access article distributed under the terms and conditions of the Creative Commons Attribution (CC BY) license (https://creativecommons.org/licenses/by/4.0/).

1. Division of Surgical Oncology, Department of Surgery, University of Colorado Anschutz Medical Campus, Aurora, CO 80045, USA; YUAN-HAW.WU@CUANSCHUTZ.EDU (Y.H.A.W.); ATSUSHI.OBA@CUANSCHUTZ.EDU (A.O.); LAUREL.BEATY@CUANSCHUTZ.EDU (L.B.); KATHRYN.COLBORN@CUANSCHUTZ.EDU (K.L.C.); SALVADOR.RODRIGUEZFRANCO@CUANSCHUTZ.EDU (S.R.F.); CHERYL.MEGUID@CUANSCHUTZ.EDU (C.M.); dan_negrini2000@yahoo.com.br (D.N.); robbie.valente@gmail.com (R.V.); STEVEN.AHRENDT@CUANSCHUTZ.EDU (S.A.); RICHARD.SCHULICK@CUANSCHUTZ.EDU (R.D.S.)
2. Department of Hepatobiliary and Pancreatic Surgery, Cancer Institute Hospital, Japanese Foundation for Cancer Research, 135-8550 Tokyo, Japan
3. Department of Biostatistics and Informatics, University of Colorado Anschutz Medical Campus, Aurora, CO 80045, USA
4. Surgical Outcomes and Applied Research Program, University of Colorado Anschutz Medical Campus, Aurora, CO 80045, USA
5. The Heart Institute, Children's Hospital Colorado, Aurora, CO 80045, USA
6. Strauss Health Sciences Library, University of Colorado Anschutz Medical Campus, Aurora, CO 80045, USA; BEN.HARNKE@CUANSCHUTZ.EDU
7. Department of Anesthesiology, Federal University of the State of Rio de Janeiro, Rio de Janeiro 21941-901, Brazil
8. Department of Surgery and Perioperative Sciences, Umeå University Hospital, 907 37 Umeå, Sweden
9. University of Colorado Cancer Center, Aurora, CO 80045, USA
* Correspondence: MARCO.DELCHIARO@CUANSCHUTZ.EDU
† These authors contributed equally to this work.

Simple Summary: Intraductal papillary mucinous neoplasms (IPMN) are common but difficult to manage since accurate tools for diagnosing malignancy are unavailable. This study evaluates the diagnostic value of main pancreatic duct (MPD) diameter for detecting IPMN malignancy, using a meta-analysis of published data. The result suggests that malignancy is highly prevalent in IPMN with ductal dilatation of >5 mm.

Abstract: Intraductal papillary mucinous neoplasms (IPMN) are common but difficult to manage since accurate tools for diagnosing malignancy are unavailable. This study tests the diagnostic value of the main pancreatic duct (MPD) diameter for detecting IPMN malignancy using a meta-analysis of published data of resected IPMNs. Collected from a comprehensive literature search, the articles included in this analysis must report malignancy cases (high-grade dysplasia (HGD) and invasive carcinoma (IC)) and MPD diameter so that two MPD cut-offs could be created. The sensitivity, specificity, and odds ratios of the two cutoffs for predicting malignancy were calculated. A review of 1493 articles yielded 20 retrospective studies with 3982 resected cases. A cutoff of ≥5 mm is more sensitive than the ≥10 mm cutoff and has pooled sensitivity of 72.20% and 75.60% for classification of HGD and IC, respectively. Both MPD cutoffs of ≥5 mm and ≥10 mm were associated with malignancy (OR = 4.36 (95% CI: 2.82, 6.75) vs. OR = 3.18 (95% CI: 2.25, 4.49), respectively). The odds of HGD and IC for patients with MPD ≥5 mm were 5.66 (95% CI: 3.02, 10.62) and 7.40 (95% CI: 4.95, 11.06), respectively. OR of HGD and IC for MPD ≥10 mm cutoff were 4.36 (95% CI: 3.20, 5.93) and

4.75 (95% CI: 2.39, 9.45), respectively. IPMN with MPD of >5 mm could very likely be malignant. In selected IPMN patients, pancreatectomy should be considered when MPD is >5 mm.

Keywords: pancreatic main duct dilatation; intraductal papillary mucinous neoplasm; high grade dysplasia; invasive carcinoma; pancreatic cystic neoplasm; pancreatic cancer; meta-analysis

1. Introduction

Pancreatic cystic lesions are common. The prevalence of these lesions is around 50% in the general population and increases with age [1]. Of these cystic lesions, pancreatic cystic neoplasm (PCN) management is challenging and important in modern pancreatology. The challenge lies in the difficulty in accurately discerning completely benign PCNs from ones with potential for malignancy progression [2–5].

Intraductal papillary mucinous neoplasm (IPMN) is a pre-cancerous lesion that accounts for at least half of all PCNs [6]. Morphologically, IPMNs can be divided into two major categories: (1) the branch-duct IPMN (BD-IPMN) that only involves the peripheral pancreatic ducts, and (2) main-duct IPMN (MD-IPMN) and mixed-type IPMN that involve the main pancreatic duct (MPD) and/or the branch ducts [7]. The morphologic and radiologic classification for identifying BD-IPMN, MD-IPMN, or mixed-type IPMN is extremely important. It is well known that BD-IPMNs have a very low risk for cancer progression; in contrast, MD- and mixed-type IPMNs are more prone to becoming cancerous [2,8]. Studies have shown that it is safe to surveil small BD-IPMNs (below 3–4 cm) that do not have any radiological features suggestive of malignancy [8–10]. In contrast, IPMNs involving the MPDs are more aggressive and generally need to be treated surgically [6,11].

The International Consensus Guidelines and the European Guidelines for managing IPMNs concordantly suggest an aggressive approach for managing MD- and mixed-type IPMNs. However, the role of MPD dilatation in deciding the indication for surgical resection of IPMN is moderately different in the two guidelines. The International Consensus Guidelines for IPMN management suggests that MD- or mixed-type IPMN with MPD dilatation of 10 mm or more should be referred for surgical treatment (high-risk stigmata) [11]. However, the same guideline suggests that surgery could still be considered for patients with 5–9.9 mm MPD (a worrisome feature), if there is the presence of mural nodule(s) ≥5 mm, cytology positivity for malignancy, or main-duct features suspicious for malignancy involvement [11]. The first European Guideline, published in 2013, recommended lowering the cutoff of MPD dilatation for surgery indication from 10 mm to 6 mm [2]. This approach was later supported by retrospective analysis that showed the implementation of MPD dilatation of 10 mm as a cutoff for surgery indication risks the possibility of IPMN undertreatment, as patients could have already developed invasive carcinoma (IC) or high-grade dysplasia (HGD) [12–14]. For better management of IPMNs, the latest evidence-based European Guidelines, published in 2018, recommends surgical resection of IPMN with MPD dilatation of 5–9.9 mm, if the patient is fit and has a long life expectancy (relative indications for surgery) [6]. This approach has also been recently supported by large retrospective surgical analyses [15].

Meanwhile, some studies have demonstrated a safe conservative approach in managing patients with suspected MD- or mixed-type IPMNs that have MPD dilatation of 5–9.9 mm [16,17]. Despite the compelling data, those studies need to be reassessed since high-volume centers have demonstrated that the accuracy of the pre-operative diagnosis of PCNs is approximately 60–80% [18–20]. Therefore, a high percentage of the suspected MD- or mixed-type IPMNs in those studies could very likely represent other more benign pancreatic diseases, such as chronic pancreatitis [18–20]. Hence, the optimal study design to analyze the disease status of PCNs is to evaluate a cohort with available histology data [21].

The role of MPD dilatation is important for establishing surgical indication. However, currently there is no consensus across existing guidelines regarding the degree of ductal dilatation that warrants pancreatectomy. This study is designed to evaluate the association of HGD and IC with ≥5 mm and ≥10 mm MPD. Sensitivity and specificity for detecting HGD and IC were calculated using the two MPD cutoffs.

2. Materials and Methods

2.1. Article Search/Selection and Outcome Assessment

This systematic review and meta-analysis was performed by following the Preferred Reporting Items for Systematic Reviews and Meta-Analyses (PRISMA) Guideline [22]. Literature search was performed on 28 February 2020 by a professional librarian at the Strauss Health Sciences Library. The following databases were queried: Ovid MEDLINE(R) ALL 1946 to 27 February 2020; Embase; Web of Science; Google Scholar. The search strategy focused on obtaining all existing literature related to MPD dilatation in IPMN and its association to malignancy. The terms including but not limited to: intraductal papillary mucinous or intraductal mucinous papillary or ipmn or ipmt; dilat or size or diameter or cut off or cutoff or mm or millimeter or milli meter were used for the systematic search. Full search strategy is provided in online Figure S1. The articles obtained from the search were uploaded to the Endnote version X9 citation management application, in which duplicated search results were eliminated. The final list of articles for initial review was uploaded to Covidence, a software designed for reviewing and selecting articles for systematic review and meta-analysis.

In the initial phase of reviewing articles, Y.H.A.W. and A.O. independently studied all records uploaded to Covidence. If the title or abstract of the articles were relevant to the topic of this study, the independent reviewers (Y.H.A.W. and A.O.) would thoroughly perform a screening of the entire article to assess for eligibility of inclusion. Non-English articles were excluded at the title/abstract review phase. Should there be a disagreement in eligibility of the included articles, D.N. would resolve the discrepancy.

Studies evaluating the association between MPD, IPMN (including BD-IPMN, MD-IPMN, or mixed-type IPMN), and malignancy were included in this study. We specifically only included studies that reported MPD ranges that could be used to create two cut-offs: ≥5 mm and ≥10 mm. Studies also had to include the counts or rates of malignancy and non-malignancy for each MPD category. We also required that included articles show histological diagnosis of lesions, specifically whether they were non-malignant or malignant. In this study, histology classification and definition are in accordance with the 2015 Baltimore Consensus Meeting Guideline [23] or the current World Health Organization guidelines [24] for IPMN. In short, HGD or IC were defined as malignancy, whereas low-grade dysplasia or moderate-grade dysplasia were defined as non-malignancy. In the event of encountering two or more publications that had identical cohorts, only the publication with the most complete dataset was included in this study.

The primary outcomes of this study were the proportion of patients with HGD, IC, or malignancy.

2.2. Data Extraction

Study characteristics and data were independently extracted by two investigators (Y.H.A.W. and A.O.) and recorded on a standardized data extraction form. Any discrepancies were resolved by other reviewers (S.F., D.N., L.B., and K.L.C.). Data extracted and used for analysis are listed in Table 1. The final extracted data were reviewed by Y.H.A.W., A.O., S.F., L.B., and K.L.C.

2.3. Risk of Bias Analysis

Y.H.A.W., S.F., and A.O. assessed the quality of the included articles by conducting an evaluation using the Risk of Bias in Non-randomized Studies of Interventions (ROBINS-I) [41]. ROBINS-1 is designed to assess an article by evaluating 7 domains of risk of bias (Table S1). The assessment will grade the 7 domains of an article with low, moderate, serious, critical, or not assessable risk. In the end, the 7 domains were collectively analyzed for every article included in this study. Additionally, Funnel plots and Egger's regression tests were used to assess publication bias (Figure S2).

Table 1. Characteristics of included articles.

Author	Year	Country	Design	<5 mm (n)		5–9 mm (n)		≥10 mm (n)	
				M	NM	M	NM	M	NM
Takanami et al. [25]	2011	Japan	Retrospective	3	2	5	5	1	0
Barron et al. [26]	2014	U.S.A.	Retrospective	17	149	74	40	40	14
Roch et al. [27]	2014	U.S.A.	Retrospective	-	-	50	64	30	27
Hackert et al. [12]	2015	Germany	Retrospective	-	-	93	64	76	27
Kang et al. [28]	2015	S. Korea	Retrospective	44	206	39	38	34	14
Kim et al. [29]	2015	S. Korea	Retrospective	15	212	19	50	4	3
Kim et al. [30]	2015	S. Korea	Retrospective	43	195	38	39	36	16
Yamada et al. [31]	2015	Japan	Retrospective	10	42	29	39	22	24
Robles et al. [32]	2016	France	Retrospective	13	57	19	25	4	2
Seo et al. [33]	2016	S. Korea	Retrospective	11	62	27	29	14	15
Sugimoto et al. [14]	2016	U.S.A.	Retrospective	-	-	22	19	42	20
Choi et al. [34]	2017	S. Korea	Retrospective	1	20	29	16	9	1
Yu et al. [35]	2017	Japan	Retrospective	39	13	14	12	3	8
Marchegiani et al. [17]	2018	Italy	Retrospective	8	43	43	126	20	32
Tsukagoshi et al. [36]	2018	Japan	Retrospective	2	17	4	4	12	3
Del Chiaro et al. [15]	2019	U.S.A./Sweden	Retrospective	65	240	134	152	107	43
Jan et al. [37]	2019	Taiwan	Retrospective	17	65	11	11	23	31
Lee et al. [38]	2019	S. Korea	Retrospective	3	36	16	16	9	6
Masaki et al. [39]	2019	Japan	Retrospective	0	0	3	6	16	4
Hwang et al. [40]	2020	S. Korea	Retrospective	25	45	11	18	18	9
Total (% *)				316 (18.4%)	1404 (81.6%)	680 (46.8%)	773 (53.2%)	520 (63.5%)	289 (36.5%)

* Percentage of cases within MPD Dilatation category; Abbreviations: M = Malignancy; NM = Non-Malignancy.

2.4. Data Synthesis and Statistical Analysis

Tests of association: Random effects models were used to estimate adjusted diagnostic odds ratios (OR) and 95% confidence intervals for the pooled data. These were estimated using the meta package in RStudio (RStudio, Boston, Massachusetts), which provides functions for diagnostic meta-analysis [42]. A continuity correction was applied to all cells in a 2 × 2 table when necessary. We evaluated the association between cutoffs of ≥5 mm and ≥10 mm and classification of HGD, IC, and malignancy. There were three primary comparisons made for the two cutoffs: (1) classification of non-malignancy and malignancy; (2) classification of non-malignancy and HGD, and (3) classification of non-malignancy and IC. Therefore, we estimated six ORs using two cutoffs and three disease classifications. Forest Plots were used to compare individual-study ORs and the pooled OR. Forest plots include OR estimates from both the fixed effects model and the random effects model. Heterogeneity amongst the included publications was assessed using Cochrane's Q test and I^2. Based on the results of these tests, this paper utilized only the random effects estimates for interpretations.

Diagnostic tests: Pooled sensitivities and specificities and 95% confidence intervals for the same six comparisons were also estimated using the mada package (R Foundation for Statistical Computing, Vienna, Austria). Using a random effects model, the mada package implements a bivariate estimation of sensitivity and specificity described by Reitsma et al. [43]. This bivariate approach is necessary because the sensitivity and specificity of a test are interrelated; therefore, univariate approaches to estimation are inappropriate. From these pooled values for sensitivity and specificity, we then estimated AUC for each comparison. The summary receiver operating characteristic (SROC) curves were plotted to assess the spread of diagnostic measures for each comparison and cutoff.

We conducted an additional analysis to evaluate the impact of including the large study by Del Chiaro et al. (senior author of this study) [15]. This was done by repeating the analyses described above excluding that study.

3. Results

The search strategy identified 3338 citations. After removing duplicated articles, 1493 were eligible for title and abstract review. Initial title and abstract review performed by two independent reviewers (Y.H.A.W. and A.O.) yielded 120 articles eligible for full-article review. Ultimately, 20 manuscripts were included for qualitative and quantitative analysis. The authors excluded one hundred manuscripts for the following reasons: 41 articles did not have MPD dilatation values; 37 articles did not have all the MPD ranges that adhered to our criteria; 8 articles had incorrect study design and did not include information needed for quantitative meta-analysis; 5 articles had vague or no histology diagnosis; 5 articles did not provide sufficient information for case number retrieval; 2 articles only used ultrasound/endoscopic ultrasound for preoperative evaluation; 1 article lacked surgical pathology results; 1 article had duplication of cohort with another included article (Figure 1).

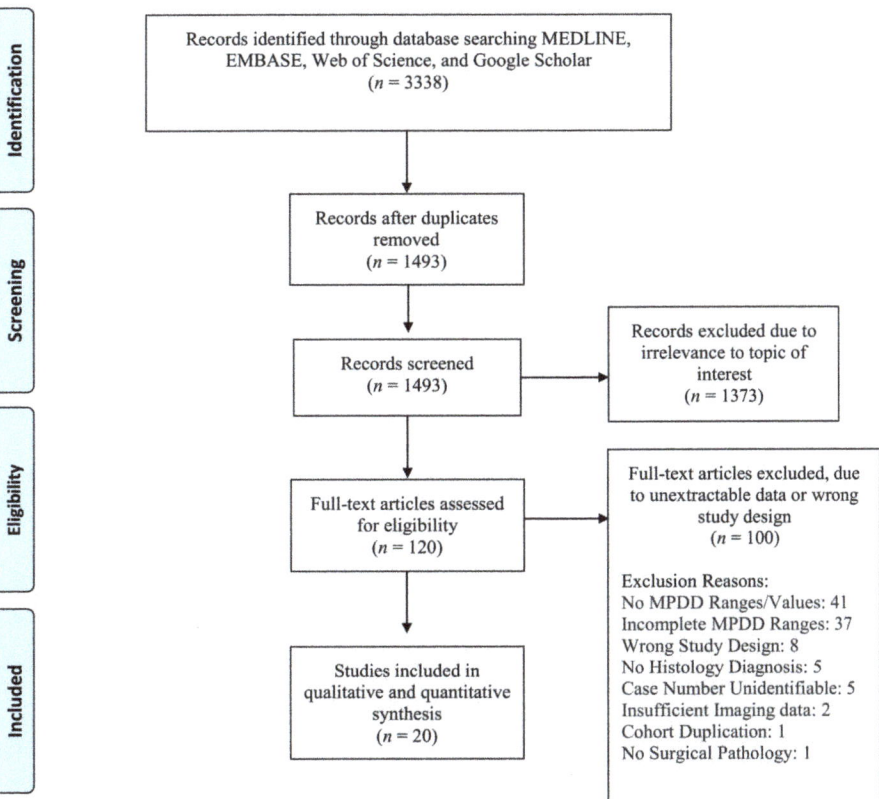

Figure 1. PRISMA flow chart showing the article selection process.

Characteristics of articles included for qualitative and quantitative analysis are listed in Tables 1 and 2. From the 20 included articles [12,14,15,17,25–31,33–40,44,45], a total of 3982 resected IPMN cases (including BD-IPMN, MD-IPMN, or mixed-type IPMN) were collected. Of the 3982 resected cases, 1516 and 2466 were malignant and non-malignant cases, respectively. Of the 1516 malignant cases, 316, 680, and 520 cases had MPD range of <5 mm, 5–9.9 mm, and ≥10 mm, respectively. Similarly, of the 2466 non-malignant cases, 1404, 773, and 289 cases had MPD range of <5 mm, 5–9.9 mm, and ≥10 mm, respectively. Ten of the 20 studies included pathologically confirmed HGD and IC cases. Of the 818 malignant cases collected from the 10 articles, 421 and 397 cases had histology diagnosis of HGD and IC, respectively. Of the 421 HGD cases, 89, 187, and 145 cases had MPD range of <5 mm, 5–9 mm, and ≥10 mm, respectively. Similarly, of the 397 IC cases, 70, 182, 145 cases had MPD range of <5 mm, 5–9.9 mm, and ≥10 mm, respectively.

Table 2. Characteristics of included article with postoperative histology diagnosis of HGD and IC.

Author	Year	Design	<5 mm			5–9 mm			≥10 mm		
			HGD	IC	NM	HGD	IC	NM	HGD	IC	NM
Takanami et al. [25]	2011	Retrospective	3	0	2	5	0	5	0	1	0
Barron et al. [26]	2014	Retrospective	10	7	149	40	34	40	27	13	14
Roch et al. [27]	2014	Retrospective	-	-	-	19	31	64	15	15	27
Kang et al. [28]	2015	Retrospective	15	29	206	17	22	38	12	22	14
Kim et al. [29]	2015	Retrospective	6	9	212	7	12	50	0	4	3
Robles et al. [32]	2016	Retrospective	8	5	57	10	9	25	4	0	2
Sugimoto et al. [14]	2016	Retrospective	-	-	-	5	17	19	18	24	20
Tsukagoshi et al. [36]	2018	Retrospective	2	0	17	3	1	4	6	6	3
Del Chiaro et al. [15]	2019	Retrospective	45	20	240	78	56	152	53	54	43
Masaki et al. [39]	2019	Retrospective	0	0	0	3	0	6	10	6	4
Total (% *)			89 (8.5%)	70 (6.7%)	883 (84.7%)	187 (24.2%)	182 (23.6%)	403 (52.2%)	145 (34.5%)	145 (34.5%)	130 (31.0%)

* Percentage of cases within MPD Dilatation category; Abbreviations: HGD, High Grade Dysplasia; IC, Invasive Carcinoma; NM, Non-Malignancy.

ROBINS-I indicated that the risk of bias of the included study was moderate in 18 [12,14,15,17,26–40] studies and serious in 2 [25,32]. The results of this analysis are provided in Table S1.

3.1. Tests of Association

Both the ≥5 mm and ≥10 mm cutoffs in resected cases were significantly associated with higher risk of malignancy compared to <5 mm and <10 mm, respectively (≥5 mm: OR = 4.36 [95% CI: 2.82, 6.75, 6.75, I^2 = 81.7%, Cochran's Q p < 0.0001]; ≥10 mm: OR = 3.18 [95% CI: 2.25, 4.49, I^2 = 68.2%, Cochran's Q p < 0.0001]). The odds of HGD were over five times higher for patients with ≥5 mm MPD {5.66 (95% CI: 3.02, 10.62, I^2 = 71.2%, Cochran's Q p = 0.002)} compared to patients with MPD < 5 mm and over four times higher for patients with ≥10 mm MPD {4.36 (95% CI: 3.20, 5.93, I^2 = 8.4%, Cochran's Q p = 0.365)} compared to patients with <10 mm. The odds of IC were over seven times higher for patients with MPD ≥5 mm {7.40 (95% CI: 4.95, 11.06, I^2 = 27.5%, Cochran's Q p = 0.2189)} compared to <5 mm and 4.7 times higher for patients with ≥10 mm duct {4.75 (95% CI: 2.39, 9.45, I^2 = 72.3%, Cochran's Q p = 0.0002)} compared to <10 mm. Forest Plots are shown in Figure 2. Summary of the odds of HGD and IC for different MPD cutoffs are in Table S2.

3.2. Diagnostic Tests

For all six comparisons, the tests for equality of sensitivities and specificities were all found to be significant (p < 0.001). This indicated heterogeneity between studies, and therefore we estimated pooled sensitivities and specificities using random effects models (Table 3). The six SROC curves from the random effects models are included in Figure 3.

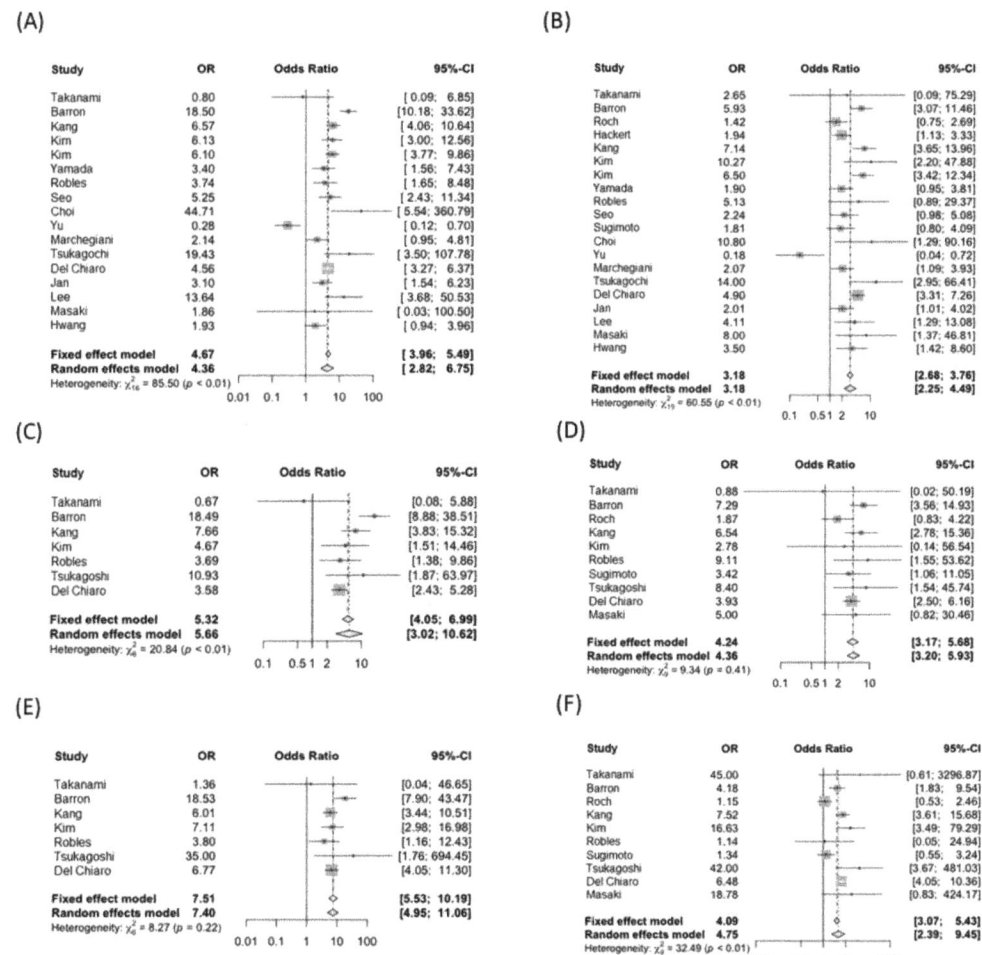

Figure 2. Meta-analysis forest plot presented in Diagnostic Odds Ratio (OR): (**A**) malignancy (M) and non-malignancy (NM), cutoff of 5 mm; (**B**) malignancy (M) and non-malignancy (NM), cutoff of 10 mm; (**C**) high-grade dysplasia (HGD) and non-malignancy (NM), cutoff of 5 mm; (**D**) high-grade dysplasia (HGD) and non-malignancy (NM), cutoff of 10 mm; (**E**) invasive carcinoma (IC) vs. non-malignancy (NM), cutoff of 5 mm; (**F**) invasive carcinoma (IC) vs. non-malignancy (NM), cutoff of 10 mm.

Table 3. Pooled sensitivity/specificity and area under the curve (AUC).

Comparisons	Dilation	Sensitivity	95% CI	Specificity	95% CI	AUC	Studies Included
Malignancy to NM	≥5 mm	74.8%	(64.6–82.2%)	58.6%	(49.0–67.6%)	0.716	17
	≥10 mm	33.8%	(27.2–41.0%)	86.4%	(79.6–91.2%)	0.586	20
High-Grade Dysplasia to NM	≥5 mm	72.2%	(62.2–80.3%)	70.1%	(60.7–78.0%)	0.769	7
	≥10 mm	35.7%	(22.3–51.9%)	88.7%	(75.8–95.1%)	0.657	10
Invasive Carcinoma to NM	≥5 mm	75.6%	(64.8–83.9%)	69.7%	(60.4–77.6%)	0.786	7
	≥10 mm	36.6%	(26.0–48.7%)	88.2%	(75.3–94.9%)	0.587	10

Abbreviations: NM, Non-Malignancy.

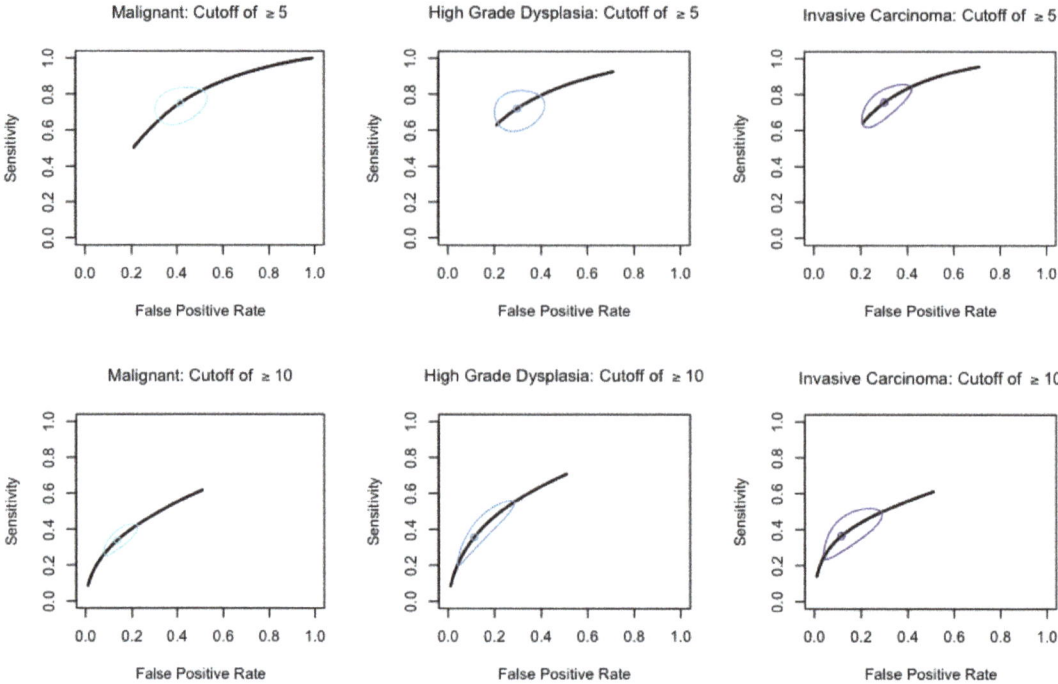

Figure 3. Summary receiver operating characteristic (SROC) curves for the bivariate diagnostic tests. Dot is point estimate that represents estimated pooled sensitivity/1-specificity for the included studies. Circle represents the confidence interval around the point estimate.

Using a cutoff point of 5 mm, specificity was 58.6% and sensitivity was 74.8% for classification of malignancy. The AUC was 0.716. For the cutoff point of 10 mm, specificity was 86.4% and sensitivity were 33.8% for classification of malignancy. The AUC was 0.586. A cutoff of 5 mm had 70.1% specificity and 72.2% sensitivity for classification of HGD. The AUC was 0.769. A cutoff of 10 mm had 88.7% specificity and 35.7% sensitivity for classification of HGD. The AUC was 0.587. A cutoff point of 5 mm had 69.7% specificity and 75.6% sensitivity for classification of IC. The AUC was 0.786. A cutoff of 10 mm had 88.2% specificity and 36.6% sensitivity for classification of IC. The AUC was 0.587 (Figure 3).

3.3. Subset Analysis Excluding Del Chiaro et al.

The analysis excluding the large study by Del Chiaro et al. [15] yielded very similar results to the overall results presented in this study. The results of this analysis are provided in Table S2.

4. Discussion

The correct clinical management of IPMNs is crucial for the prevention of pancreatic cancer [46]. An overtreatment of low-grade dysplasia lesions could result in unnecessary morbidity and mortality related to pancreatic surgery. Surgery is indicated for IPMNs in an attempt to remove IC and HGD. The latter is the optimal pre-invasive histology form and time-point for surgical intervention. Unfortunately, there is no available method that can effectively discriminate HGD from IC, except a few experimental approaches that are not yet implemented in clinical practice [15,47,48]. Recent studies reported that pancreatectomy-related mortality has decreased from 7.3% since 2000 [49], and the benchmark for postoperative mortality after pancreaticoduodenectomy published in 2019 was ≤1.6% [50], which is drastically lower than the 17–42% probability of five-year survival of resected IC [50–54]. Therefore, surgery performed on IC could be too late for extending the survival of patients, and it could be more beneficial to resect MD-IPMN while in HGD form.

According to the European evidence-based guideline for PCN management, IPMN MPD dilatation of 5–9.9 mm and ≥10 mm are relative and absolute indication for surgery, respectively [6]. Recent studies have demonstrated IPMN with MPD dilatation of ≥5 mm have a malignancy rate of 30–90% [12,15,28,33,55–59]. In this meta-analysis of 20 retrospective studies, malignancy was detected in nearly 46.8% of resected IPMN patients with 5–9.9 mm MPD and 63.5% of resected IPMN patients with ≥10 mm MPD. In total, 53.1% of resected IPMN patients with ≥5 mm MPD had malignancy. On the contrary, only 18.4% of resected cases with MPD < 5 mm were malignant IPMN. Pooled OR for malignancy calculated in this meta-analysis showed that MPD cutoff set at ≥5 mm was higher than ≥10 mm (OR = 4.4 vs. 3.2) in the resected cases. To improve the overall survival rate of malignant IPMN, HGD should be surgically removed before allowing it to progress to IC. Pooled OR from this meta-analysis showed that the odds of HGD were higher in ≥5 mm MPD than ≥10 mm MPD (OR = 5.7 vs. 4.4) in resected cases. Similarly, pooled OR for IC was also higher in ≥5 mm MPD than in ≥10 mm MPD (OR = 7.4 vs. 4.8). These data suggest that ductal dilatation of ≥5 mm should trigger the consideration for pancreatectomy.

The pooled sensitivities of ≥5 mm MPD in predicting IPMN HGD and IC were 72.2% and 75.6%, respectively. When using ≥5 mm MPD as cutoff, SROC AUC was 0.769 and 0.786 for HGD and IC, respectively, which were higher than those of ≥10 mm cutoff (AUC = 0.657 and 0.587 for HGD and IC, respectively). The predictive role of ≥10 mm MPD for malignancy is unquestionable, but ≥5 mm MPD cutoff should also be considered as a highly sensitive factor for detecting HGD and/or IC. This lower cutoff could potentially identify malignancy in advance and improve survival of IPMN patients. However, Marchegiani et al. suggested that utilization of MPD dilatation as the sole indicator for pancreatectomy could encourage unnecessary surgical procedure and that most individuals with 5–9 mm MPD should be managed expectantly, performing conversion surgery when tumor progression is identified during close, regular follow-ups [17]. In the observation arm of the same study, 3 out of 46 (6.5%) IPMN patients with 5–9 mm MPD eventually underwent surgery [17]. However, Salvia et al. reported that the diagnostic accuracy for MD-IPMNs is only approximately 80% [19], implying some of those IPMN patients who underwent conservative treatment did not actually have IPMN [21]. If a PCN were to present with mural nodule(s) or cyst(s), fine-needle aspiration (FNA) with real-time endoscopic ultrasound (EUS) could be utilized to obtain histology proof and to make a diagnosis. It is important to note that EUS can accurately identify morphologic features of PCNs but is only 51% accurate in discerning the difference between mucinous and non-mucinous lesions [60]. The accuracy would increase up to 79% if CEA measurements were obtained from cystic fluid using EUS-FNA [60]. However, mural nodules and cysts ≥40 mm have only been reported in 1.2% to 21.3% and 23.2% to 27.5% of malignant IPMNs, respectively [13,15], and FNA would not have been a possible approach if ductal dilatation were the only cross-sectional imagining finding. Studies that include resected cases disproportionately favor inclusion of more serious cases that require surgery, but at least the diagnosis could be confirmed with surgical pathology. Including only pathologically confirmed IPMN cases for analysis, this study shows that many HGD and IC patients would be missed if the decision to operate were made at MPD ≥ 10 mm associated with low sensitivity.

The results in this study underline the need for a surgical evaluation for MPD ≥5 mm and are not conclusive evidence that suggest the risk for developing cancer is higher in IPMN with 5–9.9 mm MPD. On the other hand, it could also be possible that IPMN with MPD dilatation over 10 mm are slow progressive diseases that would turn invasive when MPD reaches larger dilatation. Using ≥5 mm MPD to select surgical candidates might also identify low-grade dysplasia. Considering that the highest incidence of IC occurs with MD-IPMN, we could assume that the surgical treatment of MD-IPMN with low-grade dysplasia is perhaps not an overtreatment when compared to surgical treatment of BD-IPMN with low-grade dysplasia [21]. Nevertheless, it is important to know that the currently available information for IPMN management is not perfect, and it is important to diagnose IPMN with existing sensitive diagnostic tools to increase the overall survival rates of the patients, as the mean frequency of malignancy in MPD dilatation of ≥ 5 mm was 61.6% and that of IC IPMN was 43.1% [11].

Recognizing the potential for the Del Chiaro et al. study [15] of heavily influencing the results presented in this study given its overall size, we completed a full analysis of the data excluding this study. The results and conclusions were unchanged.

Our study has limitations related to the use of retrospective studies that lack conservatively managed cohorts as a control group. Cases could not be stratified based on the imaging modalities used. The most accurate cutoff line for MPD dilatation could not be determined in this study since data for MPD dilatation are presented in ranges. In addition, other features associated with IPMN malignancy, such as mural nodule, cytology, elevated CA 19–9, or cyst diameter, could not be included in this analysis [11]. In addition, this study includes only resected IPMNs. Therefore, the results of this study are not representative of the unresected IPMN population. However, this study was performed based on recently published study that showed MPD dilatation is currently the best predictor of HGD or IC in IPMN [15]. Although estimates of heterogeneity above 50% were observed for some of our analyses, we found no reason for publication bias based on visual inspection of the funnel plot and the results of the Egger's test (Egger Regression Model). Additionally, and as stated in the methodology, all of our statistical models were estimated using random model effects, which have previously been used successfully to account for this limitation [42]. Even with some limitations related to the retrospective nature of this study, this analysis contains the largest volume of IPMN cases analyzed and our methodological approach properly accounted for study-level variation.

5. Conclusions

MPD dilatation is an important predictive factor of IPMN malignancy and 5 mm is a highly sensitive cutoff that detects high-risk pre-cancerous or cancerous lesions in resected cases. It is important to note that this study cannot draw a conclusion for non-surgical cases. However, the need for pancreatectomy should be thoroughly evaluated in patients with ductal dilatation of ≥ 5 mm. The result of this study implies that MPD dilatation over 5 mm should trigger the referral of a patient to a high-volume center for further consultation. The decision to perform resection should only be considered after careful evaluation of multiple aspects related to the general conditions and the expectancy of life of a patient. In conjunction with new biomarkers or diagnostic modalities such as pancreatoscopy [61,62], MPD dilatation detection could improve surgical patient selection and reduce overall IPMN malignancy mortality.

Supplementary Materials: The following are available online at https://www.mdpi.com/article/10.3390/cancers13092031/s1. Figure S1: Detailed Search Strategy for Existing Online Literature, Figure S2: Funnel plot with Diagnostic Odds Ratio (DOR) and Egger's Test for publication bias assessment, Table S1: ROBINS-I Risk of Bias Assessment of included Articles, Table S2: Odds ratio, Sensitive, and Specificity for different comparisons and cutoffs.

Author Contributions: Y.H.A.W.; A.O.; L.B.; K.L.C.; and M.D.C. were involved in the study design. Y.H.A.W.; A.O., L.B.; K.L.C., and B.H. were involved in management of this study. Y.H.A.W.; A.O.; L.B.; K.L.C.; B.H.; S.F. and D.N. performed data collection, analysis, and interpretation. Y.H.A.W.; A.O.; K.L.C.; and M.D.C. were involved in the initial drafting of this manuscript. C.M.; R.V.; S.A.; S.F. and R.D.S. revised and provided important intellectual content. The authors showed no conflict in the content of this manuscript upon submission. All authors have read and agreed to the published version of the manuscript.

Funding: This research received no external funding.

Conflicts of Interest: None of the authors have any personal conflict of interest to declare, except for Del Chiaro who is a co-principal investigator on a Boston Scientific study investigating the role of intraoperative pancreatoscopy in IPMN patients. Del Chiaro has also been awarded an industry grant from Haemonetics Inc. to conduct a multicenter study that evaluates the prognostic implications and changes of thromboelastographic (TEG) in pancreas cancer patients.

References

1. Kromrey, M.-L.; Bülow, R.; Hübner, J.; Paperlein, C.; Lerch, M.M.; Ittermann, T.; Völzke, H.; Mayerle, J.; Kühn, J.-P. Prospective study on the incidence, prevalence and 5-year pancreatic-related mortality of pancreatic cysts in a population-based study. *Gut* **2018**, *67*, 138–145. [CrossRef] [PubMed]
2. Del Chiaro, M.; Verbeke, C.; Salvia, R.; Klöppel, G.; Werner, J.; McKay, C.; Friess, H.; Manfredi, R.; Van Cutsem, E.; Löhr, M.; et al. European experts consensus statement on cystic tumours of the pancreas. *Dig. Liver Dis.* **2013**, *45*, 703–711. [CrossRef]
3. Nilsson, L.N.; Keane, M.G.; Shamali, A.; Bocos, J.M.; van Zanten, M.M.; Antila, A.; Gil, C.V.; Del Chiaro, M.; Laukkarinen, J. Nature and management of pancreatic mucinous cystic neoplasm (MCN): A systematic review of the literature. *Pancreatology* **2016**, *16*, 1028–1036. [CrossRef] [PubMed]
4. Keane, M.G.; Shamali, A.; Nilsson, L.N.; Antila, A.; Bocos, J.M.; Van Zanten, M.M.; Gil, C.V.; Maisonneuve, P.; Vaalavuo, Y.; Hoskins, T.; et al. Risk of malignancy in resected pancreatic mucinous cystic neoplasms. *Br. J. Surg.* **2018**, *105*, 439–446. [CrossRef]
5. Jais, B.; Rebours, V.; Malleo, G.; Salvia, R.; Fontana, M.; Maggino, L.; Bassi, C.; Manfredi, R.; Moran, R.; Lennon, A.M.; et al. Serous cystic neoplasm of the pancreas: A multinational study of 2622 patients under the auspices of the International Association of Pancreatology and European Pancreatic Club (European Study Group on Cystic Tumors of the Pancreas). *Gut* **2015**, *65*, 305–312. [CrossRef]
6. European Study Group on Cystic Tumours of the Pancreas. European evidence-based guidelines on pancreatic cystic neoplasms. *Gut* **2018**, *67*, 789–804. [CrossRef] [PubMed]
7. Del Chiaro, M.; Verbeke, C. Intraductal papillary mucinous neoplasms of the pancreas: Reporting clinically relevant features. *Histopathology* **2017**, *70*, 850–860. [CrossRef]
8. Del Chiaro, M.; Ateeb, Z.; Hansson, M.R.; Rangelova, E.; Segersvärd, R.; Kartalis, N.; Ansorge, C.; Löhr, M.J.; Arnelo, U.; Verbeke, C. Survival analysis and risk for progression of intraductal papillary mucinous neoplasia of the pancreas (IPMN) under surveillance: A single-institution experience. *Ann. Surg. Oncol.* **2017**, *24*, 1120–1126. [CrossRef] [PubMed]
9. Lawrence, S.A.; Attiyeh, M.A.; Seier, K.; Gönen, M.; Schattner, M.; Haviland, D.L.; Balachandran, V.P.; Kingham, T.P.; D'Angelica, M.I.; DeMatteo, R.P.; et al. should patients with cystic lesions of the pancreas undergo long-term radiographic surveillance? Results of 3024 patients evaluated at a single institution. *Ann. Surg.* **2017**, *266*, 536–544. [CrossRef] [PubMed]
10. Crippa, S.; Pezzilli, R.; Bissolati, M.; Capurso, G.; Romano, L.; Brunori, M.P.; Calculli, L.; Tamburrino, D.; Piccioli, A.; Ruffo, G.; et al. Active surveillance beyond 5 years is required for presumed branch-duct intraductal papillary mucinous neoplasms undergoing non-operative management. *Am. J. Gastroenterol.* **2017**, *112*, 1153–1161. [CrossRef]
11. Tanaka, M.; Castillo, C.F.-D.; Kamisawa, T.; Jang, J.Y.; Levy, P.; Ohtsuka, T.; Salvia, R.; Shimizu, Y.; Tada, M.; Wolfgang, C.L. Revisions of international consensus Fukuoka guidelines for the management of IPMN of the pancreas. *Pancreatology* **2017**, *17*, 738–753. [CrossRef] [PubMed]
12. Hackert, T.; Fritz, S.; Klauss, M.; Bergmann, F.; Hinz, U.; Strobel, O.; Schneider, L.; Büchler, M.W. Main-duct intraductal papillary mucinous neoplasm: High cancer risk in duct diameter of 5 to 9 mm. *Ann. Surg.* **2015**, *262*, 875–880. [CrossRef] [PubMed]
13. Ateeb, Z.; Valente, R.; Pozzi-Mucelli, R.M.; Malgerud, L.; Schlieper, Y.; Rangelova, E.; Fernandez-Moro, C.; Löhr, J.M.; Arnelo, U.; Del Chiaro, M. Main pancreatic duct dilation greater than 6 mm is associated with an increased risk of high-grade dysplasia and cancer in IPMN patients. *Langenbecks Arch. Chir.* **2019**, *404*, 31–37. [CrossRef] [PubMed]
14. Sugimoto, M.; Elliott, I.A.; Nguyen, A.H.; Kim, S.; Muthusamy, V.R.; Watson, R.; Hines, O.J.; Dawson, D.W.; Reber, H.A.; Donahue, T.R. Assessment of a revised management strategy for patients with intraductal papillary mucinous neoplasms involving the main pancreatic duct. *JAMA Surg.* **2017**, *152*, e163349. [CrossRef] [PubMed]
15. Del Chiaro, M.; Beckman, R.; Ateeb, Z.; Orsini, N.; Rezaee, N.; Manos, L.; Valente, R.; Yuan, C.; Ding, D.; Margonis, G.A.; et al. Main duct dilatation is the best predictor of high-grade dysplasia or invasion in intraductal papillary mucinous neoplasms of the pancreas. *Ann. Surg.* **2019**, *272*, 1118–1124. [CrossRef]
16. Crippa, S.; Bassi, C.; Salvia, R.; Malleo, G.; Marchegiani, G.; Rebours, V.; Levy, P.; Partelli, S.; Suleiman, S.L.; Banks, P.A.; et al. Low progression of intraductal papillary mucinous neoplasms with worrisome features and high-risk stigmata undergoing non-operative management: A mid-term follow-up analysis. *Gut* **2017**, *66*, 495–506. [CrossRef]
17. Marchegiani, G.; Andrianello, S.; Morbin, G.; Secchettin, E.; D'Onofrio, M.; De Robertis, R.; Malleo, G.; Bassi, C.; Salvia, R. Importance of main pancreatic duct dilatation in IPMN undergoing surveillance. *Br. J. Surg.* **2018**, *105*, 1825–1834. [CrossRef]
18. Del Chiaro, M.; Segersvärd, R.; Mucelli, R.P.; Rangelova, E.; Kartalis, N.; Ansorge, C.; Arnelo, U.; Blomberg, J.; Löhr, M.; Verbeke, C. Comparison of preoperative conference-based diagnosis with histology of cystic tumors of the pancreas. *Ann. Surg. Oncol.* **2014**, *21*, 1539–1544. [CrossRef]
19. Salvia, R.; Malleo, G.; Marchegiani, G.; Pennacchio, S.; Paiella, S.; Paini, M.; Pea, A.; Butturini, G.; Pederzoli, P.; Bassi, C. Pancreatic resections for cystic neoplasms: From the surgeon's presumption to the pathologist's reality. *Surgery* **2012**, *152*, 135–142. [CrossRef] [PubMed]
20. Correa-Gallego, C.; Ferrone, C.R.; Thayer, S.P.; Wargo, J.A.; Warshaw, A.L.; Castillo, C.F.-D. Incidental pancreatic cysts: Do we really know what we are watching? *Pancreatology* **2010**, *10*, 144–150. [CrossRef]

21. Del Chiaro, M.; Valente, R.; Wolfgang, C. Response to comment on "Main duct dilatation is the best predictor of high-grade dysplasia or invasion in intraductal papillary mucinous neoplasms of the pancreas". *Ann. Surg.* **2019**, *270*, e109–e110. [CrossRef] [PubMed]
22. Moher, D.; Liberati, A.; Tetzlaff, J.; Altman, D.G. Preferred reporting items for systematic reviews and meta-analyses: The PRISMA statement. *J. Clin. Epidemiol.* **2009**, *62*, 1006–1012. [CrossRef] [PubMed]
23. Basturk, O.; Hong, S.M.; Wood, L.D.; Adsay, N.V.; Albores-Saavedra, J.; Biankin, A.V.; Brosens, L.A.; Fukushima, N.; Goggins, M.; Hruban, R.H.; et al. A revised classification system and recommendations from the baltimore consensus meeting for neoplastic precursor lesions in the pancreas. *Am. J. Surg. Pathol.* **2015**, *39*, 1730–1741. [CrossRef] [PubMed]
24. Adsay, N.V.; Furukawa, T.; Hruban, R.H.; Klimstra, D.S.; Klöppel, G.; Offerhaus, G.J.A.; Pitman, M.B.; Shimizu, M.; Zamboni, G. Intraductal neoplasms of the pancreas. In *WHO Classification of Tumours of the Digestive System*; IARC: Lyon, France, 2010; pp. 304–313.
25. Takanami, K.; Hiraide, T.; Tsuda, M.; Nakamura, Y.; Kaneta, T.; Takase, K.; Fukuda, H.; Takahashi, S. Additional value of FDG PET/CT to contrast-enhanced CT in the differentiation between benign and malignant intraductal papillary mucinous neoplasms of the pancreas with mural nodules. *Ann. Nucl. Med.* **2011**, *25*, 501–510. [CrossRef]
26. Barron, M.R.; Roch, A.M.; Waters, J.A.; Parikh, J.A.; DeWitt, J.M.; Al-Haddad, M.A.; Ceppa, E.P.; House, M.G.; Zyromski, N.J.; Nakeeb, A.; et al. Does preoperative cross-sectional imaging accurately predict main duct involvement in intraductal papillary mucinous neoplasm? *J. Gastrointest. Surg.* **2014**, *18*, 447–456. [CrossRef]
27. Roch, A.M.; DeWitt, J.M.; Al-Haddad, M.A.; Schmidt, I.I.C.M.; Ceppa, E.P.; House, M.G.; Zyromski, N.J.; Nakeeb, A.; Schmidt, C.M. Nonoperative management of main pancreatic duct-involved intraductal papillary mucinous neoplasm might be indicated in select patients. *J. Am. Coll. Surg.* **2014**, *219*, 122–129. [CrossRef]
28. Kang, M.J.; Jang, J.Y.; Lee, S.; Park, T.; Lee, S.Y.; Kim, S.W. Clinicopathological meaning of size of main-duct dilatation in intraductal papillary mucinous neoplasm of pancreas: Proposal of a simplified morphological classification based on the investigation on the size of main pancreatic duct. *World J. Surg.* **2015**, *39*, 2006–2013. [CrossRef]
29. Kim, Y.I.; Shin, S.H.; Song, K.B.; Hwang, D.W.; Lee, J.H.; Park, K.-M.; Lee, Y.-J.; Kim, S.C. Branch duct intraductal papillary mucinous neoplasm of the pancreas: Single-center experience with 324 patients who underwent surgical resection. *Korean J. Hepato Biliary Pancreat. Surg.* **2015**, *19*, 113–120. [CrossRef]
30. Kim, J.R.; Jang, J.Y.; Kang, M.J.; Park, T.; Lee, S.Y.; Jung, W.; Chang, J.; Shin, Y.; Han, Y.; Kim, S.W. Clinical implication of serum carcinoembryonic antigen and carbohydrate antigen 19-9 for the prediction of malignancy in intraductal papillary mucinous neoplasm of pancreas. *J. Hepatobiliary Pancreat. Sci.* **2015**, *22*, 699–707. [CrossRef]
31. Yamada, S.; Fujii, T.; Murotani, K.; Kanda, M.; Sugimoto, H.; Nakayama, G.; Koike, M.; Fujiwara, M.; Nakao, A.; Kodera, Y. Comparison of the international consensus guidelines for predicting malignancy in intraductal papillary mucinous neoplasms. *Surgery* **2016**, *159*, 878–884. [CrossRef]
32. Robles, E.P.-C.; Maire, F.; Cros, J.; Vullierme, M.-P.; Rebours, V.; Sauvanet, A.; Aubert, A.; Dokmak, S.; Lévy, P.; Ruszniewski, P. Accuracy of 2012 International Consensus Guidelines for the prediction of malignancy of branch-duct intraductal papillary mucinous neoplasms of the pancreas. *United Eur. Gastroenterol. J.* **2016**, *4*, 580–586. [CrossRef]
33. Seo, N.; Byun, J.H.; Kim, J.H.; Kim, H.J.; Lee, S.S.; Song, K.B.; Kim, S.C.; Han, D.J.; Hong, S.M.; Lee, M.G. Validation of the 2012 International Consensus Guidelines using computed tomography and magnetic resonance imaging: Branch duct and main duct intraductal papillary mucinous neoplasms of the pancreas. *Ann. Surg.* **2016**, *263*, 557–564. [CrossRef]
34. Choi, S.-Y.; Kim, J.H.; Yu, M.H.; Eun, H.W.; Lee, H.K.; Han, J.K. Diagnostic performance and imaging features for predicting the malignant potential of intraductal papillary mucinous neoplasm of the pancreas: A comparison of EUS, contrast-enhanced CT and MRI. *Abdom. Radiol.* **2017**, *42*, 1449–1458. [CrossRef]
35. Yu, S.; Takasu, N.; Watanabe, T.; Fukumoto, T.; Okazaki, S.; Tezuka, K.; Sugawara, S.; Hirai, I.; Kimura, W. Validation of the 2012 Fukuoka Consensus Guideline for intraductal papillary mucinous neoplasm of the pancreas from a single institution experience. *Pancreas* **2017**, *46*, 936–942. [CrossRef]
36. Tsukagoshi, M.; Araki, K.; Saito, F.; Kubo, N.; Watanabe, A.; Igarashi, T.; Ishii, N.; Yamanaka, T.; Shirabe, K.; Kuwano, H. Evaluation of the international consensus guidelines for the surgical resection of intraductal papillary mucinous neoplasms. *Dig. Dis. Sci.* **2017**, *63*, 860–867. [CrossRef]
37. Jan, I.-S.; Chang, M.-C.; Yang, C.-Y.; Tien, Y.-W.; Jeng, Y.-M.; Wu, C.-H.; Chen, B.-B.; Chang, Y.-T. Validation of indications for surgery of european evidence-based guidelines for patients with pancreatic intraductal papillary mucinous neoplasms. *J. Gastrointest. Surg.* **2020**, *24*, 2536–2543. [CrossRef] [PubMed]
38. Lee, J.E.; Choi, S.-Y.; Min, J.H.; Yi, B.H.; Lee, M.H.; Kim, S.S.; Hwang, J.A.; Kim, J.H. Determining malignant potential of intraductal papillary mucinous neoplasm of the pancreas: CT versus MRI by using revised 2017 international consensus guidelines. *Radiology* **2019**, *293*, 134–143. [CrossRef] [PubMed]
39. Masaki, Y.; Koshita, S.; Noda, Y.; Kanno, Y.; Ogawa, T.; Masu, K.; Sawai, T.; Ito, K. Should we regard all main duct type intraductal papillary mucinous neoplasms of the pancreas (MD-IPMN) as an indication of surgery? A retrospective study in 29 patients with MD-IPMN showing mural nodules. *Pancreatology* **2019**, *19*, 352–359. [CrossRef] [PubMed]
40. Hwang, J.A.; Choi, S.-Y.; Lee, J.E.; Kim, S.S.; Lee, S.; Moon, J.Y.; Heo, N.H. Pre-operative nomogram predicting malignant potential in the patients with intraductal papillary mucinous neoplasm of the pancreas: Focused on imaging features based on revised international guideline. *Eur. Radiol.* **2020**, *30*, 3711–3722. [CrossRef]

41. Sterne, J.A.; Hernán, M.A.; Reeves, B.C.; Savović, J.; Berkman, N.D.; Viswanathan, M.; Henry, D.; Altman, D.G.; Ansari, M.T.; Boutron, I.; et al. ROBINS-I: A tool for assessing risk of bias in non-randomised studies of interventions. *BMJ* **2016**, *355*, i4919. [CrossRef]
42. Balduzzi, S.; Rücker, G.; Schwarzer, G. How to perform a meta-analysis with R: A practical tutorial. *Evid.-Based Ment. Health* **2019**, *22*, 153–160. [CrossRef]
43. Reitsma, J.B.; Glas, A.S.; Rutjes, A.W.; Scholten, R.J.; Bossuyt, P.M.; Zwinderman, A.H. Bivariate analysis of sensitivity and specificity produces informative summary measures in diagnostic reviews. *J. Clin. Epidemiol.* **2005**, *58*, 982–990. [CrossRef] [PubMed]
44. Kawaguchi, Y.; Yasuda, K.; Cho, E.; Uno, K.; Tanaka, K.; Nakajima, M. Differential diagnosis of intraductal papillary-mucinous tumor of the pancreas by endoscopic ultrasonography and intraductal ultrasonography. *Dig. Endosc.* **2004**, *16*, 101–106. [CrossRef]
45. Yamaguchi, T.; Baba, T.; Ishihara, T.; Kobayashi, A.; Nakamura, K.; Tadenuma, H.; Ito, H.; Miyazaki, M.; Saisho, H. Long-term follow-up of intraductal papillary mucinous neoplasm of the pancreas with ultrasonography. *Clin. Gastroenterol. Hepatol.* **2005**, *3*, 1136–1143. [CrossRef]
46. Del Chiaro, M.; Segersvard, R.; Lohr, M.; Verbeke, C. Early detection and prevention of pancreatic cancer: Is it really possible today? *World J. Gastroenterol.* **2014**, *20*, 12118–12131. [CrossRef] [PubMed]
47. Gaiser, R.A.; Pessia, A.; Ateeb, Z.; Davanian, H.; Moro, C.F.; Alkharaan, H.; Healy, K.; Ghazi, S.; Arnelo, U.; Valente, R.; et al. Integrated targeted metabolomic and lipidomic analysis: A novel approach to classifying early cystic precursors to invasive pancreatic cancer. *Sci. Rep.* **2019**, *9*, 1–12. [CrossRef]
48. Gaiser, R.A.; Halimi, A.; Alkharaan, H.; Lu, L.; Davanian, H.; Healy, K.; Hugerth, L.W.; Ateeb, Z.; Valente, R.; Moro, C.F.; et al. Enrichment of oral microbiota in early cystic precursors to invasive pancreatic cancer. *Gut* **2019**, *68*, 2186–2194. [CrossRef]
49. Finks, J.F.; Osborne, N.H.; Birkmeyer, J.D. Trends in hospital volume and operative mortality for high-risk surgery. *N. Engl. J. Med.* **2011**, *364*, 2128–2137. [CrossRef]
50. Sánchez-Velázquez, P.; Muller, X.; Malleo, G.; Park, J.; Hwang, H.; Napoli, N.; Javed, A.; Inoue, Y.; Beghdadi, N.; Kalisvaart, M.; et al. Benchmarks in pancreatic surgery. A novel tool for unbiased outcome comparisons. *Ann Surg.* **2019**, *270*, 211–218. [CrossRef]
51. Woo, S.M.; Ryu, J.K.; Lee, S.H.; Yoo, J.W.; Park, J.K.; Kim, Y.T.; Yoon, Y.B. Survival and prognosis of invasive intraductal papillary mucinous neo-plasms of the pancreas: Comparison with pancreatic ductal adenocarcinoma. *Pancreas* **2008**, *36*, 50–55. [CrossRef]
52. Poultsides, G.A.; Reddy, S.; Cameron, J.L.; Hruban, R.H.; Pawlik, T.M.; Ahuja, N.; Jain, A.; Edil, B.H.; Iacobuzio-Donahue, C.A.; Schulick, R.D.; et al. Histopathologic basis for the favorable survival after resection of intraductal papillary mucinous neoplasm-associated invasive adenocarcinoma of the pancreas. *Ann. Surg.* **2010**, *251*, 470–476. [CrossRef]
53. Chari, S.T.; Yadav, D.; Smyrk, T.C.; DiMagno, E.P.; Miller, L.J.; Raimondo, M.; Clain, J.E.; Norton, I.A.; Pearson, R.K.; Petersen, B.T.; et al. Study of recurrence after surgical resection of intraductal papillary mucinous neoplasm of the pancreas. *Gastroenterology* **2002**, *123*, 1500–1507. [CrossRef] [PubMed]
54. McMillan, M.T.; Lewis, R.S.; Drebin, J.A.; Teitelbaum, U.R.; Lee, M.K.; Roses, R.E.; Fraker, D.L.; Vollmer, C.M. The efficacy of adjuvant therapy for pancreatic invasive intraductal papillary mucinous neoplasm (IPMN). *Cancer* **2015**, *122*, 521–533. [CrossRef] [PubMed]
55. Abdeljawad, K.; Vemulapalli, K.C.; Schmidt, C.M.; Dewitt, J.; Sherman, S.; Imperiale, T.F.; Al-Haddad, M. Prevalence of malignancy in patients with pure main duct intraductal papillary mucinous neoplasms. *Gastrointest. Endosc.* **2014**, *79*, 623–629. [CrossRef] [PubMed]
56. Ogawa, H.; Itoh, S.; Ikeda, M.; Suzuki, K.; Naganawa, S. Intraductal papillary mucinous neoplasm of the pancreas: Assessment of the likelihood of invasiveness with multisection CT. *Radiology* **2008**, *248*, 876–886. [CrossRef] [PubMed]
57. Shin, S.H.; Han, D.J.; Park, K.T.; Kim, Y.H.; Park, J.B.; Kim, S.C. Validating a simple scoring system to predict malignancy and invasiveness of intraductal papillary mucinous neoplasms of the pancreas. *World J. Surg.* **2010**, *34*, 776–783. [CrossRef] [PubMed]
58. Jun, D.Y.; Kwon, H.J.; Kim, S.G.; Kim, S.H.; Chun, J.M.; Kwon, Y.B.; Yoon, K.J.; Hwang, Y.J.; Yun, Y.K. Predictive factors for invasive intraductal papillary mucinous neo-plasm of the pancreas. *Korean J. Hepatobiliary Pancreat. Surg.* **2011**, *15*, 237–242. [CrossRef]
59. Kawakubo, K.; Tada, M.; Isayama, H.; Sasahira, N.; Nakai, Y.; Takahara, N.; Uchino, R.; Hamada, T.; Miyabayashi, K.; Yamamoto, K.; et al. Disease-specific mortality among patients with intra-ductal papillary mucinous neoplasm of the pancreas. *Clin. Gastroenterol. Hepatol.* **2014**, *12*, 486–491. [CrossRef]
60. Brugge, W.R.; Lewandrowski, K.; Lee-Lewandrowski, E.; Centeno, B.A.; Szydlo, T.; Regan, S.; del Castillo, C.F.; Warshaw, A.L. Diagnosis of pancreatic cystic neoplasms: A report of the cooperative pancreatic cyst study. *Gastroenterology* **2004**, *126*, 1330–1336. [CrossRef]
61. Arnelo, U.; Siiki, A.; Swahn, F.; Segersvärd, R.; Enochsson, L.; del Chiaro, M.; Lundell, L.; Verbeke, C.S.; Löhr, J.M. Single-operator pancreatoscopy is helpful in the evaluation of suspected intraductal papillary mucinous neoplasms (IPMN). *Pancreatology* **2014**, *14*, 510–514. [CrossRef] [PubMed]
62. Tyberg, A.; Raijman, I.; Siddiqui, A.; Arnelo, U.; Adler, D.G.; Xu, M.M.; Nassani, N.; Sejpal, D.V.; Kedia, P.; Nah Lee, Y.; et al. Digital pancreaticocholangioscopy for mapping of pancreaticobiliary neoplasia: Can we alter the surgical resection margin? *J. Clin. Gastroenterol.* **2019**, *53*, 71–75. [CrossRef] [PubMed]

MDPI
St. Alban-Anlage 66
4052 Basel
Switzerland
Tel. +41 61 683 77 34
Fax +41 61 302 89 18
www.mdpi.com

Cancers Editorial Office
E-mail: cancers@mdpi.com
www.mdpi.com/journal/cancers

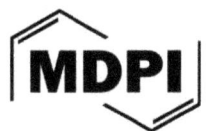

www.ingramcontent.com/pod-product-compliance
Lightning Source LLC
LaVergne TN
LVHW070416100526
838202LV00014B/1471